Fundamentals of Clinical Psychiatry

"Fundamentals of Clinical Psychiatry: A Practical Handbook is an invaluable resource for both seasoned psychiatrists and those learning the specialty. This comprehensive guide distils complex psychiatric concepts into practical, accessible advice, making it a helpful reference for daily clinical practice. The authors cover a wide range of topics, from diagnosis to treatment strategies, ensuring that readers are well equipped to handle diverse patient needs. The emphasis on evidence-based approaches and real-world applications distinguishes this handbook, fostering confidence in decision-making. Rich with clinical and practical information, it serves as a crucial companion in navigating the challenges of psychiatric care. I highly recommend this handbook to anyone seeking to enhance their understanding and skills in clinical psychiatry."

Allan Young
Chair of Mood Disorders and Director, Centre for Affective Disorders,
Institute of Psychiatry, Psychology and Neuroscience, King's College London

Fundamentals of Clinical Psychiatry

A Practical Handbook

Edited by

Marsal Sanches

Professor of Psychiatry and Behavioral Sciences, The University of Texas Health Science Center at Houston (UTHealth Houston), McGovern Medical School

Jair C. Soares

Professor and Chair, Department of Psychiatry and Behavioral Sciences, The University of Texas Health Science Center at Houston (UTHealth Houston), McGovern Medical School

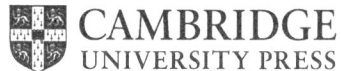

CAMBRIDGE
UNIVERSITY PRESS

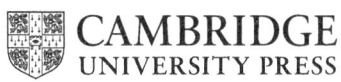

Shaftesbury Road, Cambridge CB2 8EA, United Kingdom

One Liberty Plaza, 20th Floor, New York, NY 10006, USA

477 Williamstown Road, Port Melbourne, VIC 3207, Australia

314–321, 3rd Floor, Plot 3, Splendor Forum, Jasola District Centre, New Delhi – 110025, India

103 Penang Road, #05–06/07, Visioncrest Commercial, Singapore 238467

Cambridge University Press is part of Cambridge University Press & Assessment, a department of the University of Cambridge.

We share the University's mission to contribute to society through the pursuit of education, learning and research at the highest international levels of excellence.

www.cambridge.org
Information on this title: www.cambridge.org/9781009334747

DOI: 10.1017/9781009334730

First published 2025

A catalogue record for this publication is available from the British Library

Library of Congress Cataloging-in-Publication Data
Names: Sanches, Marsal, editor. | Soares, Jair C., editor.
Title: Fundamentals of clinical psychiatry : a practical handbook / edited by Marsal Sanches, Jair C. Soares.
Description: Cambridge, United Kingdom ; New York, NY : Cambridge University Press, 2025. | Includes bibliographical references and index.
Identifiers: LCCN 2024030148 (print) | LCCN 2024030149 (ebook) | ISBN 9781009334747 (paperback) | ISBN 9781009334730 (epub)
Subjects: MESH: Mental Disorders | Psychiatry | Handbook
Classification: LCC RC454 (print) | LCC RC454 (ebook) | NLM WM 34 | DDC 616.89–dc23/eng/20240724
LC record available at https://lccn.loc.gov/2024030148
LC ebook record available at https://lccn.loc.gov/2024030149

ISBN 978-1-009-33474-7 Paperback

Contents

Contributors

Ali Abbas Asghar-Ali
Baylor College of Medicine, Houston, TX, USA

Dean J. Atkinson
The University of Texas Health Science Center at Houston (UTHealth Houston), McGovern Medical School. Houston, TX, USA

Gabriela Austgen
Baylor College of Medicine, Houston, TX, USA

Taiwo T. Babatope
University of Texas Health Science Center at Houston (UTHealth), Houston, TX, USA

Anita Barrera
The University of Texas Health Science Center at Houston (UTHealth Houston), McGovern Medical School. Houston, TX, USA

Robert J. Boland
The Menninger Clinic/Baylor College of Medicine, Houston, TX, USA

John M. Bouras
Geode Health, Houston, TX, USA

Marcelo J. A. A. Brañas
National Institute of Developmental Psychiatry for Children and Adolescents; Universidade de Sao Paulo, Sao Paulo, SP, Brazil

Lois W. Choi-Kain
Harvard Medical School, Boston, MA, USA

Stephen Conway
Brigham and Women's Hospital, Harvard Medical School, Boston, MA, USA

Marcos S. Croci
National Institute of Developmental Psychiatry for Children and Adolescents; Universidade de Sao Paulo, Sao Paulo, SP, Brazil

Parnaz Daghighi
The University of Texas Health Science Center at Houston (UTHealth Houston), McGovern Medical School. Houston, TX, USA

Morgan T. Deal
University of Colorado School of Medicine, Denver, CO, USA

Jennifer R. Gatchel
Baylor College of Medicine, Houston, TX, USA

Marcelo Bruno Generoso
Faculty of Medical Sciences of Santa Casa de São Paulo, Sao Paulo, SP, Brazil

Nisha Giridharan
Baylor College of Medicine, Houston, TX, USA

Wayne K. Goodman
Baylor College of Medicine, Houston, TX, USA

Silvia Hafliger
The University of Texas Health Science Center at Houston (UTHealth Houston), McGovern Medical School. Houston, TX, USA

Abdul Haseeb
The University of Texas Health Science Center at Houston (UTHealth Houston), McGovern Medical School. Houston, TX, USA

Amanda Helminiak
Optum, Inc., subsidiary of UnitedHealth Group USA

Karen Horn
The University of Texas Health Science Center at Houston (UTHealth Houston), McGovern Medical School. Houston, TX, USA

Julia Jurist
McLean Hospital, Belmont, MA, USA

Grace Kim
The University of Texas Health Science Center at Houston (UTHealth Houston), McGovern Medical School. Houston, TX, USA

Nermin Koch
The University of Texas Health Science Center at Houston (UTHealth Houston), McGovern Medical School. Houston, TX, USA

Ryan E. Lawrence
New York - Presbyterian Hospital and Columbia University Medical Center, New York, NY, USA

Claudia Lex
KABEG Hospital, Villach; Alpen-Adria University of Klagenfurt, Austria

Priscilla Granja Machado
Independent Researcher, Brazil

Rodrigo Machado-Vieira
The University of Texas Health Science Center at Houston (UTHealth Houston), McGovern Medical School. Houston, TX, USA

Sanjay J. Mathew
Baylor College of Medicine, Houston, TX, USA

Carrie J. McAdams
University of Texas Southwestern Medical School, Dallas, TX, USA

Jeffrey McBride
The University of Texas Health Science Center at Houston (UTHealth Houston), McGovern Medical School. Houston, TX, USA

Caroline W. McCool
Vanderbilt University Medical Center, Nashville, TN, USA

Thomas D. Meyer
The University of Texas Health Science Center at Houston (UTHealth Houston), McGovern Medical School. Houston, TX, USA

Nidal Moukaddam
Baylor College of Medicine, Houston, TX, USA

Margo Nathan
University of North Carolina at Chapel Hill, Chapel Hill, NC, USA

Olaoluwa Okusaga
Baylor College of Medicine, Houston, TX, USA

Carolina Olmos
The University of Texas Health Science Center at Houston (UTHealth Houston), McGovern Medical School. Houston, TX, USA

Antonio F. Pagán
The University of Texas Health Science Center at Houston (UTHealth Houston), McGovern Medical School. Houston, TX, USA

Natalie R. Parks
The University of Texas Health Science Center at Houston (UTHealth Houston), McGovern Medical School. Houston, TX, USA

Riah Patterson
University of North Carolina at Chapel Hill, Chapel Hill, NC, USA

Maria Carolina Pedalino Pinheiro
Faculty of Medical Sciences of Santa Casa
de São Paulo, Sao Paulo, SP, Brazil

Lindsey S. Pershern
Baylor College of Medicine, Houston, TX,
USA

Grace S. Pham
Baylor College of Medicine, Houston, TX,
USA

Edward Poa
Baylor College of Medicine, Houston, TX,
USA

Olusegun Adebisi Popoola
Baylor College of Medicine, Houston, TX,
USA

Joao Quevedo
The University of Texas Health Science
Center at Houston (UTHealth Houston),
McGovern Medical School. Houston, TX,
USA

Julia N. Riddle
University of North Carolina at Chapel
Hill, Chapel Hill, NC, USA

Anne Ruminjo
University of North Carolina at Chapel
Hill, Chapel Hill, NC, USA

Marsal Sanches
The University of Texas Health Science
Center at Houston (UTHealth Houston),
McGovern Medical School. Houston, TX,
USA

Salih Selek
The University of Texas Health Science
Center at Houston (UTHealth Houston),
McGovern Medical School. Houston, TX,
USA

Sudhakar Selvaraj
Intracellular-Therapies, Inc, USA

Lokesh Shahani
The University of Texas Health Science
Center at Houston (UTHealth Houston),
McGovern Medical School. Houston, TX,
USA

Syed Shahzeb Ayaz
Baylor College of Medicine Houston, TX,
USA

Sameer A. Sheth
Baylor College of Medicine, Houston, TX,
USA

Jair C. Soares
The University of Texas Health Science
Center at Houston (UTHealth Houston),
McGovern Medical School. Houston, TX,
USA

Juan J. Sosa
University of Texas Southwestern Medical
Center, Dallas, TX, USA

Cesar A. Soutullo
The University of Texas Health Science
Center at Houston (UTHealth Houston),
McGovern Medical School. Houston, TX,
USA

Jordan T. Stiede
Baylor College of Medicine, Houston, TX,
USA

Eric A. Storch
Baylor College of Medicine, Houston, TX,
USA

Emily R. Strouphauer
Baylor College of Medicine, Houston, TX,
USA

Antonio L. Teixeira
University of Texas Health Science Center
at San Antonio, TX, USA

Vaishali Tirumalaraju
The University of Texas Health Science
Center at Houston (UTHealth Houston),

McGovern Medical School. Houston, TX, USA

Erika S. Trent
University of Houston, Houston, TX, USA

Thanh Thuy Truong
Baylor College of Medicine, Houston, TX, USA

Michael Weaver
University of Texas Health Science Center at Houston (UTHealth), Houston, TX, USA

Heather Webber
University of Texas Health Science Center at Houston (UTHealth), Houston, TX, USA

Laura M. Welch
University of Texas Health Science Center at Houston (UTHealth), Houston, TX, USA

Andrew D. Wiese
Baylor College of Medicine, Houston, TX, USA

Luis A. Wische-Fernandez
The University of Texas Health Science Center at Houston (UTHealth Houston), McGovern Medical School. Houston, TX, USA

Cristian Patrick Zeni
The University of Texas Health Science Center at Houston (UTHealth Houston), McGovern Medical School. Houston, TX, USA

Foreword

I was delighted and honored when asked to contribute a foreword to this much-needed textbook developed by Marsal Sanches and Jair Soares. As they specify in their preface, this text is devoted specifically to "making the information easy to understand and clinically useful for trainees." It is designed to help those learners interested in, but still early in their learning about, mental health problems both to feel the humanistic elements of psychiatry and to appreciate the robust but developing basic and clinical science of our exciting and nuanced field.

Dr. Sanches has long embodied an extraordinary combination of educational, clinical, and research interests and ability. His multiple accomplishments as an academic physician are clearly reflected in the organization of this textbook. Dr. Soares, a leader in academic psychiatry and a pioneer in mood disorders research in the United States, has a long list of accomplishments in and contributions to the field of psychiatry, many of which are also reflected in this book.

The editors' emphasis on promoting faculty engagement with learners can be found in many chapters. For example, Chapter 4 helpfully describes the complexity and multidisciplinary requirements for the classification of mental illness, as well as the clinical need to continuously review and update the clinical formulation. The chapter's authors also emphasize that the formulation is established by the clinician but shared and developed collaboratively with the individual patient. As they point out, this is a daunting but intriguing work, in part because of the lack of biomarkers for most of our illnesses. Therefore, there exists the need to embrace a biopsychosocial – and even to appreciate a spiritual – approach to those we are privileged to treat. This chapter also emphasizes that although the diagnostic process is phenomenological, with many pathways for arriving at a single diagnosis, that diagnosis also allows understanding – and therefore healing (i.e., restoration to a community) – individual patients who have often felt alienated or ostracized because of their differences. This rich approach continues in other chapters, such as Chapter 16, which describes various categories of depression and how different pathways of those biopsychosocial determinants can lead to a depressive diagnosis. The authors also emphasize that the patient's history and circumstances as well as their more objective biological and behavioral findings must all be taken into account when developing and implementing treatment options.

Chapter 9 is another example of a concise and clear description of complex and practically important materials that learners must quickly appreciate. It succinctly covers the basic principles and certain key exceptions (confidentiality vs. dangerousness to others) often encountered early in the practitioners' careers. It also addresses the complexity of dual relationships that the learners will find helpful and that should lead to important conversations with their faculty.

Directors of education in medical, nursing, psychology, and social work schools will find this textbook a useful aid to nurture the interest of students exploring our field. Postgraduate education leaders in all disciplines will also recommend this textbook to their learners who are getting started on what will be a rewarding and meaningful career but may feel a bit overwhelmed by their new levels of responsibility and need key information presented in a clear and clinically useful language.

James W. Lomax, MD
Distinguished Emeritus Professor of Psychiatry, Karl Menninger Chair of Psychiatric Education, Menninger Department of Psychiatry and Behavioral Sciences, Baylor College of Medicine

Preface

Over the course of our careers as academic psychiatrists, we often have been asked by students, residents, and trainees from different areas about reading materials we could recommend to help them build their knowledge base and become properly introduced to the fascinating field of psychiatry. While there is no shortage of manuals, textbooks, and other publications authored by experts in their respective fields, some of them lack the ability to connect with the learning mind due to their complexity. Few of the available manuals are able to speak a common language, accessible to trainees at different stages of their learning process. This book aims to fill that gap.

The last several decades have observed a marked growth in the interest in psychiatry and mental health. The better understanding of the pathophysiological basis of mental disorders has consolidated psychiatry's place among medical specialties [1]. At the same time, the growing awareness of the negative impact mental health conditions have on individuals' functioning and well-being, as well as the alarming increases in suicide rates, has drawn attention to the importance of mental health treatment [2–3]. In the United States, the passage of the Affordable Care Act and the Mental Health Parity and Addiction Equity Act has expanded coverage for mental health services for a large portion of the population [4]. Nevertheless, access to psychiatric treatment remains an issue. More than half of the US counties experience consequential shortage in psychiatric care [5]. Despite recent trends that point to increases in the interest for psychiatry as a medical specialty among medical students, the shortage of psychiatrists is likely to worsen over the next several years, indicating an urgent need for more psychiatrists and other qualified mental health professionals, aiming at addressing the increased demand for mental health care [6].

Containing contributions by authors highly regarded for their work as clinicians, researchers, and educators, this book aims to provide the reader with a solid basis on the practical aspects of clinical psychiatry. Initially, general themes of high importance for psychiatry and mental health care are discussed. Subsequently, practical aspects related to the diagnosis and management of specific psychiatric syndromes and conditions are addressed in concise, structured chapters comprising an introduction, clinical and nosological consideration, brief pathophysiological aspects, management, and prognosis of the respective conditions.

During the planning and preparation of this book, a specific emphasis was placed on making the information easy to understand and clinically useful for trainees. This is not meant to be a comprehensive psychiatry textbook in which experts can look for the most recent evidence-based recommendations on the management of mental disorders or the latest findings on mental health research. Instead, authors strived to convey their individual clinical experience practicing psychiatry, as well as certain underlying theoretical constructs of importance for the basic understanding of psychiatry and mental health from an academic point of view. We expect this book to be of great interest to medical students, psychiatry residents, psychology trainees, general practitioners, and other health care workers aiming at expanding their knowledge base in the fields of psychiatry and mental health.

References

1. M. Sanches, On being a psychiatrist in the XXI century. (2019). https://med.uth.edu/psychiatry/2019/07/31/psychopathology-life-and-society-on-being-a-psychiatrist-in-the-xxi-century.

2. P. K. Chaudhury, K. Deka, & D. Chetia, Disability associated with mental disorders. *Indian Journal of Psychiatry*, **48** (2006) 95–101. https://doi.org/10.4103/0019-5545.31597.

3. M. F. Garnett & S. C. Curtin, Suicide mortality in the United States, 2001–2021. *NCHS Data Brief*, **464** (2023) 1–8.

4. K. Beronio, S. Glied, & R. Frank, How the Affordable Care Act and Mental Health Parity and Addiction Equity Act greatly expand coverage of behavioral health care. *Journal of Behavioral Health Services & Research*, **41** (2014) 410–428. https://doi.org/10.1007/s11414-014-9412-0.

5. J. S. Gardner, B. E. Plaven, P. Yellowlees, & J. H. Shore, Remote telepsychiatry workforce: a solution to psychiatry's workforce issues. *Current Psychiatry Reports*, **22** (2020) 8. https://doi.org/10.1007/s11920-020-1128-7.

6. P. F. Buckley & H. A. Nasrallah, The psychiatry workforce pool is shrinking: what are we doing about it? *Current Psychiatry*, **15** (2016) 23–24, 95.

Introduction

Marsal Sanches and Jair C. Soares

This book aims at providing the reader with an introduction to psychiatry and to the study of mental disorders. While still addressing basic theoretical concepts of importance for the understanding of psychiatry as a specific field of knowledge, its main focus is not an extensive discussion or a comprehensive review of research findings. Instead, whenever possible, the different topics are addressed from a practical point of view, allowing the reader not only to expand their base knowledge but, most importantly, to obtain a good picture of how patients experiencing these conditions usually present themselves in clinical contexts. Moreover, the treatment of mental disorders is addressed in an object-ive, straightforward way, based on the respective authors' own clinical experience in the management of a high number of patients, in different settings.

The chapters are sorted into two distinct portions. The first half of the book (Chapters 2–15) comprises general topics of interest for psychiatrist and mental health workers. Themes such as the psychiatric interview, psychopathology and the mental status exam, diagnostic and classification in psychiatry, and introduction to psychosocial aspects of psychiatric care, along with the biological basis of mental illnesses, are provided. Specific chapters focusing on transcultural and ethico-legal aspects of psych-iatry, as well as the practice of psychiatry in special populations (children and adoles-cents, geriatric patients, and women in reproductive age), are also included. Two chapters address biological treatments in psychiatry (psychopharmacology and neuro-stimulation techniques). The last two chapters of this section focus on suicide and psychomotor agitation utilizing a syndromic approach, given the importance of these conditions in psychiatric practice and their transdiagnostic nature.

In contrast, Chapters 16–32 address specific conditions or groups of disorders most commonly seen in psychiatric practice. Most chapters in this portion of the book are organized in the same way, with different sections contemplating general considerations, pathophysiological aspects, clinical presentation, and therapeutic aspects of each disorder or groups of disorders. Nonetheless, in the description of clinical features and diagnostic considerations, the contributors were given full discretion to utilize a more systematic, criteria-based approach (according to contemporary international classifications) or to use a more generic clinical framework, based on their own preference and the approach usually adopted by them in their respective daily practices. Despite the popularity and importance of systematic classifications in psychiatry, the goal of this book is not to provide a comprehensive list of diagnostic categories and criteria for every single condition hereby discussed, and the reader primarily interested in detailed information on such criteria should consult specific diagnostic manuals or books primarily focused on systematic classifications of mental illnesses [1–3].

Last, despite all the efforts made by the authors in providing accurate and up-to-date information in the present book, the field of psychiatry is constantly evolving. The authors, editors, and publisher make no warranties that the information included in this book is totally free from error. The data included in this book with regards to the diagnosis and management of patients with mental disorders (including medication risks, benefits, and side effects) are not meant to be comprehensive, and providers should consider consulting additional resources (including information provided by manufacturers, in the case of medications) before making treatment decisions. Ultimately, providers carry the responsibility for treatment decisions made in the management of patients under their care, and the authors, editors, and publisher disclaim any responsibility for the continued currency of this information and disclaim all liability for any and all damages (including direct or consequential damages) that might result from the use of information contained in this book.

References

1. American Psychiatric Association, ed., *Diagnostic and statistical manual of mental disorders: DSM-5-TR*, 5th ed., text rev. (Washington, DC: American Psychiatric Association Publishing, 2022).

2. World Health Organization, ed., *The ICD-10 classification of mental and behavioural disorders: clinical descriptions and diagnostic guidelines* (Geneva: World Health Organization, 1992).

3. P. Tyrer, ed., *Making sense of the ICD-11: for mental health professionals* (Cambridge University Press, 2023). https://doi.org/10.1017/9781009182232.

The Psychiatric Interview

Dean J. Atkinson and Amanda Helminiak

2.1 Introduction

The psychiatric interview is of paramount importance in the field of psychiatry, allowing the clinician to connect with the patient and to collect sufficient information to guide treatment. Once concluded, the interviewer should be able to describe the patient's complaints, appearance, and situation in a manner that informs diagnostic and therapeutic decisions [1]. Some of the complexities faced include conducting a mental status exam while trying to establish therapeutic rapport, soothing the patient's suffering, interviewing for diagnostic criteria, and arranging a treatment plan. It is often assumed that the skills for this crucial assessment will be "learned on the job," but this approach is fraught with possibilities for developing bad habits and failures at rapport-building. Instead, by dedicating attention to this topic, trainees may be empowered to meet these challenges as confident and effective interviewers. While some variables may prove unpredictable at times, the interviewer may bring order to the encounter through the deliberate application of learned skills. Continuous self-reflection is essential for improvement and is important for both trainees and seasoned veterans alike. This chapter will discuss the mindful preparation, execution, and assessment of effective interviews.

2.2 Before the Interview

In preparing for the interview, it is important to consider the environment in which it will take place. This includes the physical location (i.e., office environment vs emergency room), the presence of distractors, and general ambience. There will be substantial differences between a patient encounter in a quiet, planned, office visit compared with the loud, unpredictable, and chaotic nature of a high-acuity psychiatric inpatient unit. The interviewer should strive to minimize any challenges inherent to their individual setting and create a calm environment for the patient. Whenever possible, interviews should provide as much privacy as possible while maintaining safety. It is also worth noting that the patient's emotional state can have significant implications for the quality of the assessment. It is quite difficult to obtain a valid history from an acutely agitated and aggressive patient or from a profoundly depressed patient with little speech output. Other patients may be guarded due to paranoia, anxiety, or skepticism toward health care workers, which can also impair data collection. In some cases, these factors may be modifiable within a reasonable time frame, which would make a brief postponement acceptable. In other circumstances, the interviewer may not have this luxury and will have to proceed as able. In the hospital setting, it is also best to avoid interruptions to sleep, meals, and recreational activities so as to minimize frustration and distraction.

Before engaging any patient in a clinical interview, some effort should be made to collect any pertinent and available data relevant to the situation. This information will highlight important topics and inform the interviewer about potential pitfalls. The amount of information might be very limited, such as that obtained during a walk-in emergency department encounter, or it could be extensive, such as when detailed notes have been provided by a transferring facility. Past records can be particularly illuminating, especially if current symptoms bear some similarity to prior presentations. A word of caution: Though this chart review can be quite helpful, it may be incorrect for a variety of reasons. Similarly, it is also not uncommon for collateral information to be inaccurate, even if well intended. One must therefore maintain an air of skepticism and flexibility, avoiding a rigid path of exploration.

After reviewing the information, it is worthwhile to identify which interview topics are best to prioritize; for example, assessing suicide risk factors in a patient with depression will be of greater importance than their educational history. This is not to say that a full initial history is unimportant, but rather to point out that some triage may be necessary, due to time limitations or other constraints. The bottom line is to review the available information, get a basic impression of what the interview will entail, and formulate a strategy for proceeding accurately and in a timely manner.

The components of a typical psychiatric interview include the Chief Complaint, History of Present Illness, Review of Systems, Past Psychiatric History, Past Medical History, Family History, Social History, and the Mental Status Examination. In the following section, a variety of techniques for structuring and navigating through the psychiatric interview will be discussed in more detail.

2.3 During the Interview

To emphasize the unique nature of the psychiatric interview, consider the similarity to the services of a locksmith. Clients seek the services of a locksmith to help them gain access to something important that they cannot unlock on their own. Slight tension or pressure can help focus and gently guide patients toward progress, but too much pressure will be disruptive and counterproductive. Psychiatrists must attend closely to each step in the interview, assessing the response to individual lines of questioning and adapting their approach to find the next best step, focusing on using the right tool for the job.

To unlock a complex patient history, the first focus should be on building good rapport with the patient. Patients who like their clinicians feel more comfortable sharing intimate details of their lives and are more likely to follow treatment recommendations. To achieve a strong therapeutic alliance is a challenging and nuanced art form and requires thoughtful intention. Renowned psychologist Carl Rogers advocated for a client-centered approach to this task, emphasizing the principles of Genuineness, Unconditional Positive Regard, and Accurate Empathy [2]. **Genuineness** entails the interviewer being authentic and honest, even if this means not representing a model of perfection. At times this may inadvertently lead to conflict or may compromise the perceived authority inherent in the clinician's role; however, relatability and accessibility are predominantly more beneficial. With **Unconditional Positive Regard**, the interviewer strives to be accepting of the client for who they are and to refrain from judgment. Finally, **Accurate Empathy** involves the ability to understand emotions from the patient's perspective while maintaining appropriate professional distance. In addition, this principle requires the ability to communicate this understanding effectively to the patient.

From the field of motivational interviewing, the use of simple and complex reflections may be of great utility to this end [3]. **Simple Reflections** comprise the patient's own words or very similar verbiage and involve the clinician merely repeating them to demonstrate listening. **Complex Reflections**, by contrast, are those in which the psychiatrist has added their own interpretation to more fully imply their understanding of what the patient has expressed. For example, if a patient says, "I have been feeling so angry at my spouse," the clinician may demonstrate a simple reflection by stating, "You've been really upset." Alternatively, the clinician may utilize a complex reflection, bringing in their perceived alternate viewpoint. For example, they could reply, "You have been feeling unappreciated lately." Here, the interviewer is using an educated guess, potentially unlocking the true underlying sentiment at hand, which may not yet be in the patient's conscious awareness.

In engaging with the patient, body language is also critical to keep in mind; for example, arm-crossing and leaning away from the patient may lead to disengagement, while open body language and leaning forward in an interested way can allow the patient to feel more at ease. Conversely, the interviewer may attend to the patient's body language as an indicator of their engagement.

Much like the approach a locksmith must take to an unyielding door, the interviewer should be strategic and flexible, employing a variety of tools to achieve their goal. To tackle the interview with a rote checklist would be metaphorically similar to gaining entrance to a locked room by way of a sledgehammer. This is not guaranteed to be effective and may cause irreparable harm. In reality, the ideal interview is one that does not feel much like an interview. With sufficient practice, the experience should feel more like a conversation, but one that is subtly targeted and focused without seeming rigid or overtly structured [1]. Questions are adapted from the context of the interview and follow the patient's narrative while providing opportunities to redirect and ask for additional details. While the locksmith has a variety of picks at their disposal, one toolbox available to the interviewer comes in the form of so-called **Gates**, as described by internationally acclaimed psychiatrist Shawn Christopher Shea [4]. Gates are devices to transition between topics or areas of exploration during the encounter. In other words, when used effectively, they allow an interview to feel more conversational. Though not an exhaustive list, three of the most powerful examples are the Spontaneous Gate, the Referred Gate, and the Natural Gate.

A **Spontaneous Gate** occurs when the patient changes topic and the interviewer does not redirect. If the topic change is beneficial, then this is an easy win; if this happens too often, however, it will lead to wandering. The most important thing to learn is how to recognize when the patient is changing topics and to decide how best to respond. Here is an example of a Spontaneous Gate:

CLINICIAN: "Is this the first time you've seen a mental health professional?"

PATIENT: "Oh no, I've been seeing a psychiatrist off and on since I was a teenager. The last one told me I had bipolar disorder and put me on a bunch of different meds. My mom used to take meds for bipolar too."

CLINICIAN: "Tell me a bit more about that."

In the above example, the Spontaneous Gate occurred when the patient stopped discussing their own psychiatric history and switched to family history instead, a change that was supported by the clinician. If the clinician felt the switch was premature, this could have been redirected with a short statement such as, "Before we move on to that, could you tell me which medications you've tried in the past?" If not redirected, the interviewer will likely have to come back to this topic later to obtain the remaining unknown information.

A **Referred Gate** occurs when the clinician utilizes previous content from the interview as a way to change the topic. This is fairly flexible and can be used at nearly any time, provided the interviewer has a good working memory of the conversation that has transpired. In the prior example, let's assume that the interviewer had redirected the patient away from the family history section so that they could elicit a complete past psychiatric history. If they now wish to change the topic to family history, they might say something like this:

PATIENT: "That's about all I remember about my past treatment."

CLINICIAN: "You mentioned earlier that your mother had also been treated for bipolar disorder, what about other family members?"

PATIENT: "Actually yes – my brother . . . and my mom's sister too."

The interviewer above has now smoothly changed subjects by referencing a bit of information the patient has already disclosed. With this technique in mind, it is good to be cognizant of what the patient is saying at all times, tucking away opportunities to be used in future parts of the interview.

A **Natural Gate** occurs when the interview uses a patient's recent statement as a springboard, asking a transition question to switch the topic. These require some creativity, but once mastered, they are extraordinarily powerful.

PATIENT: "I've been seeing a psychiatrist off and on since I was a teenager. The last one told me I had bipolar disorder and put me on a bunch of different meds."

CLINICIAN: "Does anyone else in the family have bipolar disorder?"

In this example, the interviewer is choosing to initiate a transition from the patient's past psychiatric history into family history. With practice, this technique has an enormous potential for flexibility.

By utilizing the above transitions, an interviewer can learn to smoothly guide the progression of the encounter in a conversational manner while retaining control over the direction and content discussed.

When engaging with a patient, it is important for an interviewer to monitor not only the content of their speech but also their manner of speaking [5]. The tone of a statement can dramatically affect the way it is perceived, even when the content is identical. Consider the difference in emphasis between "Oh, that makes sense" (said with a thoughtful facial expression) and "Oh, THAT makes sense" (said with a slight smirk). The first would likely be perceived as supportive, while the latter could be interpreted as sarcastic. While the tone of voice is certainly important, facial expression and overall demeanor can have a significant impact as well. **Affect Matching** is a term used to describe the efforts made on the part of the interviewer to slightly mirror the patient [3]. If they are speaking with a low volume and tone of voice, such as is often seen in depression, the interviewer would be wise to lower their own volume and tone to more closely approximate that of the patient. This should be evaluated on a case-by-case basis and is not always appropriate, but generally speaking, patients will be more comfortable sharing information with someone whose manner does not contrast sharply with their own.

It is also important to avoid jargon and to speak at the level of your patient, something that can occasionally be achieved by incorporating their own language into your own [5, 6]. Medical terminology often enters into the general public's lexicon and cannot always be trusted to convey an accurate message (e.g., bipolar, OCD).

Special attention should also be given to phrasing in a nonjudgmental manner, if the interviewer wishes to obtain accurate data. For example, consider the differences between asking "How far did you **go** in school?" and "How far did you **get** in school?" The first is a fairly benign historical question that entails a choice on behalf of the patient. The second can be perceived as condescending, almost as if to say, "How far did you get before you couldn't get any farther?" Interviewers may find patients more willing to share about sensitive topics like substance use by asking about "experimentation" with "recreational drugs" rather than asking about "abuse" of "illegal drugs."

In addition to avoiding judgmental statements, it is important to be flexible when screening for psychiatric symptomatology. A common error among trainees and seasoned clinicians alike is to lapse into routine forms of screening questions. Too often, for instance, the only screen for auditory hallucinations in every patient seems to be: "Are you hearing things that other people don't hear?" or "Are you hearing any voices?" There are numerous problems with this. The first is that these questions will feel contrived when used in a rote manner and not adapted to the patient's own unique experience. The second is that many patients will perceive the question incorrectly. Patients experiencing hallucinations rarely characterize them as "hallucinations," since this would mean they are not real, when to the patient they are experienced as very real indeed. Patients who have substantial history speaking with mental health professionals know all too well that the term "voices" really means "hallucinations." The third issue is that these questions are too specific. Although auditory hallucinations in the form of a voice are fairly common, this represents only one type of auditory hallucination that could be experienced. Clinicians should continuously monitor their phrasing, searching for areas to optimize in a patient-centered manner. Any demonstrable pattern that does not incorporate the individual patient's clinical picture and history should be looked upon with great scrutiny and preferably transformed into a more nuanced screening question whenever possible. Any phrasing that could be misconstrued as judgmental or is otherwise off-putting should be adjusted accordingly.

Another nonverbal area that warrants attention is the application of body language. Clinicians should attend to their own facial expressions, body position, and posture. Some facial reactivity is expected when patients divulge details to communicate empathy, though too much can be counterproductive. For example, it would be inappropriate to have no reaction to a patient's recounting of a substantial past trauma, but if the interviewer's reaction communicates discomfort or shock, this may cause a patient to stop sharing additional information. Concerning the rest of the body, an effort should be made to meet the patient on their level, preferably both parties sitting and turned at an angle. An interviewer who stands over the patient may be perceived as looking down on them, in congruence with their physical state. It is also helpful to maintain an open stance, avoiding the crossing of arms (even if the room is cold). For paranoid patients, great care must be taken to keep hands visible at all times rather than clasped behind the back or stuffed into pockets. An engaged interviewer will find themselves leaning in toward the patient in a listening stance rather than sitting far back in their chair in an unconscious attempt to escape from the conversation. Some notetaking is appropriate, as it demonstrates attentiveness, though if patients appear uncomfortable, this should be minimized.

2.4 After the Interview

In order to continue developing improved interview skills over time, it is necessary to be intentional about self-reflection following patient encounters. Tracking the length of time spent on the interview, any lapses in information gathering, and the quality of therapeutic alliance achieved are important. It is also reasonable to seek the guidance of more seasoned practitioners in determining areas for optimization. Some licensing programs require periodic graded patient encounters to be performed, during which the observers rate the interviewer on the success of data collection, the ability to develop a rapport with the patient, and subsequent presentation skills.

2.5 Conclusion

With dedication and practice, both locksmiths and mental health clinicians alike can solve even the most intricate puzzles using the right tools. The clinician must be appropriately empathic and nonjudgmental, even paying attention to their own body language so as to convey active listening and alliance with the patient. In their discussion with the patient, a skilled interviewer should masterfully employ techniques such as Gates to acquire important information with finesse. Finally, continual growth should be sought over time through self-assessment, or through external assessment options when available. It is by this process that clinicians may develop into excellent interviewers who are more readily able to help their patients. Although important, historically there has been a lack of directed educational initiatives to improve interviewing skills [7]; emphasizing these with an intentional curriculum may serve future mental health clinicians.

References

1. J. Nordgaard, L. A. Sass, and J. Parnas. The psychiatric interview: validity, structure, and subjectivity. *Eur Arch Psychiatry Clin Neurosci* **263**, 353–364 (2013). https://doi.org/10.1007/s00406-012-0366-z.

2. C. Rogers. The necessary and sufficient conditions of therapeutic personality change. *J Consult Psychol* **21**(2), 95–103 (1957).

3. W. Miller and S. Rollnick. *Motivational Interviewing: Helping People Change.* 3rd ed. Guilford Press, 2013.

4. S. Shea. *Psychiatric Interviewing: The Art of Understanding – A Practical Guide for Psychiatrists, Psychologists, Counselors, Social Workers, Nurses, and Other Mental Health Professionals.* 3rd ed. Elsevier, 2017.

5. J. Morrison. *The First Interview.* 4th ed. Guilford Press, 2014.

6. D. Carlat. *The Psychiatric Interview.* 4th ed. Wolters Kluwer, 2017.

7. E. Lenouvel, C. Chivu, J. Mattson, et al. Instructional design strategies for teaching the mental status examination and psychiatric interview: a scoping review. *Acad Psychiatry* **46**, 750–758 (2022). https://doi.org/10.1007/s40596-022-0161.

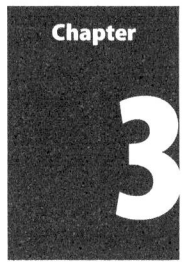

Chapter 3

Psychopathology and the Mental Status Examination

Marsal Sanches

3.1 Introduction

Based on the current standards established for the practice of psychiatry, a formal psychiatric evaluation must include a detailed, itemized description of the mental status exam (MSE). Despite considerable variations with regards to its structure and the terminology utilized in its description, the MSE carries considerable weight from a clinical, decision-making, and even legal perspective.

The MSE, in its current format, was conceived as the psychiatric equivalent of the physical examination. For purposes of documentation, it is considered, by most practitioners, the "objective" portion of the psychiatric assessment, in contrast with history data (obtained from the patient and from other sources), which comprise the "subjective" part of the examination. Nonetheless, except for some of its portions, which require specific questions for purposes of clarification, most of the MSE is performed concomitantly to the process of history taking and is based on the observations of the psychiatrist during the interview.

This process of formulation of the MSE is closely related to the concept of psychopathology itself. Psychopathology, in a more basic sense, is the study of the experiences reported by the patient that deviate from normality, acquiring a pathological meaning [1]. Obviously, defining what is "normal" in psychiatry is not an easy task, as a certain behavior or experience can be considered normal or pathological depending on different factors, including the patient's cultural context, the degree of suffering experienced by the patient as a result of the experience or behavior, and the functional impact of the behavior in question, among others. Because of that, the MSE is based on the so-called phenomenological approach [2]. This means that, during the interview, the psychiatrist critically analyzes the experiences reported by the patient, as well as the behaviors displayed during the assessment, and reaches conclusions regarding their nature, by trying to "place themselves in the patient's shoes" and comparing those experiences with their own and with similar experiences reported by other individuals the interviewer has previously interacted with. In addition, the interviewer should take into account other elements, such as the context of the interview and the sociocultural environment in which the patient is immersed. A conclusion regarding the nature of the elements reported or displayed by the patient is then eventually reached [3]. The different psychopathological elements identified through this process will then become a key element for the formulation of the patient's psychiatric diagnosis (Figure 3.1).

The present chapter provides a succinct description of the MSE and of the main psychopathological concepts of interest.

Table 3.1 The Mental Status Examination

1. General Appearance and Presentation

2. Psychomotricity

3. Speech

4. Thought Process

5. Thought Content

6. Mood

7. Affect

8. Sensoperception

9. Insight and Judgement

10. Cognition

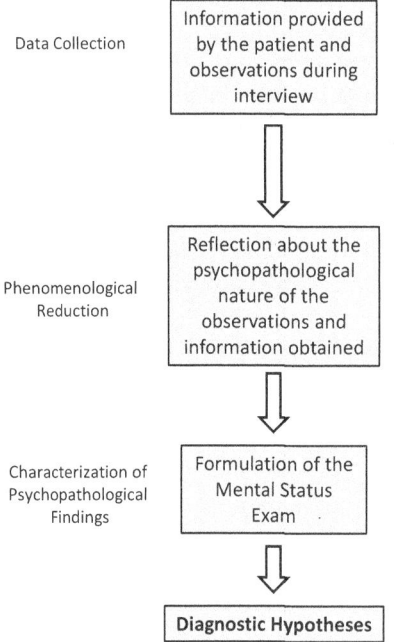

Figure 3.1 Obtaining the diagnosis – a flow chart.

3.2 Structure of the Mental Status Exam

There are different ways to organize the mental status exam. The structure presented below (also repeated in Table 3.1) is among the most popular ones and tries to avoid the overlap of elements for which a more objective description is feasible (e.g., general appearance) with others, which are based on inferences regarding the patient's inner state and specific mental functions (e.g., thought process).

Table 3.2 Most common abnormal movements observed during the mental status exam

Abnormal Movement	Description	Diagnostic Value*
Tremors	Shaking, rhythmic movements	Neurological conditions Essential tremor Substance withdrawal Side effects of medications
Diskinetic movements	Writhing movements of the trunk, limbs, or face	Tardive dyskinesia Neurological conditions
Tics	Repetitive, noncontinuous movements or vocalizations in limited muscle groups	Tourette's syndrome Tic disorders
Mannerisms	Peculiar/unusual movements, behaviors, or postures, often with purpose	Psychotic disorders Catatonia Autism spectrum disorders
Stereotypies	Repetitive, frequent movements with no purpose/goal	Psychotic disorders Catatonia Autism spectrum disorder
Motor compulsions	Repetitive movements with variable degrees of complexity, aiming at relieving the anxiety associated with obsessive thoughts	Obsessive-compulsive disorder

* List is not supposed to be exclusive

1. General Appearance and Presentation

    This item includes not only objective aspects of the encounter with the patient, such as their appearance, grooming, dressing, and facial expression, but also general subjective impressions gathered by the interviewer over the course of the examination. How does the patient look? Is the patient uncooperative (negativism)? Do they look guarded, suspicious, or uncomfortable? Was the interview easy to perform? Curiously, even the more objective items related to the patient's appearance and behavior should be considered in accord with the context where the interview takes place. A patient who looks poorly groomed or wearing a peculiar set of clothes should be analyzed in according with their cultural and socioeconomic status before a pathological meaning is attributed to it by the examiner.

2. Psychomotor Aspects

    In this item, we usually include motor aspects of the patient's presentation, which are translated into movements or lack thereof. Is the patient agitated, restless, or physically violent? Are they gesticulating to emphasize their point of view? How does the patients gait look? Are any abnormal movements noticed, such as tremors, diskinetic movements, tics, mannerisms, or stereotypies [4]? (See also Table 3.2). Is the patient displaying any compulsions, that is, repetitive acts associated with obsessive thoughts (see Point 5 below)? Are there any signs of psychomotor slowness or inhibition? Patients in catatonic states classically (but not always) present with immobility, mutism, stereotypies, waxy flexibility (tendency to keep limbs immobile, in the position they are placed by the examiner), and echolalia (tendency to repeat words or phrases) [5].

3. Speech

Speech, as an item of the mental status exam, is often described according to its rate, volume, and tone. Rate corresponds to the speed of the speech ("normal," increased, or decreased). As for the volume, the speech is described as increased (loud), "normal," or decreased. The speech's tone is described as "normal," angry, flat, or sad (among others). This item also includes qualitative changes in speech such as echolalia and coprolalia (involuntary tendency to use obscene or socially inappropriate words) [6].

Please note that, despite its apparent objectivity and easiness to describe, the inclusion of speech as an independent item of the mental status exam can be questioned from a phenomenological standpoint. In many patients, the characterization of speech overlaps with other items of the mental status exam, including psychomotor aspects, thought process, mood, affect, and cognition.

4. Thought Process

Thought process indicates how the patient's ideas are connected and how the patient shifts from one topic to another. Most individuals have an *organized* or *linear* thought process: The ideas are well connected, and changes in the topic of the speech happen in a gradual and easy-to-follow way. In *flight of ideas*, the patient shifts from topic to topic quickly, although it is still possible for the interviewer to follow the patient as the topic shifts take place. Patients with *looseness of associations* do not show smooth transition from one topic to the other, which can present in several different degrees, ranging from mildly derailed thought process to disorganized thought process, which in its extreme presentation is sometimes called "word salad." In another spectrum of the thought process, we can find descriptions of thought *circumstantiality* and *tangentiality*. These abnormalities in thought process correspond to the opposite of disorganized thought process, in the sense that the patient has difficulties switching to a different topic and reverberates around the same focus (perseveration), often unable to distinguish what is essential from what is dispensable in their report (prolixity) [3].

5. Thought Content

This item comprises the report of the patient's inner experiences, most commonly transmitted to us through speech. More than a mere description of the experiences themselves, an accurate characterization of the thought content implicates a careful analysis of the form of the experience itself, and not only of their content. This allows the inference of different subtypes of inner experiences, as follow:

a) *Delusions*: classically conceptualized as unreal experiences that are not affected by logical arguments in contrary [7–9], delusions are classified according to their theme including, among others, paranoid, grandiose, nihilistic, religious, erotic, and somatic. From a phenomenological standpoint, it is useful to explore how the patient reached certain conclusions regarding an experience before characterizing it as delusional [8]. That is particularly important in the case of non-bizarre delusions, where the search for collateral data aiming at confirming the lack of veracity of a non-bizarre belief might be inconclusive or not feasible.

b) *Obsessions*: obsessions correspond to intrusive, repetitive, and ego-dystonic beliefs that are recognized by the patient as their own thoughts [10]. Patients experiencing obsessions are aware of the pathological nature of the thoughts in question but feel compelled to experience them. An obsession has been sometimes compared to a "mental foreign body", to illustrate the patient's repetitive and mostly unsuccessful efforts to remove it from their mind. The most common types of obsessions are related to contamination, harming others, and control. Obsessions are frequently accompanied by compulsions, which are repetitive acts aiming at decreasing the anxiety associated with an obsessive thought. It is important to note that compulsions are not part of the thought content, and can be included in the subjective history data or in the psychomotor aspects item of the MSE (if observed during the assessment). Although the classic description of obsessions characterizes them as, by definition, ego-dystonic, that feature is not always apparent, and the most recent edition of DSM-5 included a poor insight specifier in the obsessive-compulsive disorder diagnostic category.

c) *Overvalued or prevailing ideas*: these are ego-syntonic ideas that, due to their emotional content, tend occupy most of the patient's thought content and influence their behaviors [11–12]. For instance, patients in grief states or adjustment disorders often present with overvalued ideas

d) *Other elements of thought content*: there are virtually no limits on the different types of thought content a patient can experience. Suicidal thoughts, homicidal thoughts, and thoughts related to life circumstances are some examples. Ideas associated with current mood state are thoughts that seem to be in congruence with the mood state experienced by the individual during the interview. For example, patients with depressed mood will often report depressive thoughts, while patients with anxious or irritable mood may describe thought contents associated with those feelings (anxious or angry thoughts). Similarly, patients with elated mood may report thoughts related to overconfidence and some degree of grandiosity, as well as excessive plans for the future. In case an apparently mood-related thought seems to be delusional in nature, it should be classified as a delusional thought and not as a mood-associated thought. A common source of confusion in the description of the thought content is the difference between suicidal thoughts and passive death thoughts. The distinction between these two elements is of great importance, as the former may be an indicator of imminent risk of suicide. If a patient reports passive death thoughts, they express wishes to be dead but has no deliberations, intent, or plan related to taking their own life. On the other hand, suicidal ideation designates thoughts involving some degree of planning or deliberation related to causing their own death, with or without intent to put those actions into practice. It is important to emphasize that, according to this conceptualization, the terms "passive suicidal ideation" or "passive suicidal thoughts" seem inappropriate from a phenomenological standpoint and should, therefore, be avoided during the description of the mental status exam.

6. Mood and Affect

Although usually described as two independent items of the mental status exam, mood and affect are discussed here as a single topic due to the considerable variation in the terminology and concepts adopted for their description [13–15]. Both correspond to the emotional aspects of the patient during the interview. A popular way to distinguish between mood and affect establishes that mood corresponds to the word the patient utilizes to describe their inner emotional state. As such, it should always be documented between quotes. Affect, on the other hand, would correspond to the emotion the patient seems to be displaying, based on the interviewer's judgment. According to this concept, a patient might subjectively describe their mood as "depressed" while actually displaying a happy emotional state (incongruent affect) or displaying little or no emotions (constricted or flat affect), or quickly shifting across different emotions (labile affect). An alternative approach would be describing mood as the emotion that, based on the interviewer's observations, seems to prevail during the interview, while affect would correspond to the totality of the emotional experiences exhibited by the patient during the assessment. Following this model mood would be described as euthymic ("normal"), depressed, manic, anxious, or irritable. Affect, on the other hand, would be described according to its congruence (as congruent or incongruent, according to whether or not the displayed emotions match the thought content reported by the patient), its stability (as stable or labile, according to how quickly emotions seem to shift during the interview), and its modulation (as modulating, constricted, or flat/blunted, according to how clearly emotions are displayed during the interview).

7. Sensoperception

The description of experiences associated with environmental stimuli (captured through the sensorial organs) and their inner reconstruction are usually included in this item of the mental status exam [16–18]. The classic examples of sensoperceptional abnormalities include perceptual distortions involving external visual stimuli, such as distortions related to size (micropsias, macropsias), color (xanthopsia), distance, or shape of external objects. In the case of illusions (a term usually utilized to describe visual experiences), an external object is perceived as a totally different one. Individuals with perceptual distortions may have different degrees of insight associated with the experiences in questions, sometimes recognizing them as unreal and other times not having full awareness of the abnormal nature of those perceptions.

Even though this could be questioned from a phenomenological standpoint, hallucinations are commonly included in the sensoperception section of the mental status exam because they are perceived by the patient as sensoperceptive abnormalities. In the case of a hallucination, there is no external object to be perceived, and the mind, pathologically, creates a mental element that is *erroneously recognized by the patient* as resulting from an external stimulus. There are different types of hallucinations:

a) *Visual hallucinations*: those can vary in terms of how structured they are. Less elaborate visual hallucinations may include shadows, shapes, or dysmorphic elements. More structured visual hallucinations include people, animals, fantastic entities, and others. Visual hallucinations are usually considered a "red flag" for psychotic disorders secondary to a medical condition, although they can be present in nonorganic medical disorders as well. The suspiciousness for an organic (medical) etiology for the hallucinations is raised when the visual hallucination is not accompanied by delusions, does not include an associated auditory component (e.g., human figures that do not talk to the patient), or is accompanied by disorientation / decreased level of consciousness.

b) *Auditory hallucinations*: a hallmark of psychiatric conditions, auditory hallucinations can have different presentations. Dialogue hallucinations correspond to voices speaking directly to the patient, who feels compelled to engage in conversation with them. Command auditory hallucinations are experienced as orders heard by the patient. Third-person auditory hallucinations correspond to one or more voices usually making derogatory comments about the patient without addressing him/her directly. Thought echo is experienced as a voice reproducing the content of the patient's thoughts in real time, usually verbatim. The diagnostic importance of true auditory hallucinations is undeniable as an indicator of psychosis, and can be present in different conditions, including manic states, severe depression, and schizophrenia. Specifically, third-person auditory hallucinations were classically considered first-rank symptoms of schizophrenia, meaning that they were highly suggestive (although not pathognomonic) of that condition.

c) *Hallucinatory-like phenomena with intact reality testing*: several other experiences perceived by the patient as secondary to sensoperceptional stimuli can resemble hallucinations if taken based on face value, but lack the impaired judgment component. In other words, they are recognized by the patient as unreal, even though they can be associated with different levels of distress. The term "organic hallucinosis" has been utilized in such situations, when the experience in question is clearly secondary to a medical etiology or is substance induced [19]. Similarly, patients with borderline personality disorder or posttraumatic stress disorder, among other conditions, may experience quasi-hallucinatory experiences that resemble true hallucinations but are not accompanied by impaired judgment (i.e., patients knows they are not real) and may show some incongruence with other findings of the mental status exam.

8. Insight and Judgment

These two items of the mental status exam are often described together. There is considerable variation in their conceptualization and the way clinicians assess them, with both terms frequently used interchangeably. Both have to do with the patient's awareness of the natures of their own experiences and how normal or pathological they are regarded by the patient. A simple way to conceptualize these terms is to consider judgment as the patient's general awareness of the abnormal or dysfunctional nature of their experiences, while insight would be related to whether or not the patient would recognize those behaviors as a result of a mental disorder. Following this concept, impairments in insight and judgment are usually closely connected (that is, if a patient has impaired judgment, insight is also impaired), although there are exceptions to that rule. In contrast, in many academic departments, insight is described as the patient's own awareness of the pathological nature of his/her behaviors, beliefs, or other experiences, while judgment is restricted to what is named "hypothetical judgment": the patient is presented with a hypothetical situation and asked to describe what would be his/her course of action if he/she were the one facing the situation in question. Some examples include the classic questions such as "What would you do if you were in a movie theater and someone suddenly yells 'Fire!'" or "How would you proceed if you were driving and a ball came bouncing from the sidewalk onto the middle of the street?" These questions may illicit interesting content, able to provide valuable information on the patient's mental functioning but work more as a measure of judgment in the general sense, not in the phenomenological sense.

9. Cognition

This item of the mental status exam includes several different functions that are directly or indirectly connected. While the MSE includes an assessment of cognition, a specific cognitive screening (e.g., the Mini-Mental State Examination or the Montreal Cognitive Assessment) [20–21] or a full neuropsychological evaluation should be considered when primary cognitive disorders (e.g., dementia) are suspected.

a) *Consciousness*: in classic phenomenology, consciousness is regarded as having a vertical axis, or the "level of consciousness," and a horizontal axis, or the "field of consciousness" [22]. Abnormalities in consciousness are usually related to decreases in those axis. In the vertical axis, consciousness can be described as ranging from full alertness to coma. Between those two poles there may be several intermediate degrees of impairment in the level of consciousness, with considerable variations in the terms utilized to describe them. Patients with an impaired level of consciousness usually show decreased responsiveness to external stimuli as well as psychopathological findings related to other mental functions, such as attention, orientation, and thought process. In the horizontal axis, on the other hand, consciousness is assessed with respect to its amplitude. Changes in the horizontal axis of consciousness are difficult to characterize from a phenomenological standpoint. Enlargement in the field of consciousness is usually described in association with the use of psychedelic drugs and meditation-induced altered states of consciousness. In contrast, when experiencing a narrowing in the field of consciousness, patients present with trance-like states. During such states they are able to perform certain acts in an automatic way, with little or no subsequent recall, as observed in certain types of epilepsy and dissociative states.

b) *Orientation*: orientation indicates the patient's ability to situate themselves with regards to themselves (identity or orientation to self) and to external elements (time, place, and situation) [23]. Disturbances in orientation can be an indicator of psychosis (e.g., patients who are delusional may have abnormal orientation to self) or, more commonly, of impairments in other cognitive functions. For example, patients with a decreased level of consciousness or memory impairment often present with disorientation regarding time, space, or situation. Often, orientation data are implicitly obtained by the interviewer during the conversation with the patient. If necessary, specific questions about orientation can be asked.

c) *Attention*: this function represents the patient's ability to direct their mental activity toward one specific stimulus (tenacity) and to shift it to new stimuli (vigilance) [3–24]. In some conditions (e.g., severe depression) both can be impaired, but as a general rule, they alternate. In other words, conditions or states with increased focus (hypertenacity) are associated with decreased vigilance. On the other hand, states of hypervigilance (distractibility) will be accompanied by decreases in the ability to focus (hypotenacity). During the patient's examination, attention can be inferred through the patient's ability to participate in the interview and the quality of their interaction with the interviewer, or can be specifically tested by asking the patient to repeat a certain sequence (e.g., numbers, days of the week, months of the year) forward and then backward.

d) *Memory*: memory is one of the most important mental functions, and a detailed description of the various modalities of memory (e.g., episodic, semantic, procedural, and working memory) [24] and their diagnostic value is beyond the scope of the present chapter. In the MSE, the item "memory" is used as a rough estimation of the patient's episodic memory: that is, their ability to retain and recall facts, events, or other specific data with which they are provided. According to the temporal distance between the stimulus and the recall, memory can be classified as *immediate*, *recent*, and *remote*. Practically speaking, a simple way to test the patient's memory is asking them to repeat three numbers (or three words). The ability to promptly repeat the information is a measure of *immediate memory*, which, if impaired, is actually an indicator of attentional problems. After the patient has repeated the numbers/words, the interviewer should apply a distractor (e.g., talk with the patient about past events, which can be used as a way to measure the patient's *remote memory*). Finally, after at least 5 minutes have elapsed, the interviewer should ask the patient to recall the three words or numbers they were previously asked to repeat. That should be adopted as an estimation of the patient's *recent memory*. While memory impairment may be an indirect result of disturbances in other mental functions and may be present in many mental disorders (e.g., mood disorders, anxiety disorders, and psychotic disorders), primary deficits in memory are typically found in neuropsychiatric conditions such as traumatic brain injuries and neurocognitive disorders.

e) *Other cognitive functions*: although not routinely included in the MSE, these functions and their abnormalities can be tested when the suspicion for neuropsychiatric or cognitive disorders is high. Those include the assessment and description of calculation abilities, language, visuospatial functioning, and executive functioning [22–24].

3.3 Conclusions

This chapter provided a practical approach for the description of the MSE, based on concepts from classic psychopathology. While it is possible that the MSE, in its current structure, becomes obsolete as new diagnostic approaches and novel nosological systems are adopted, a sound knowledge of psychopathology will always remain pivotal for the proper diagnosis and management of psychiatric conditions. For example, it is unlikely that an algorithm or a biological marker will ever be able to master the subtle processes involved in distinguishing culturally endorsed conditions from psychiatric disorders. That should continue to be the job of mental health professionals.

References

1. G. Stanghellini, The meanings of psychopathology. *Current Opinion in Psychiatry*, **22** (2009) 559–564. https://doi.org/10.1097/YCO.0b013e3283318e36.

2. H. Häfner, Descriptive psychopathology, phenomenology, and the legacy of Karl Jaspers. *Dialogues in Clinical Neuroscience*, **17** (2015) 19.

3. M. Sanches, A. P. Marques, S. Ortegosa, A. Freirias, R. Uchida, & S. Tamai, The mental status exam: can it be standardized? *Arquivos Médicos dos Hospitais e da Faculdade de Ciências Médicas da Santa Casa de São Paulo*, **50** (2005) 18–23.

4. Y. Mahgoub, S. Sarwar, & A. Francis, Catatonic stereotypies and mannerisms vs.

tics: not everything that quacks is a duck! *Psychosomatics*, **61** (2020) 307–308. https://doi.org/10.1016/j.psym.2019.11.005.

5. C. Kaufmann, N.Agalawatta, & G. S. Malhi, Catatonia: stereotypies, mannerisms and perseverations. *Australian and New Zealand Journal of Psychiatry*, **52**(4) (2018) 391–393.

6. R. G. Shavitt, A. G. Hounie, M. C. R. Campos, & E. C. Miguel, Tourette's syndrome. *Pshyciatric Clinics of North America*, **29**(2) (2006) 471–486.

7. C. Allen, The nature of delusions. *Nature*, **179** (1957) 719–720. https://doi.org/10.1038/179719b0.

8. C. Kiran & S. Chaudhury, Understanding delusions. *Industrial Psychiatry Journal*, **18** (2009) 3–18. https://doi.org/10.4103/0972-6748.57851.

9. M. Maj, Karl Jaspers and the genesis of delusions in schizophrenia. *Schizophrenia Bulletin*, **39** (2013) 242–243. https://doi.org/10.1093/schbul/sbs190.

10. A. R. Rasmussen & J. Parnas, What is obsession? Differentiating obsessive-compulsive disorder and the schizophrenia spectrum. *Schizophrenia Research*, **243** (2022) 1–8. https://doi.org/10.1016/j.schres.2022.02.014.

11. R. Mullen & R. J. Linscott, A comparison of delusions and overvalued ideas. *The Journal of Nervous and Mental Disease*, **198** (2010) 35–38. https://doi.org/10.1097/NMD.0b013e3181c818b2.

12. P. J. McKenna, Disorders with overvalued ideas. *British Journal of Psychiatry*, **145** (1984) 579–585.

13. L. Baldaçara, C. R. Bueno, D. S. Lima, L. P. C. Nóbrega, & M. Sanches, Mood and affect: how to define them? *Arquivos Médicos dos Hospitais e da Faculdade de Ciências Médicas da Santa Casa de São Paulo*, **52**(3) (2007) 108–113.

14. S. Pridmore, Mood and affect. *Psychiatry and Clinical Neurosciences*, **73** (2019) 347. https://doi.org/10.1111/pcn.12836.

15. M. Serby, Psychiatric resident conceptualizations of mood and affect within the mental status examination. *American Journal of Psychiatry*, **160** (2003) 1527–1529. https://doi.org/10.1176/appi.ajp.160.8.1527.

16. E. Miller, The affective nature of illusion and hallucination. *Journal of Neurology, Neurosurgery & Psychiatry*, **1–8** (1927) 1–8. https://doi.org/10.1136/jnnp.s1-8.29.1.

17. J. D. Blom, Auditory hallucinations. In *Handbook of Clinical Neurology* (Elsevier, 2015), pp. 433–455. https://doi.org/10.1016/B978-0-444-62630-1.00024-X.

18. M. Manford, Complex visual hallucinations: clinical and neurobiological insights. *Brain*, **121** (1998) 1819–1840. https://doi.org/10.1093/brain/121.10.1819.

19. J. R. Cornelius, J. Mezzich, H. Fabrega, M. D. Cornelius, J. Myers, & R. F. Ulrich, Characterizing organic hallucinosis. *Comprehensive Psychiatry*, **32** (1991) 338–344. https://doi.org/10.1016/0010-440X(91)90083-O.

20. Z. S. Nasreddine, N. A. Phillips, V. Bédirian, S. Charbonneau, V. Whitehead, I. Collin, J. L. Cummings, & H. Chertkow, The Montreal Cognitive Assessment, MoCA: a brief screening tool for mild cognitive impairment. *Journal of the American Geriatrics Society*, **53** (2005) 695–699. https://doi.org/10.1111/j.1532-5415.2005.53221.x.

21. E. Mossello & M. Boncinelli, Mini-Mental State Examination: a 30-year story. *Aging Clinical and Experimental Research*, **18** (2006) 271–273. https://doi.org/10.1007/BF03324660.

22. M. R. Louzã Neto, Da Motta, Telma, Wang, Yuan-Pang, & Helkis, Helio, *Psiquiatria basica* (Artes Medicas, 1995).

23. A. DeLong, Phenomenological space-time: toward an experiential relativity. *Science*, **213** (1981) 681–683. https://doi.org/10.1126/science.7256273.

24. P. D. Harvey, Domains of cognition and their assessment. *Dialogues in Clinical Neuroscience*, **21** (2019) 227–237. https://doi.org/10.31887/DCNS.2019.21.3/pharvey.

Chapter

4

Classifications and the Diagnostic Process in Psychiatry

Marcelo Bruno Generoso and Marsal Sanches

4.1 The Diagnostic Process

The diagnostic process is a core feature of medical practice and may be understood as the path a clinician takes starting from listening to the complaint reported by a patient until the definition of a specific construct selected from a predefined set of categories agreed upon by the medical community to designate a specific condition. This will, ideally, summarize the symptoms experienced by the patient, facilitating the proper communication between health care providers and enabling the proper treatment of the condition [1]. Depending on the complexity of each health problem, this process may take from a few minutes to several months or even years. While sometimes a diagnostic formulation can be straightforward, for example when diagnosing a patient with classic symptoms of delirium in a medical inpatient unit, in other situations the diagnosis is not immediately clear. In certain situations, due to psychopathological issues and limited insight, patients are only able to provide limited information during an initial assessment, and the involvement of the family and other sources of collateral data become critical.

The task of performing an accurate diagnosis is undoubtedly challenging, and a stepwise approach may be useful. The first step consists of information gathering with patients, their families, and other health care professionals or caregivers if applicable. At this step, interviewing skills play a decisive role to ensure proper rapport and precise understanding of what is being said. The second step corresponds to the mental status examination. The third step is the integration of a preliminary diagnostic hypothesis with laboratory or medical imaging data, when appropriate. The fourth step includes consultations with other specialties if necessary; the fifth and final step comprises data integration and interpretation, allowing a specific diagnosis to be formulated [2, 3]. In reality, this is commonly an ongoing process, in which the clinicians often revisit some steps to better understand critical data, evaluate new findings, and even review or update previously established hypotheses.

Moreover, the diagnostic process is intrinsically related to clinical reasoning itself, which can be defined as the cognitive process involved in evaluating and managing a patient's clinical presentation [4]. The current understanding of clinical reasoning is anchored in a dual-process model that proposes two systems guiding this mental effort. System 1 works as a pattern recognition program in which the physician intuitively and automatically recognizes the presented set of data and correlates it to a series of similar situations trying to fit it into a box of previously known experiences. System 2, also described as the analytical system, is required for complex or novel situations or for a diagnosis revision, for example, and can be understood as meticulous critical thinking in which each possible hypothesis will have to be exhaustively scrutinized [5–7].

System 1 is faster but riskier than system 2, since it is more tendentious and biased, but it is an excellent tool in emergency situations that require prompt action. On the other hand, system 2 is slow and requires conscious and arduous reasoning that follows strict scientific thinking and is very useful in excluding, validating, or revisiting possible diagnoses or following a line of treatment by analyzing all the possible variables involved. These systems can be seen as complementary strategies in the decision-making process, and it is important to be mindful of their existence as well as the advantages and disadvantages of each one so that the diagnostic process can be optimized [8].

In summary, reaching a psychiatric diagnosis is a considerable challenge, since it relies essentially on the description of symptoms and facts reported by patients or their families and behavior observation. Our specialty still lacks reliable biological markers or laboratory tests to confirm mental disorders such as major depressive disorder or anxiety disorders. Laboratory and imaging medicine are mostly used to exclude possible organic causes of the symptoms observed or reported by the patient; therefore, the diagnosis of mental illness remains primarily based on symptoms and course [9].

4.2 The Importance of the Diagnosis in Psychiatry

A psychiatric diagnosis is basically a name agreed upon and approved by medical societies for a set of symptoms, signs, and complaints displayed and reported by a patient. Diagnoses provide a common language and facilitate communication among health care professionals, define prognoses, help determine possible interventions or treatments with the best chance of success, enable prevention strategies, and facilitate medical teaching and research [10, 11]. The diagnosis is also of great importance for the patient, as it not only provides a common denomination for the symptoms experienced by a patient but also helps delineate a therapeutic and prognostic pathway.

4.3 Understanding Mental Illness

According to the American Psychiatric Association (APA), a mental illness is a health condition that changes a person's thinking, feelings, or behavior accompanied by distress or difficulty in functioning in work, family, or social activities [12]. In a broader sense, we can understand mental illnesses as the product of a complex interaction between predisposing, precipitating, perpetuating, and protective factors. Those factors include not only biological aspects but also psychological issues related to the patient's personal life history, as well as environmental and social factors [13].

Mental illnesses are traditionally distinguished from neurological conditions such as epilepsy or Parkinson's disease, as the biological basis of the former has not yet been completely elucidated. This scenario will probably change in the future with research advances providing a progressively better understanding of the pathophysiology of mental illnesses.

4.4 The Development of Diagnostic Systems in Psychiatry

We can trace diagnostic classifications for mental disorders back to Hippocratic writings (around 400 BC). Hippocrates disconnected mental disorders from supernatural factors, sorting them out into mania, melancholy, panic, phrenitis, insanity, disobedience, paranoia, epilepsy, and hysteria [14]. Nonetheless, modern psychiatric nosology started to become better defined in the 19th century, when different authors (such as Philip Pinel and his disciple, Jean-Étienne Esquirol) proposed their own diagnostic classification systems. Still, a turning point in psychiatry nosology was the publication of Emil Kraepelin`s *Lehrbuch der Psychiatrie* or *Manual of Psychiatry*, in 1899. Kraepelin proposed two main categories based on course and outcome: manic-depressive insanity, which included the conditions currently called mood disorders, with a fluctuating course and full recovery between episodes; and the so-called *dementia precox* (later named schizophrenia), which would start in adolescence or early adulthood and show progressive worsening, with residual symptoms and deficits [15]. Kraepelin was a brilliant clinician, and his classification was based on meticulous observation and written records of thousands of patients and their clinical condition.

Nowadays, there are two diagnostic manuals that are largely used in psychiatry: the Diagnostic and Statistical Manual of Mental Disorders (DSM) published by the APA, currently in its fifth version with one text revision (DSM-5-TR); and the International Classification of Diseases and Related Health Problems (ICD) published by the World Health Organization (WHO), currently in its eleventh version (ICD-11). While ICD encompasses all health conditions and diseases, DSM focuses only on mental disorders.

4.5 The Diagnostic and Statistical Manual of Mental Disorders

The DSM aims at classifying mental disorders and improving diagnostic reliability. First published by the APA in 1952 in the context of important geopolitical changes following World War II, the manual was strongly influenced by Adolf Meyer, a Swiss-American psychiatrist and neurologist who is considered one of the fathers of scientific psychiatry in the United States.

The first edition of DSM (DSM-I) evolved from psychiatrist William Menninger`s technical bulletin "Medical 203" released in 1943, an Armed Forces classification manual for mental disorders guided by Sigmund Freud's and Adolf Meyer's theories, and from the *Statistical Manual of the Use of Hospitals for Mental Disease* of the hospitalized population in the United States, published by the APA (at the time American Medico-Psychological Association). To better embase the publication, drafts of the proposal were circulated among 520 American and Canadian psychiatrists, and 241 replies were received [16]. This first version of DSM classified mental disorders into those caused by an organic brain dysfunction and those secondary to social-environmental stressors on an individual's biological constitution and inability to adapt – in other words, occurring without evidence of organic brain findings [17].

While the second version of the manual, published in 1968, remained mainly guided by psychodynamic understanding, the third version (DSM-III), published in 1980, was an important milestone in the history of psychiatry. It was developed in the 1970s, a time when psychopharmacotherapy, symptoms assessment scales, and behaviorist psychotherapy approaches were in ascension. DSM-III offered a paradigm shift in modern psychiatry for its atheoretical or aetiological nature, as it did not intend to explain the cause of mental disorders through psychoanalytical formulations and relied on symptom description, diagnostic criteria, and differential diagnoses. It also underwent reliability testing through field trials to calibrate mental disorders criteria. After its publication, DSM-III moved psychiatry closer to other medical specialties with a more scientific orientation and a palatable understanding of mental disorders and their diagnostic process. Quickly, the majority of scientific publications started to utilize DSM-III criteria and diagnostic categories, providing a common language among researchers and contributing to advancements in clinical research. Medical schools also started to adopt DSM-III as the standard psychiatric classification for academic purposes.

DSM-III-R, a text revision, was published in 1987. That was followed by DSM-IV in 1994 and its text revision in 2000. DSM-5, published in 2013, was a product of the contribution of more than 400 experts from different fields of medicine and psychology and a series of 13 international conferences, which resulted in a manual with 22 main categories and including more than 150 mental disorders. Last, in 2022, the text revision of DSM-5 was published (DSM-5-TR).

4.5.1 DSM-5-TR

In addition to the detailed description of the minimal criteria necessary for the diagnosis of mental disorders, including duration of symptoms, DSM-5-TR provides data related to registry procedures, specifiers, related characteristics that support diagnosis, prevalence, development and course, risk factors and prognosis, culture and gender related aspects, differential diagnosis, and comorbidity, among others. Moreover, relevant laboratory or physical exam findings can be included in the diagnostic formulation if appropriate. The manual is divided into three major sections: section 1 is an introductory section and provides instructions on how to use the manual; section 2 is composed of the descriptions of mental disorders and relevant information on them; and section 3 encompasses conditions of interest for further research and assessment. Compared to DSM-5, it underwent a comprehensive literature review of diagnostic criteria and specifiers, with great attention given to cultural and ethnic diversity as well as sex and gender disparities. The manual maintains 22 categories of disorders (Table 4.1).

Table 4.1 DSM-5-TR disorders categories

- Neurodevelopmental Disorders
- Schizophrenia Spectrum and Other Psychotic Disorders
- Bipolar and Related Disorders
- Depressive Disorders
- Anxiety Disorders
- Obsessive-Compulsive and Related Disorders
- Trauma- and Stressor-Related Disorders
- Dissociative Disorders
- Somatic Symptom and Related Disorders
- Feeding and Eating Disorders
- Elimination Disorders
- Sleep–Wake Disorders
- Sexual Dysfunctions
- Gender Dysphoria
- Disruptive, Impulse-Control, and Conduct Disorders
- Substance-Related and Addictive Disorders
- Neurocognitive Disorders
- Personality Disorders
- Paraphilic Disorders
- Other Mental Disorders and Additional Codes
- Medication-Induced Movement Disorders and Other Adverse Effects of Medication
- Other Conditions That May Be a Focus of Clinical Attention

4.6 International Classification of Diseases

The first internationally standardized classification system for diseases, focused on causes of death, is considered to be the Bertillon Classification, named after its main author Jacques Bertillon in 1893, and was adopted by the International Statistical Institute. In 1948, after several reviews, the recently founded WHO published the renamed International Classification of Diseases (ICD-6), including not only causes of death but also morbidity, with the addition of a specific section for mental disorders. The main objectives were to provide a global medical common language to improve international cooperation and understanding, as well as to facilitate the standardization of records for epidemiological purposes [18]. ICD-10, published in 1994, embraced the atheoretical classification of mental and behavioral disorders proposed by DSM-III and eliminated terms such as "endogenous depression" and "neurotic depression," emphasizing symptom descriptions rather than offering theoretical explanations for the disorders.

4.6.1 ICD-11

ICD-11, approved in the 72nd World Health Assembly in 2019 and effective since January 1, 2022, brings significant restructuring, with a feasible digital framework interface for data storing and a management software, as well as the possibility for tailored composition of disease coding and correlations among them. Each disease can be coded on its own diagnostic stem with extension codes as well as clustered with other stem codes for better understanding [19]. For example, in a suicide attempt (stem code) with overdose, the substance used can be specified (extension code). Extension code topics are presented in Table 4.2.

Further, ICD-11 focuses on global validity and practical utility; provides codes for mortality causes reporting and allows coding of diseases, disorders, and other health-related conditions contributing for governments strategic plans concerning public health; and is the adopted classification for health care payments and billing. It also includes designations of severity, course, and specific symptoms when suitable.

There are four main chapters of interest in ICD-11 for mental health professionals; mental, behavioral, and neurodevelopmental disorders; sleep–wake disorders; diseases of

Table 4.2 Topics of extension codes in ICD-11

- Severity scale value
- Temporality
- Aetiology
- Topology scale value
- Anatomy and topography
- Histopathology
- Dimensions of injury
- Dimensions of external causes
- Consciousness
- Substances
- Diagnosis code descriptors
- Capacity or context
- Health devices, equipment, and supplies

Table 4.3 ICD-11 mental, behavioral, and neurodevelopmental disorders groups

- Neurodevelopmental disorders
- Schizophrenia and other primary psychotic disorders
- Catatonia
- Mood disorders
- Anxiety and fear-related disorders
- Obsessive-compulsive and related disorders
- Disorders specifically associated with stress
- Dissociative disorders
- Feeding and eating disorders
- Elimination disorders
- Disorders of bodily distress and bodily experience
- Disorders due to substance use and addictive behaviours
- Impulse control disorders
- Disruptive behaviour and dissocial disorders
- Personality disorders
- Paraphilic disorders
- Factitious disorders
- Neurocognitive disorders
- Mental and behavioural disorders associated with pregnancy, childbirth and the puerperium
- Psychological and behavioural factors affecting disorders or diseases classified elsewhere
- Secondary mental or behavioural syndromes associated with disorders or diseases classified elsewhere

the nervous system; and conditions related to sexual health. There was a significant effort from the WHO and the APA to find common ground between DSM-5 and ICD-11 to improve compatibility. A list of essential features of each disorder is provided but, unlike DSM-5, a specific number of symptoms and their duration are avoided unless there is widespread agreement on these topics for certain disorders, which may be useful to increase clinical utility through different cultures and countries [20]. The mental, behavioral, and neurodevelopmental disorders chapter encompasses 21 disorder groups (Table 4.3) and adds 15 new diagnoses (Table 4.4).

4.7 Conclusion

As presented, the diagnosis is a crucial step in a patient's assessment and treatment plan and is a result of the process of clinical reasoning that encompasses two complementary strategies, one based on pattern recognition and the other on meticulous thinking and data scrutinization.

We currently have at our disposal two main diagnostic manuals (DSM-5-TR and ICD-11) that, despite facing challenges and limitations, are the two best tools for that end so far. They are far from perfect and still rely on the patient's history, symptoms presentation, and the fulfillment of criteria in a descriptive manner. Mostly, they still lack reliable biomarkers, leading to potential issues related to the validity of their different diagnostic categories, but they are essential for communication among health care professionals, patients, and their families, as well as for clinical research.

Table 4.4 New diagnoses in the mental, behavioral, and neurodevelopmental disorders chapter of ICD-11

- Catatonia
- Bipolar Type II Disorder
- Body Dysmorphic Disorder
- Olfactory Reference Disorder
- Hoarding Disorder
- Excoriation Disorder
- Complex PTSD
- Prolonged Grief Disorder
- Binge Eating Disorder
- Avoidant/Restrictive Food Intake Disorder
- Body Integrity Dysphoria
- Gaming Disorder
- Compulsive Sexual Behaviour Disorder
- Intermittent Explosive Disorder
- Premenstrual Dysphoric Disorder

References

1. Jutel, A. Sociology of diagnosis: a preliminary review. *Sociol Health Illn.* 2009;31(2):278–299.

2. Kassirer, JP. Teaching clinical reasoning: case-based and coached. *Acad Med.* 2010;85(7):1118–1124.

3. Committee on Diagnostic Error in Health Care; Board on Health Care Services; Institute of Medicine; National Academies of Sciences, Engineering, and Medicine. *Improving Diagnosis in Health Care,* Balogh EP, Miller BT, Ball JR, eds. National Academies Press; 2015.

4. Barrows, HS, Tamblyn, RM. *Problem-Based Learning: An Approach to Medical Education.* Springer Publishing Company; 1980.

5. Stanovich, KE, West, RF. Individual differences in reasoning: Implications for the rationality debate? *Behav Brain Sci.* 2001;23(5):645–665.

6. Hogarth, RM. *Deciding Analytically or Trusting Your Intuition? The Advantages and Disadvantages of Analytic and Intuitive Thought. The Routines of Decision Making.* Lawrence Erlbaum Associates Publishers; 2005.

7. Kahneman, D. *Thinking, Fast and Slow.* Farrar, Straus and Giroux; 2011.

8. Balogh, EP, Miller, BT, Ball, JR, eds. *Improving Diagnosis in Health Care.* National Academies Press; 2015.

9. Möller, H-J. The consequences of DSM-5 for psychiatric diagnosis and psychopharmacotherapy. *Int J Psychiatry Clin Pract.* 2014;18(2):78–85.

10. Frances A. *Essentials of Psychiatric Diagnosis: Responding to the Challenge of DSM-5®.* Revised ed. Guilford Press; 2013.

11. Johnstone, L, ed. *A Straight Talking Introduction to Psychiatric Diagnosis.* PCCS Books; 2014.

12. American Psychiatric Association. Mental Illness [Internet]. 2022 [accessed Sep 9, 2023]. Available from: https://www.psychiatry.org/patients-families/what-is-mental-illness.

13. Winters, NC, Hanson, G, Stoyanova, V. The case formulation in child and adolescent psychiatry. *Child Adolesc Psychiatr Clin N Am.* 2007;16(1):111–132.

14. Kleisiaris, CF, Sfakianakis, C, Papathanasiou, IV. Health care practices in ancient Greece: the Hippocratic ideal. *J Med Ethics Hist Med.* 2014;7:6.

15. Kendler, KS. The development of Kraepelin's concept of dementia praecox: a close reading of relevant texts. *JAMA Psychiatry.* 2020;77(11):1181–1187.

16. Surís, A, Holliday, R, North, CS. The evolution of the classification of psychiatric disorders. *Behav Sci (Basel).* 2016;6(1):5.

17. Kawa, S, Giordano, J. A brief historicity of the Diagnostic and Statistical Manual of Mental Disorders: issues and implications for the future of psychiatric canon and practice. *Philos Ethics Humanit Med.* 2012;7:2.

18. Moriyama, IM, Loy, RM, Robb-smith, AHT, Rosenberg, HM, Hoyert, DL, eds. *History of the Statistical Classification of Diseases and Causes of Death.* National Center for Health Statistics; 2011.

19. Harrison, JE, Weber, S, Jakob, R, Chute, CG. ICD-11: an international classification of diseases for the twenty-first century. *BMC Med Informatics Decision Making.* 2021;21(6):206.

20. Gaebel, W, Stricker, J, Kerst, A. Changes from ICD-10 to ICD-11 and future directions in psychiatric classification. *Dialogues Clin Neurosci.* 2020;22(1):7–15.

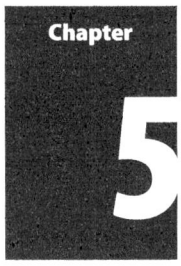

Neurobiology of Mental Disorders

Karen Horn, Anita Barrera, Abdul Haseeb, and Rodrigo Machado-Vieira

5.1 Introduction

Psychiatric disorders are mostly multifactorial and have the potential to disrupt an individual's perception of reality, affecting their mood, sleep, appetite, thought content and processing, and a wide range of behavioral, cognitive, and social interactions. The neurobiology of mental disorders involves a complex interplay between brain structure and brain function, as well as human psychological manifestations and behaviors. While psychological and environmental factors contribute to the development of mental disorders, the intricate neurobiological mechanisms underlying these conditions provide invaluable insight to understanding and treating them. Mental disorders encompass a wide range of conditions including mood disorders, psychotic disorders, and anxiety disorders (Figure 5.1). Here, we briefly discuss the neural circuitry, neurotransmitter systems, genetics, and structural and functional brain changes that contribute to the development of different mental disorders [1, 2, 3].

5.2 Neurobiology of Psychosis

The main feature of psychotic disorders is psychosis, characterized by the presence of hallucinations, delusions, as well as disorganized thought and behaviors. Psychotic disorders include schizophrenia spectrum disorders, delusional disorder, and psychosis due to substances or underlying medical conditions, among others. However, psychosis can also be a feature in other mental disorders such as bipolar disorder, major depressive disorder, and some personality disorders. Research into the neurobiology of psychotic disorders aims to elucidate the underlying mechanisms, paving the way for improved understanding, early detection, and targeted interventions for individuals affected by these conditions [1, 2, 3].

5.2.1 Genetics of Psychosis

Genetics plays a significant role in the development of mental disorders [4]. While the precise genetic contributions to mental disorders are still being studied, research has shown that a combination of genetic and environmental factors influences the risk of developing these conditions. Here are some key points regarding the genetics of mental disorders. Twin studies have found that the lifetime risk for schizophrenia is about 1%; 6.5% in first-degree relatives of patients, 12.5% for dizygotic twins, and about 50% for monozygotic twins, suggesting a strong genetic component in the development of these disorders [1]. Several mutated genes are thought to contribute to psychotic disorders. The majority of genetic advancement that has taken place in psychiatry is largely due to genome-wide association

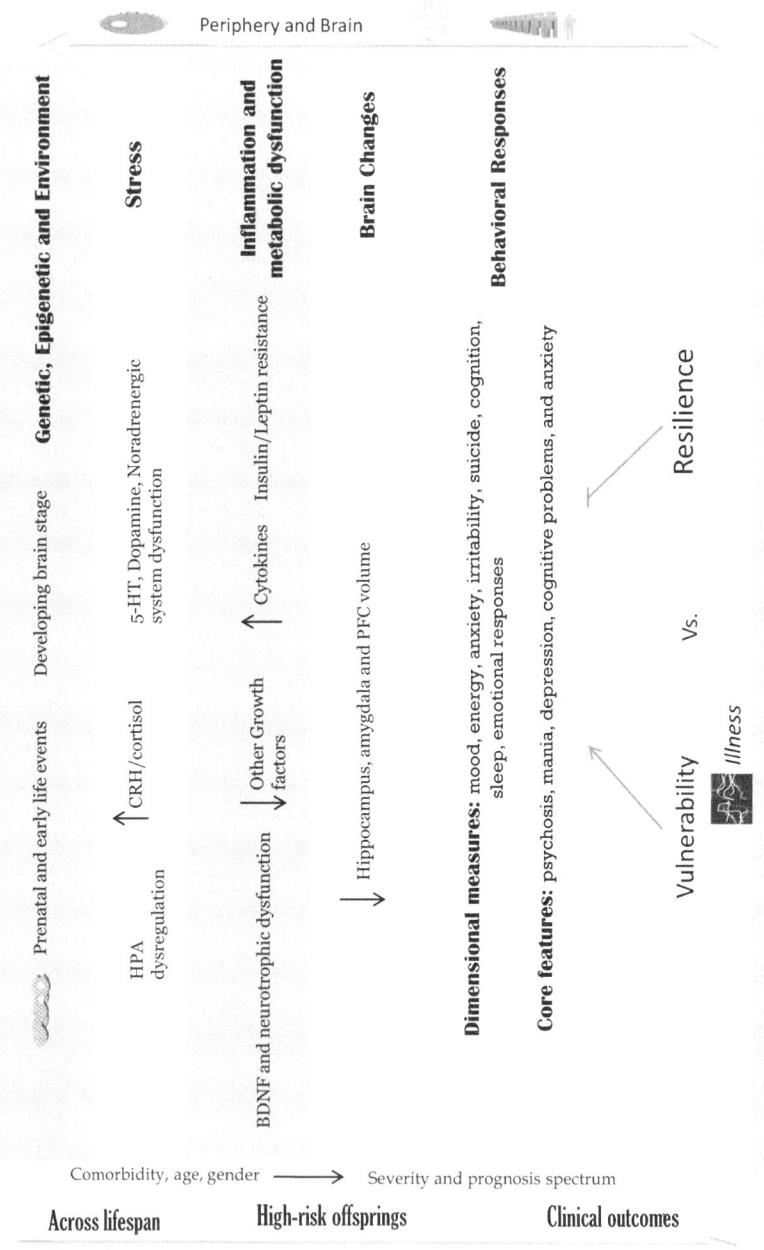

Neurobiology of Psychiatric Disorders

Figure 5.1 The neurobiology of psychiatric disorders involves a wide range of biomarkers at multiple levels, including genetic, stress-related, environmental, inflammatory, and behavioral response that can trigger mood-related symptoms and psychosis.

studies (GWAS). GWAS aim to identify genetic variations through the use of genetic markers known as single nucleotide polymorphisms (SNPs). In schizophrenia, thousands of distinct genetic loci with more than 100 common alleles have been identified through GWAS. Each gene is only thought to increase vulnerability by small increments, and susceptibility is conferred by overlapping sets of genes. Therefore, it may be useful to conceptualize a spectrum of clinical phenotypes when considering psychosis.

Evidence in both human studies and animal models suggest that alteration in dopaminergic function presents a strong susceptibility factor for the development of schizophrenia. GWAS found a significant linkage at locus 1q42 along with a suggestive linkage at 22q1, relating to genes DISC1 (disrupted-in-schizophrenia 1) and COMT (catechol-o-methyltransferase), respectively. These genes are involved in both presynaptic dopamine and its metabolism [2]. Other genes involved in the regulation of dopamine have been associated with schizophrenia, providing insight into the relationship between dopaminergic transmission and the development of psychosis [5].

Meta-analyses of individual genetic linkage studies have shown evidence of a connection between schizophrenia and bipolar disorder through regions containing many genes, although no specific names for these regions have been recognized. Still, several independent studies have implicated CACNA1C – a gene that codes for the α-1C subunit of L-type voltage-gated calcium channel. This channel is involved in neuronal activity and synaptic plasticity. CACNA1C has been associated with increased risk of psychosis in major depressive, bipolar, and schizoaffective disorders, as well as schizophrenia [3, 4].

Two genes linked to schizophrenia are of particular interest: the dystrobrevin-binding protein 1(DTNBP1) gene, also known as dysbindin, and the neuregulin 1 (NRG1) gene. Both genes are expressed at central nervous system synapses and are involved in glutamate transmission [6]. It has been reported that individuals with the dysbindin risk haplotype of DTNBP1 were more likely to display the negative symptoms of schizophrenia (i.e., anhedonia) [5]. Studies of chromosomal structural copy number variants (CNVs) demonstrate an increased susceptibility to psychotic disorders linked to microdeletions on chromosome 22q11. Notably, CNVs associated with schizophrenia have also shown involvement in neurodevelopmental disorders such as autism and generalized epilepsy [2].

Other findings of schizophrenia studies show multiple correlated variants in the major histocompatibility complex (MHC), associated with acquired immunity [6]. MHC genes have been found in brain regions associated with learning and cognition. Although no clear relationship has been established, it is now believed that altered immune system and inflammatory mechanisms could also be implicated in the development of schizophrenia.

Currently, there is no genetic testing available for different mental illnesses because the link between multiple genes and specific DNA or protein alterations involved in their etiologies has yet to be identified. Future research should be aimed at exploring genetic epidemiology suitable for family and twin studies. The study of candidate genes in psychiatric disorders is still in its early stages, and for each currently identified, further investigation is warranted.

5.2.2 Neurotransmission in Psychosis

Our knowledge about the pathophysiology of psychosis is largely based on studies showing alteration of neurotransmitters and their function. The primary symptoms observed in schizophrenia have been attributed to abnormalities in many neurotransmitter systems. This connection was established, in part, because antipsychotics work by altering the levels and/or actions of neurotransmitters in the brain [7].

An important feature of psychosis is subcortical dopamine dysfunction. Excessive dopamine activity in the mesolimbic system, involved in reward and motivation, has been implicated with the positive symptoms of psychosis [7]. Positive symptoms include hallucinations and delusions. Recently, studies have suggested a strong association between presynaptic dopamine dysfunction in the associative striatum, and abnormalities in dopamine synthesis, synaptic levels, and release [8]. Individuals at high risk of developing schizophrenia show comparable abnormal dopaminergic function in the associative striatum, even before the onset of psychotic symptoms. Elevated levels of dopamine synthesis and release have also been associated with the age of onset in psychosis [9].

The cause of the increased activity of dopaminergic neurons in the striatum is largely unknown, but some theories propose variations in hippocampal control, cortical input to dopamine systems, or inherent abnormalities of dopaminergic neurons. It has been suggested that disrupted interactions between the thalamus, the cerebral cortex, and the striatum are associated with hallucinations and delusions [6]. Auditory hallucinations in schizophrenia have also been linked to altered connectivity and function in the thalamus, hippocampus, and striatum [8].

Decreased activity of the glutamate N-methyl-D-aspartate (NMDA) receptor is also potentially involved in the pathophysiology of psychosis [10]. The NMDA receptor antagonists ketamine and phencyclidine (PCP) are known to cause cognitive dysfunction in healthy individuals. PCP has shown to decrease dopamine activity in the prefrontal cortex, subsequently increasing dopamine activity in the mesolimbic system. These effects are associated with the negative symptoms of schizophrenia as well as psychosis [6, 10, 11]. Distinct imaging and functional studies in subjects with schizophrenia show evidence of decreased function of NMDA [10]. Moreover, studies suggest a correlation between decreased NMDA receptor activity and dysfunction of gamma-aminobutyric acid (GABA) interneurons in areas of the hippocampus, prefrontal cortex, and cingulate cortex. NMDA receptor blockade has also shown to reduce GABA transmission in these areas. Postmortem studies in schizophrenia subjects support these findings by showing decreased GABA levels in the prefrontal cortex, specifically in the parvalbumin class of GABA interneurons.

Brain-derived neurotrophic factor (BDNF) signaling supports neuronal growth and development. It also has been shown to mediate glutamatergic and GABAergic transmission. Theories suggest that decreased BDNF expression may be related to the dysfunction within the prefrontal cortex along with the disruption in cognitive function and working memory observed in schizophrenic patients [12]. Negative symptom medications for schizophrenia include D-serine, glycine, and sarcosine because of their ability to modulate the NMDA receptors.

5.2.3 Neuroanatomical Changes in Psychosis

When patients present with new-onset psychosis, brain scans were once thought necessary to rule any somatic causes. This practice has lost favor in clinical practice because of the lack of evidence to support its use in the absence of overt neurological signs in psychotic patients [13, 14]. Furthermore, although structural abnormalities were commonly found, they typically did not require any intervention, as psychosis was rarely thought to be associated with them [15].

While brain imaging might be unnecessary for clinical practice, the obtained from brain scans showed that individuals who experience psychosis indeed exhibit profound gray matter loss in the prefrontal, medial and superior temporal lobes. Volume loss in the superior and medial temporal lobes, as well as the thalamus, is believed to be associated with the negative symptoms observed in patients with schizophrenia [16]. CT scans have also demonstrated ventricular enlargement, specifically in the lateral and third ventricle, along with a higher rate of cortical thinning in the prefrontal cortex [17, 18]. One possible distinguishing feature between schizophrenia and other psychotic disorders lies in hippocampal size. Data have shown that decreased bilateral hippocampal volume is associated with chronic schizophrenia. In contrast, patients with mood disorders with psychotic features or otherwise unspecified psychosis showed normal hippocampal size. Of note, amygdala volumes in this group of patients were significantly increased when compared to schizophrenia patients [19].

A reduced number and size of oligodendrocytes have also been found in the prefrontal cortex and thalamus of schizophrenia patients when compared to healthy individuals [20]. Moreover, working memory and cognitive decline in schizophrenia may be due to abnormal glial cell differentiation and increased demyelination [21]. Decreased executive functioning relates to structural abnormalities in the striatum, thalamus, cerebellum, anterior cingulate gyrus, hippocampus, medial temporal lobe, medial frontal cortex, and posterior parietal cortex [17]. Other findings showed that proinflammatory cytokines could predict the activation of microglia leading to tissue loss. This possibly indicates that psychosis is immune-related and that neuroinflammation may be a key contributing factor [6, 22]. Very few studies have reported the effects of psychotic disorders on white matter, but one study suggested a reduction in white matter as schizophrenia progresses to a chronic state [23, 24]. The relationship between white matter and cognitive function has not been fully investigated.

Scientists continue to explore the biological mechanisms underlying psychotic disorders in order to improve our understanding and help develop more effective treatments.

5.3 Neurobiology of Mood Disorders

Mood disorders, also known as affective disorders, are psychiatric conditions characterized by significant disturbances in a person's emotional state, with symptoms ranging from persistent, overwhelming hopelessness to extremely elevated mood. Major depressive disorder (MDD), its various subtypes—such as persistent depressive disorder and premenstrual dysphoric disorder—as well as the bipolar disorders (BPD) comprise the category of mood disorders. These conditions affect millions of people worldwide, causing considerable distress and impairing daily function. Several factors, including psychological influences, play a crucial role in the development of mood disorders, and extensive research has been done to investigate the underlying neurobiology contributing to their pathophysiology.

5.3.1 Genetics of Mood Disorders

Analyses of the latest large-scale genome-wide association studies on major depressive disorder (MDD), bipolar disorder (BD), and other affective disorders have sought to identify genetic variants linked to increased susceptibility for mood disorders. Findings of SNPs analyses have suggested that the affective disorders exist on a spectrum, and that there is a significant genetic relationship between the mood disorders.

Twin studies have aimed to assess the heritability of major depression. Data suggest that 30–40% of susceptibility to MDD is accounted for by genetic factors. These studies also identified specific variants involved in neurotransmitter pathways, neuroplasticity, and stress response [26]. GWAS of MDD and other depressive variants have identified several loci of genes involved with various biological pathways including excitatory neurotransmission, synaptic function, and immune response. Some of the identified genes, such as the sortilin-related VPS10 domain containing receptor 3 (SORCS3), dopamine receptor D2 (DRD2), and calcium binding protein 1 (CABP1), are linked to glutamate release at excitatory synapses. As in other mental disorders [10], the balance of excitatory and inhibitory pathways appears to be altered in depressive mood disorders [25].

For BD, GWAS have identified at least 30 significant loci, including genes involved in biological processes such as calcium signaling (CACNA1C), ion channels and transporters (SCN2A, SLC4A1), neurotransmitter receptors (GRIN2A), and synaptic function (RIMS1, ANK3) [27]. Other pathways involved include insulin secretion and endocannabinoid signaling. Notably, these studies found no overlapping loci with those associated with depression; however, they highlighted shared genetic risks between BD and schizophrenia.

Genetic connections between BD and MDD have continued to be explored. Findings suggest a significant genetic component—60%–80%—in the heritability of BD, indicating a higher heritability of BD when compared to MDD. Data from twin studies exploring associating genetic factors of mania (in BD) and depression indicate that the majority of genetic variance (71%) is specific to mania and not related to depression [28]. SNPs analyses have suggested that bipolar disorder type 2 is the bridge between the two poles of MDD and schizophrenia-like bipolar disorder type 1, indicating the existence of a spectrum of affective disorders [24]. However, heritability studies have rejected this model, indicating a more complex explanation to the genetic relationship and the considerable clinical heterogeneity exhibited in mood disorders [28].

5.3.2 Neurotransmission in Mood Disorders

The pathophysiology of mood disorders involves complex interactions between biological, genetic, and environmental factors [25, 26, 28]. While the exact mechanisms are still being explored, current data provides valuable insight into the underlying processes involved in mood disorders. Alterations of the neurotransmitter systems involved with mood regulation, including serotonin, norepinephrine, and dopamine, have shown to contribute to the depressive symptoms observed in MDD [29]. Synaptic plasticity is disrupted by altered signaling pathways, leading to maladaptive changes in mood regulation and contributing to the susceptibility of depression. Exposure to trauma and stress can influence epigenetic modifications in the hypothalamic-pituitary-adrenal (HPA) axis, also affecting synaptic structure and function [30, 31]. Additionally, alterations in growth factors, such as brain derived neurotrophic factor (BDNF), inflammatory cytokines, insulin metabolism, and sex steroids, are also thought to affect neuronal function and brain plasticity [32]. These effects may explain the reduced volume of the prefrontal cortex and hippocampus often seen in mood disorders, as well as its relationship to disease severity.

In BP, studies have implicated the CACNA1C gene, suggesting aberrant calcium signaling is a contributing factor to its pathophysiology. Pharmacotherapy with calcium channel blockers such as pregabalin and lamotrigine, as well as mood stabilizers such as lithium, further support the involvement of calcium dysregulation in the underlying mechanism of BD [33]. Variations at CACNA1C have also been linked to schizophrenia and unipolar depression [4]. Dysregulation in BDNF signaling, neural growth, and synaptic plasticity have been associated with the structural abnormalities observed in bipolar disorder, further highlighting the implication of many related mechanisms in the development of various mental disorders.

5.3.3 Neuroanatomical Findings in Mood Disorders

Neuroimaging, neuropathology, and lesion analysis studies have helped identify neural networks and areas associated with regulating emotional behavior, and their role in the pathophysiology of mood disorders. The medial prefrontal cortex (MPFC), located in the anterior part of the prefrontal cortex, plays a crucial role in mood regulation and emotional processing. The MPFC interacts with the amygdala, hippocampus, and other limbic structures to form complex neural circuits that appraise emotional stimuli, helping determine appropriate emotional responses [29]. Through inhibitory connections, the MPFC can modulate the activity of the amygdala, reducing the expression of fear and anxiety. This process is essential for maintaining emotional balance and preventing excessive emotional responses. Studies suggest that heightened reactivity and increased connectivity in the amygdala may underlie the exaggerated emotional responses commonly seen in depression [29, 34, 37]. Dysfunction in the MPFC can also lead to deficits in reward processing and anhedonia, a core symptom of mood disorders.

Another region of interest is the subgenual anterior cingulate cortex (sgACC), located below the genu of the corpus callosum. Increased sgACC activity correlates with more severe depression [29]. Studies have also implicated the sgACC in the anxiety symptoms observed in mood disorders [35]. Reduced gray matter volume in the left sgACC and decreased white matter in the corpus callosum have been observed in both MDD and BD [29, 36]. Interestingly, decreased right cerebellar gray matter was common in BD and MDD, as well as schizophrenia [36].

A comprehensive analysis of studies on structural MRI noted that BD affects both cortical and subcortical areas, with reduced right hippocampal volume being part of these observations [37]. In individuals with depression, the hippocampus may also exhibit reduced volume and altered function [29, 37]. Postmortem pathological studies have demonstrated several volumetric changes of gray matter that correlate with findings in neuroimaging studies in MDD and BD. Histological abnormalities also include decreased glial cells and synapses in areas of the anterior cingulate cortex, the prefrontal cortex, and the amygdala [29]. Overall, these neuroanatomical and structural changes provide insights into the underlying pathophysiology of mood disorders. They highlight the involvement of specific brain regions and neural circuits in mood regulation and emotional processing, offering potential targets for future research and therapeutic interventions. It is important to note that these neuroanatomical abnormalities are not specific to mood disorders and can be present in other psychiatric conditions as well. Additionally, individual differences and heterogeneity within these disorders make it challenging to establish universal neuro-anatomical markers. Further research is needed to better understand the precise relationships between neuroanatomy and mood disorders.

5.4 Other Mental Disorders

Our previous discussion aimed to provide a closer look at the neurobiological mechanisms of some of the most devastating psychiatric disorders. However, the psychotic and mood disorders are only a fraction of a wide range of disorders that affect mental health. There are more than 200 types of mental illnesses that can present at any point in a person's life, manifesting with effects ranging from minor to severely debilitating symptoms that impact every aspect of daily life. A brief overview of some of the findings in other common mental disorders follows.

5.4.1 Anxiety Disorders

Anxiety disorders are characterized by persistent or excessive fear and worry that often interfere with normal function. These disorders include generalized anxiety disorder (GAD), panic disorder, social anxiety disorder, and specific phobias. Although comprising its own group, research has linked the genetic susceptibility of anxiety disorders to other mental health conditions [11, 41].

Panic disorder has shown the largest heritability, with several genes implicated, including COMT, adenosine 2A receptor, 5HT2A receptor, and monoamine oxidase-A. Genome-wide analyses of social anxiety disorder have also implicated genes encoding the norepinephrine transporter, COMT, CRF, and SERT. Notably, these findings further demonstrate the involvement of monoamine function in the development of various types of mental disorders [38].

The limbic system plays a crucial role in emotion regulation and fear responses. Limbic structures associated with anxiety disorders include the amygdala, the hippocampus, the hypothalamus, and the anterior cingulate cortex [38]. In individuals with anxiety disorders, the amygdala may show increased activity and sensitivity. The interplay between the hippocampus and the hypothalamus, and its effects on the HPA axis, have also been implicated in the development of anxiety and mood disorders [30, 38].

Neurotransmitter pathway dysfunction is also believed to play a role in anxiety disorders, as a key mechanism of anxiolytic therapy involves the modulation of mono-aminergic systems.

5.4.2 Personality Disorders

Ten distinct personality disorders (PD) have been recognized by the DSM-5 and are divided into three clusters. Cluster A includes paranoid PD, schizoid PD, and schizotypal PD. Cluster B consists of antisocial PD, borderline PD, histrionic PD, and narcissistic PD. Finally, Cluster C includes avoidant PD, dependent PD, and obsessive-compulsive PD. These disorders tend to emerge during adolescence or early adulthood, and are typically deeply ingrained and inflexible, contributing to both the distress experienced by the patients and the burden on society as a whole.

Research has suggested some heritability in personality disorders. For cluster A, heritability estimates may be as high as 60%. For cluster B, heritability ranged between

25% and 38%, although twin studies have estimated up to 77% heritability in some cases. Cluster C personality disorders showed heritability of around 60%. Studies have high-lighted genetic overlap and shared familial risk between cluster A PDs and schizophrenia. Additionally, avoidant PD occurs more frequently in relatives of individuals with schizophrenia [39]. Borderline PD and MDD have also shown to share familial risk factors. These findings suggest an overlap between many mental conditions, as well as the genetic vulnerabilities that contribute to the development of these disorders.

The pathophysiology of personality disorders involves multiple factors that interact to make way to their development. Neuroimaging studies reveal structural and functional abnormalities in areas associated with emotion regulation, impulse control, and decision-making. The impulsive aggression observed in borderline PD has been attributed to reduced metabolism in the frontal lobe and hyperactivity in the amygdala [40]. Decreased serotonergic activity has also been observed in borderline PD, as well as other PDs that display aggression. Imbalanced glutamatergic excitation and GABAminergic inhibition are also thought to be involved in dysregulation of the limbic system and emotional response. Studies have shown that bilateral hippocampal volume is reduced in borderline PD [37]. In patients with schizotypal PD, structural abnormalities appear as reduced volume in the temporal and prefrontal cortex, similar to schizophrenia patients. However, these changes are not as pronounced, and schizotypal patients retain higher levels of executive and cognitive functions. Increased dopamine metabolites have also been observed in the CSF of schizotypal PD patients. Cluster C is also known as the "anxious cluster." In efforts to avoid uncomfortable and anxiety-producing situations, these patients adopt behaviors that impair their relationships and quality of life [41]. Disruptions in dopamine and serotonin activity are closely associated with anxiety disorders and are thought to also be a factor in cluster C PD.

Importantly, environmental factors and childhood experiences are thought to play a key role in the development of PD, and contribute to maladaptive traits in genetically vulnerable individuals [40, 41]. Yet, there is significant variation among their pathophysiology, and each disorder shows unique characteristics as well as symptom presentation. In all, the neurobiology of personality disorders is not fully understood. More research is needed to understand the underlying mechanisms and develop effective interventions to improve the quality of life for patients with personality disorders. It is important to note that the neurobiology of mental disorders is complex and multifactorial, and our understanding of their biomarkers and pathways involved is still evolving. These are just some of the key factors that have been studied in relation to mental disorders. Future research may uncover additional mechanisms and provide a more comprehensive understanding of these conditions.

5.5 Conclusions and Perspectives

The study of the neurobiology of mental disorders involves multiple perspectives and approaches to gain a comprehensive understanding of these complex conditions. Key perspectives commonly employed in this field may include additional studies with molecular and cellular mechanisms underlying mental disorders. It involves studying genetic and epigenetic factors, molecular pathways, neurotransmitter systems, receptor function, and intracellular signaling pathways. This approach could help identify specific molecular targets and potential therapeutic interventions. Also, the study of systems and brain circuitry related to connectivity and communication between different brain regions, and how disruptions in these circuits contribute to the symptoms of mental disorders, may represent a valuable tool to provide new insights. Furthermore, studies on neurodevelopmental variables, cognitive processes, emotional regulation, decision-making, and social functioning in individuals with mental disorders are warranted. This perspective aims to integrate findings from various levels of analysis, such as molecular, cellular, circuitry, and behavioral, to help develop a deeper understanding of mental disorders. It recognizes the complex interactions between genetic, neural, and environmental factors and seeks to bridge different perspectives to provide a holistic view of these disorders.

References

1. C. L. Narayan, D. Shikha, S. Shekhar. Schizophrenia in identical twins. *Indian J Psychiatry.* 2015;**57**(3):323–324.

2. T. C. Uzuneser, J. Speidel, G. Kogias. Disrupted-in-schizophrenia 1 (DISC1) overexpression and juvenile immune activation cause sex-specific schizophrenia-related psychopathology in rats. *Front Psychiatry.* 2019;**10**:222.

3. T. Kircher, M. Wöhr, I. Nenadic, et al. Neurobiology of the major psychoses: a translational perspective on brain structure and function. *Eur Arch Psychiatry Clin Neurosci.* 2019;**269**:949–962.

4. N. Craddock, M. C. O'Donovan, M. J. Owen. Psychosis genetics: modeling the relationship between schizophrenia, bipolar disorder, and mixed (or "schizoaffective") psychoses. *Schizophr Bull.* 2009;**35**(3):482–490.

5. R. E. Straub, Y. Jiang, C. J. MacLean, et al. Genetic variation in the 6p22.3 gene DTNBP1, the human ortholog of the mouse dysbindin gene, is associated with schizophrenia. *Am J Hum Genet.* 2002;**71**:337–348.

6. E. Luvsannyam, M. S. Jain, M. K. L. Pormento, et al. Neurobiology of schizophrenia: a comprehensive review. *Cureus.* 2022;**14**(4):e23959.

7. M. W. Lochmann van Bennekom, H. J. Gijsman, F. G. Zitman. Antipsychotic polypharmacy in psychotic disorders: a critical review of neurobiology, efficacy, tolerability and cost effectiveness. *J Psychopharmacol.* 2013;**27**(4):327–336.

8. J. P. Kesby, D. W. Eyles, J. J. McGrath, et al. Dopamine, psychosis and schizophrenia: the widening gap between basic and clinical neuroscience. *Transl Psychiatry.* 2018;**8**(1):30.

9. O. D. Howes, J. Kambeitz, E. Kim, et al. The nature of dopamine dysfunction in schizophrenia and what this means for treatment. *Arch Gen Psychiatry.* 2012;**69**(8):776–786.

10. J. T. Coyle. Glutamate and schizophrenia: beyond the dopamine hypothesis. *Cell Mol Neurobiol.* 2006;**26**(4–6):365–384.

11. J. Y. Tsou. Intervention, causal reasoning, and the neurobiology of mental disorders: pharmacological drugs as experimental instruments. *Stud Hist Philos Biol Biomed Sci.* 2012;**43**(2):542–551.

12. W. T. O'Connor, S. D. O'Shea. Clozapine and GABA transmission in schizophrenia disease models: establishing principles to guide treatments. *Pharmacol Therapeutics.* 2015;**150**:47–80.

13. B. K. Bain. CT scans of first-break psychotic patients in good general health. *Psychiatr Serv.* 1998;**49**(2):234–235.

14. B. Strahl, Y. K. Cheung, S. L. Stuckey. Diagnostic yield of computed tomography of the brain in first episode psychosis. *J Med Imaging Radiat Oncol.* 2010;**54**(5):431–434.

15. M. Forbes, D. Stefler, D. Velakoulis, et al. The clinical utility of structural neuroimaging in first-episode psychosis: a systematic review. *Aust N Z J Psychiatry.* 2019;**53**(11):1093–1104.

16. K. H. Karlsgodt, D. Sun, T. D. Cannon. Structural and functional brain

abnormalities in schizophrenia. *Curr Dir Psychol Sci.* 2010;**19**(4):226–231.

17. B. Dietsche, T. Kircher, I. Falkenberg. Structural brain changes in schizophrenia at different stages of the illness: a selective review of longitudinal magnetic resonance imaging studies. *Austral N Z J Psychiatry.* 2017;**51**(5):500–508.

18. B. Birur, N. V. Kraguljac, R. C. Shelton, et al. Brain structure, function, and neurochemistry in schizophrenia and bipolar disorder: a systematic review of the magnetic resonance neuroimaging literature. *NPJ Schizophrenia.* 2017;**3**:15.

19. C. Pantelis, M. Yücel, S. J. Wood, et al. Structural brain imaging evidence for multiple pathological processes at different stages of brain development in schizophrenia. *Schizophr Bull.* 2005;**31**(3):672–696.

20. N. Uranova, D. Orlovskaya, O. Vikhreva, et al. Electron microscopy of oligodendroglia in severe mental illness. *Brain Res Bull.* 2001;**55**:597–610.

21. A. G. Dietz, S. A. Goldman, M. Nedergaard. Glial cells in schizophrenia: a unified hypothesis. *Lancet Psychiatry.* 2020;**7**(3):272–281.

22. T. D. Cannon, Y. Chung, G. He, et al. Progressive reduction in cortical thickness as psychosis develops: a multisite longitudinal neuroimaging study of youth at elevated clinical risk. *Biol Psychiatry.* 2015;**77**(2):147–157.

23. S. M. Lawrie, A. M. McIntosh, J. Hall, et al. Brain structure and function changes during the development of schizophrenia: the evidence from studies of subjects at increased genetic risk. *Schizophr Bull.* 2008;**34**(2):330–340.

24. J. R. Coleman, H. A. Gaspar, J. Bryois, et al. The genetics of the mood disorder spectrum: genome-wide association analyses of more than 185,000 cases and 439,000 controls. *Biol Psychiatry.* 2020;**88**(2):169–184.

25. D. M. Howard, M. J. Adams, M. Shirali, et al. Genome-wide association study of depression phenotypes in UK Biobank identifies variants in excitatory synaptic pathways. *Nat Comm.* 2018;**9**:1470.

26. P. F. Sullivan, M. C. Neale, K. S. Kendler. Genetic epidemiology of major depression: review and meta-analysis. *Am J Psychiatry.* 2000;**157**(10):1552–1562.

27. E. A. Stahl, G. Breen, A. J. Forstner, et al. Genome-wide association study identifies 30 loci associated with bipolar disorder. *Nat Genetics.* 2019;**51**:793–803.

28. P. McGuffin, F. Rijsdijk, M. Andrew, et al. The heritability of bipolar affective disorder and the genetic relationship to unipolar depression. *Arch Gen Psychiatry.* 2003;**60**(5):497–502.

29. W. C. Drevets, J. L. Price, M. L. Furey. Brain structural and functional abnormalities in mood disorders: implications for neurocircuitry models of depression. *Brain Struct Funct.* 2008;**213**(1–2):93–118.

30. G. Bonacina, A. Carollo, G. Esposito. The genetic side of the mood: a scientometric review of the genetic basis of mood disorders. *Genes (Basel).* 2023;**14**(2):352.

31. F. F. Zhang, W. Peng, J. A. Sweeney, et al. Brain structure alterations in depression: psychoradiological evidence. *CNS Neurosci Ther.* 2018;**24**(11):994–1003.

32. R. Duman, G. Aghajanian, G. Sanacora, et al. Synaptic plasticity and depression: new insights from stress and rapid-acting antidepressants. *Nat Med.* 2016;**22**:238–249.

33. P. J. Harrison, J. R. Geddes, E. M. Tunbridge. The emerging neurobiology of bipolar disorder. *Trends Neurosci.* 2018;**41**(1):18–30.

34. J. P. Gray, V. I. Müller, S. B. Eickhoff, et. al. Multimodal Abnormalities of Brain Structure and Function in Major Depressive Disorder: A Meta-Analysis of Neuroimaging Studies [published correction appears in *Am J Psychiatry.* 2022; **179**(9):691]. *Am J Psychiatry.* 2020; **177**(5):422-434.

35. F. Iorfino, I. B. Hickie, R. S. C. Lee, et al. The underlying neurobiology of key functional domains in young people with mood and anxiety disorders: a systematic review. *BMC Psychiatry.* 2016;**16**:156.

36. W. Zhang, J. A. Sweeney, L. Yao, et al. Brain structural correlates of familial risk

for mental illness: a meta-analysis of voxel-based morphometry studies in relatives of patients with psychotic or mood disorders. *Neuropsychopharmacology*. 2020;**45**(8):1369–1379.

37. J. B. Ding, K. Hu. Structural MRI brain alterations in borderline personality disorder and bipolar disorder. *Cureus*. 2021;**13**(7):e16425.

38. E. I. Martin, K. J. Ressler, E. Binder, et al. The neurobiology of anxiety disorders: brain imaging, genetics, and psychoneuroendocrinology. *Psychiatr Clin North Am*. 2009;**32**(3):549–575.

39. T. Reichborn-Kjennerud. Genetics of personality disorders. *Clin Lab Med*. 2010;**30**(4):893–910.

40. M. Goodman, A. New, L. Siever. Trauma, genes, and the neurobiology of personality disorders. *Ann N Y Acad Sci*. 2004;**1032**:104–116.

41. L. J. Siever, L. N. Weinstein. The neurobiology of personality disorders: implications for psychoanalysis. *J Am Psychoanal Assoc*. 2009;**57**(2):361–398.

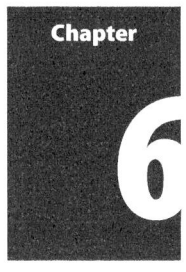

Psychosocial Theories and Their Implications for Psychiatry

Claudia Lex and Thomas D. Meyer

6.1 Introduction

Psychiatry and psychology are closely related disciplines but come from different origins. Psychiatry developed from medicine, specifically neurology, and is defined as a medical branch concerned with the study, diagnosis, and treatment of mental illness [1]. Psychology, on the other hand, has its roots in philosophy. It is defined as the study of mind and behavior covering not only mental illness but the whole spectrum of mental life, human experience, and behavior [1]. Because of this broad focus, psychology overlaps with many other disciplines, such as economics, sociology, and medicine. Obviously, psychology influences and is influenced particularly by psychiatry. For example, many clinical psychologists use psychiatric manuals to diagnose mental health problems. Vice versa, psychiatrists often rely on psychological tools for assessments given the lack of physiological tests or biomarkers to diagnose conditions such as pain or psychosis. In this chapter, we will introduce five basic psychological theories that have been historically most influential and that we regard as useful for psychiatry. Finally, we will present two more global, overarching theories: the stress-vulnerability model, which provides a general model of the etiology of almost all psychiatric disorders and illnesses; and humanistic psychology, which could be considered as a fundamental approach of how to build and maintain therapeutic relations focusing on the specific needs of the individual.

6.2 Psychoanalysis

The Austrian neurologist Sigmund Freud developed psychoanalysis at the beginning of the 20th century. Even though Freud was a physician, psychoanalysis is regarded as a psychological theory. The original version and its modifications have since substantially influenced the work of many health professionals. Freud thought that the mind consisted of two major parts reflecting functional structures that do not have any anatomical representation. First, the "conscious mind" is the operating mind. Everybody is naturally aware of feelings, thoughts, experiences, and behaviors related to this part of the mind. However, according to psychoanalysis, the more powerful part of the mind is the "unconscious mind." The unconscious contains the instinctual drives and repressed thoughts and feelings. The assumption is that individuals usually cannot actively access the contents of their subconscious. There is also the "preconscious" that represents the thoughts and feelings that are not present everyday but people can actively retrieve them as needed [2]. In psychoanalytic treatments, therapists help patients to bring contents of the unconscious to a conscious level. This supposedly enables the person to reflect the subconscious contents and facilitates catharsis (healing of the person). Later, Freud revised his ideas and created a personality theory comprising three components: the Id, the Ego, and the Superego. The Id contains primitive impulses and drives, whereas the Superego comprises moral forces, internalized voices of the parents, and feelings of guilt and shame. The Ego stands between the Id and the Superego and tries to balance these two conflicting forces [3]. These three parts are in permanent struggle because each part has a different primary aim. When a conflict is too burdensome or anxiety-provoking, people use so-called defense mechanisms. For example, one defense mechanism is repression, meaning that the Ego excludes the threatening content from the consciousness; another one is projection, where one's own unacceptable feelings or thoughts are perceived in someone else [4]. In addition, Freud developed a theory about children's psychosexual development that is intertwined with the above-listed concepts.

Since its formulation, Freud's theories have been passionately discussed, reviewed, and extended. These debates have led different psychoanalysts to develop new ideas and schools: for example, Melanie Klein was interested in treatments for children, Jacques Lancan set up Freudian Schools in France, and Otto Kernberg developed a theory about the neurotic, borderline, and psychotic personality organization that influenced the psychodynamic therapy of patients with borderline personality [5]. It is important to note, however, that Kernberg's concept of borderline personality structure goes beyond and is not the same as the formal diagnosis of borderline personality disorder. Finally, psychoanalysis has more or less directly influenced different treatment approaches and research areas, such as Bowlby's attachment theory [6, 7] or Klerman and Weissman's interpersonal psychotherapy [8, 9].

6.3 Behaviorism

In the second half of the 19th century, there was a movement to establish psychology as a separate discipline from philosophy. Many thought that philosophy was insufficient to explain the human mind because it seemed too subjective, not based on experimental science, and its theories could be neither proved nor disproved. Therefore, psychologists, such as Wilhelm Wundt in Germany and William James in the United States, started to apply more scientific methods and founded experimental laboratories to explore the effects of different stimuli on physical, cognitive, and emotional responses. These experimental approaches set the stage for "behaviorism," which is sometimes called the first wave of psychology, especially when referring to the therapeutic models or strategies derived from it.

A highly relevant person and one of the early pioneers of behaviorism is Ivan Pavlov, a Russian physiologist, who received the Nobel Prize for his behavioral experiments with dogs in 1904. He discovered the learning principles that are subsumed under the term *classical conditioning*. He started his studies by presenting food to his dogs. The food ("unconditioned stimulus") provoked salivation in the dogs ("unconditioned response"). In the next step, he presented the "unconditioned stimulus" (food) jointly with a "neutral stimulus" (ringing a bell) to the dogs. He discovered that, after a few trials, it was sufficient to ring the bell (without presenting the food) to trigger salivation. Thus, the ringing of a bell as an originally "neutral stimulus" became a "conditioned stimulus" and triggered a "conditioned response" (salivation) [10, 11].

As a logical extension of these studies, two psychologists, John B. Watson and Rosalie Rayner, tested whether the principles of classical conditioning also apply to humans.

In order to examine this question, they conducted a series of studies, the most famous one with a 9-month-old baby, who was referred to as "Little Albert" [12]. They started the experiment by showing objects and live animals, such as a white furry rats to the baby. They observed that the baby was curious about them, tried to reach out for them, and did not show any signs of anxiety. Obviously, these animals and objects symbolized "neutral stimuli." Then, on a different occasion, they introduced the "unconditioned stimulus" in form of a loud noise that stressed the baby and made him cry ("unconditioned response"). They then repeatedly presented the rat combined with the noise. After a few weeks, the rat had become a "conditioned stimulus" that provoked on its own a "conditioned response" (crying) in the baby boy, even if the rat was presented without the noise. Moreover, Little Albert's fear seemed to have generalized because he showed signs of fear when confronted with other furry animals such as rabbits. Although these experiments raise serious ethical concerns, they demonstrated that principles of classical conditioning are applicable to humans.

The Harvard psychologist B. F. Skinner and his experiments led to what is now known as operant conditioning or operant leaning principles [13]. For example, he placed rats in specially prepared cages called Skinner boxes. Rats naturally explore such a box and may by accident press a lever in the box that provides some food (sugar). After a few trials, the rats learned to press the lever in order to get the food. Skinner called this form of learning "positive reinforcement." In contrast, "negative reinforcement" happens if the rat learns to push a lever to avoid or stop negative stimuli. Nowadays this is considered one of key mechanisms how avoidance behavior (e.g., in the context of anxiety) is learned and maintained. Therefore, the original basic rationale of desensitization and exposure therapy as part of behavior therapy is to help individuals unlearn the association between a conditioned stimulus (e.g., dog, dentist, needle) and the conditioned response (e.g., fear, nausea). *Positive punishment* is the term used to describe when an aversive consequence (e.g., electric shock) is introduced to decrease the likelihood that an unwanted behavior is displayed, and *negative punishment* is the removal of a positive consequence to make a behavior less frequent (e.g., removing a favored toy).

Many psychological models and therapy strategies are rooted in classical and operant learning principles. For example, Lewinsohn [14] conceptualized depression as the consequence of an accumulating loss of positive reinforcements. Following this line, behavior activation therapy for depression [15] analyzes antecedents and consequences of behaviors and their link to depressive symptoms. Also consistent with the operant learning theory is positive activity scheduling that is one of the core strategies in psychological depression treatment [16]. Nock and Prinstein [17] have developed a behavioral model of self-mutilative behavior. Nonsuicidal self-mutilative behavior can be observed in various psychiatric disorders but also in the general population, especially in adolescents. The model postulates that negative reinforcement occurs when the self-injury's function is used to remove a negative internal state (e.g., boredom, emotional pain) or to avoid an unwanted social encounter. Positive reinforcement takes place when self-injury is used to create a desired internal state (e.g., distraction, feeling grounded by the physical pain), or when the person expects or gets extra care and attention from others. Finally, classical conditioning can be useful to understand addictive behaviors [18]. Usually, a psychotropic substance such as alcohol is an unconditioned stimulus that provokes an unconditioned response (e.g., relaxation, less inhibition/shyness). Over time, neutral stimuli, such as seeing a beer glass, certain friends, or a liquor store, are paired with the unconditioned stimulus, which for humans can now include even mental images of alcohol as a form of generalization. Neutral stimuli can therefore become conditioned stimuli that trigger a conditioned response (e.g., either drinking or craving a drink). Thus, to overcome addictions, it is an important step for people to understand these mechanisms to be better able to analyze their behavior and to prevent relapse.

6.4 Cognitive Theory

The second wave of psychology or psychotherapy, the "cognitive revolution," emerged around 1960 in the United States. At that time, some began to criticize behavioral psychology because they felt that it was only concerned with observable behavior as units that can be experimentally and scientifically studied. They argued that behaviorism ignored internal states and processes (e.g., attributions, interpretations, thoughts). When we referred in the previous section to mental images of alcohol in the context of addiction treatment, introducing this term already refers to the inclusion of cognitive concepts into behavioral models. In addition to the evolution of modern cognitive psychology, some psychiatrists and psychologists began to question the effectiveness of psychoanalysis that was the main therapeutic approach at that time. Among them was Aaron Beck. He was trained as a psychoanalyst but, based on his clinical experience, he turned to cognitive and behavioral psychology to develop a new model of depression [19, 20]. He postulated that in most situations humans do not simply react after stimuli presentations like the animals in behavioristic experiments; rather, they individually evaluate these stimuli based on their attitudes and beliefs formed by experiences (e.g., "If I make a mistake, people will look down on me"; "Everybody has to like me"; "You cannot really trust anyone"). These evaluations or appraisals then strongly influence their behavior. Following this theory, patients with depression tend to view neutral stimuli as negative for the self and, therefore, get even more depressed. For example, a depressed patient who hears the ringing of an incoming phone call might express negative thoughts: "I cannot pick up the phone because I don't know what to talk about to my friend, and therefore she will turn away from me." This view leads to a behavior that is similar to avoidance, namely ignoring the call. Consequently, these appraisals and behaviors lead to even more social isolation, anxiety, and depression.

Attribution theories represent another important cognitive perspective in psychology. Originally, Martin Seligman and his team conducted behavioral experiments with dogs [21]. They put dogs in conditions where they had no chance to avoid adverse stimuli (e.g., electric shocks). The dogs soon gave up finding solutions, surrendering to the aversive situation. Unexpectedly, when the experimenter changed the conditions by adding a chance to escape, the dogs did not use the new opportunities but stayed in the cage. Seligman and his team named their observations "learned helplessness." Later, this theory was reformulated by adding a cognitive component to the model and focusing on the symptom of hopelessness in depression [22, 23]. The basic model emphasizes that it matters to what extent we attribute our experience to internal versus external, stable versus variable, global versus specific causes. For example, it was found that depressive patients attribute their perceived failures more to global and stable causes (e.g., "I am stupid"; "I am not meant to find happiness") rather than to specific and variable causes (e.g. "This test was just too difficult"; "I did not put enough effort into it this time").

These cognitive models and their specifications are still highly influential ways of thinking in psychiatry and clinical psychology to date. The original cognitive models have been modified for many different psychiatric disorders [24], have been integrated with biological theories [25], and have been used to understand the etiology of disorders and to develop treatment strategies. One example of these developments is the cognitive model for psychosis [26]. Individuals who are vulnerable to psychosis (e.g., genetically) often develop underlying beliefs that the external world is threatening and tend to attribute negative events to external factors. For instance, a vulnerable person might by chance catch a look from a fellow passenger on a bus. This glance might activate underlying beliefs relating to danger. Consequently, the activated apprehension related to the perceived danger will intensify monitoring of the situation and the self, which will increase the likelihood of noticing random things that suddenly acquire a meaning. Thus, the glance of that person might be interpreted as predictor for a bad catastrophe or that the other people on the bus might be watching or being after them. The person might even show some behavior that attracts other people's attention, therefore reinforcing and confirming what the person feared in the first place. In this way vulnerable individuals can develop paranoid ideas or even delusions.

6.5 Social Cognitive Theory

The social cognitive theory (SCT) was formulated by Albert Bandura as an advancement of his social learning theory. Initially, the social learning theory [27] suggested that children learn by observing and imitating of other peoples' behavior. In their famous "Bobo Doll" experiments, Bandura and his team showed that children learn social behavior – in this case, aggression – through watching a film demonstrating a person's aggressive behavior toward a doll [28, 29]. However, the social learning theory could not explain how people develop more complex behaviors, feelings, and thoughts. In addition, people usually have cognitive control over their behavior and do not imitate every behavior they observe. In order to respond to this critique and to emphasize the cognitive aspect of his theory, Bandura [30] extended his theory and renamed it to SCT. For example, SCT takes into account the reciprocal interactions between the individual and the environment, negative and positive reinforcements, past experiences, and expectations of the individual. Most importantly, the concept of self-efficacy was introduced and is now regarded as a key construct of SCT. Self-efficacy refers to the level of confidence one has to succeed in his or her desired goal.

Since its formulation, SCT has been applied to diverse areas such as education, public health, business, mass communication, and global problems [31, 32]. In psychiatric contexts, SCT has been used to promote health-related behavior [33] and to provide treatments to different disorders and symptoms, such as cannabis use disorder [34] and negative symptoms of psychosis [35]. Finally, there is evidence that online treatment programs based on SCT are effective [36].

6.6 Mindfulness-Based and Metacognitive Concepts

Behavioral and cognitive models and treatments have been effectively used to this day, but they also have their limitation; for example, the classic cognitive-behavioral therapy, which focuses on changing behaviors and thoughts, does not work for everyone. This has resulted in additional, new ways to think about psychiatric disorders and psychological interventions. Since a few decades ago, health care professionals have become interested in Far Eastern philosophies and started to implement meditation and mindfulness into treatments. The mindfulness-based stress reduction (MBSR) [37] and the dialectic behavioral therapy (DBT) [38] were pioneer programs in this context. One central idea of these treatments is to combine cognitive-behavioral elements with paying mindful attention to inner states such as feelings, physical sensations, and thoughts. Patients are taught to attend to these inner states in a nonjudgmental way, trying to accept inner states rather than to evaluate them or to change them. Both MBSR and DBT have been shown to be effective in treatment [39, 40].

On a more abstract level, some have focused on "metacognition" defined as thoughts people have about their thoughts or, more generally, about their cognitive systems. For example, it refers to appraisals individuals make about quality and frequency of their own thoughts, but also to their perceived ability to control their thoughts. Metacognition influences the development, maintenance, and decrease of a variety of psychiatric symptoms [41]. Interventions based on these concepts include the acceptance and commitment therapy (ACT) [42] and the mindfulness-based cognitive therapy (MBCT) [43].

In addition to treatment approaches, there are also etiological metacognitive models related to different psychiatric disorders. One example is the metacognitive model of rumination and depression [44–46]. The model is based on the finding that specific cognitive styles, such as rumination, are linked to onset and chronicity of affective episodes [47]. Furthermore, it suggests that rumination and its link to depression are affected by beliefs people hold about rumination – in other words, their metacognitive beliefs. Specifically, there are two different sets of rumination-related metacognition. First, an individual might express his or her positive beliefs about rumination ("Rumination is useful because I will find solutions to my problem"). Second, there are negative beliefs emphasizing the threat of ruminations ("I cannot control my rumination, it makes me sick") and its negative interpersonal consequences ("My friends will no longer like me because I ruminate all the time"). According to the metacognitive model of rumination and depression, a trigger (e.g., an argument with a friend) can activate positive metacognitions about the effectiveness of rumination, and the person starts to ruminate. However, rumination is rarely helpful for solving problems or overcoming negative feelings; rather, it leads to even more negative thoughts. Consequently, these negative thoughts activate negative metacognition about rumination that further increases depressive symptoms. Based on these assumptions, Wells [48] developed the metacognitive therapy, which is an effective treatment for current, recurrent, and persistent depression [49].

6.7 Stress-Vulnerability Model

Most mental health professionals are concerned with why a person becomes ill and how that person can be effectively treated. In the 1970s, psychologists Joseph Zubin and Bonnie Spring tried to find an answer to the question of why some individuals seemed to have an increased risk for schizophrenia and some did not. However, they could find only partial answers in the etiological models that were popular at that time. Therefore, they came up with a new model they termed the *stress-vulnerability model*, sometimes also called the stress-diathesis model [50]. While the model originally focused on schizophrenia, it has since become a template for most mental health problems and even physical illnesses such as hypertension or cancer. The model suggests that people have a certain degree of vulnerability to develop specific illnesses or conditions. For example, genetic factors or prenatal infections might increase the vulnerability. When individuals with increased vulnerabilities are exposed to stressful events later in life (or accumulative stress), they will develop symptoms associated with that condition or typical for that illness more likely than individuals with low vulnerabilities. Protective factors such as competences and coping abilities influence this process. Since then the stress-vulnerability model has been further advanced, adding cognitive, neurological, neurochemical, neurostructural, and emotional components [51], and it has been widely applied [52].

In contrast to the aforementioned theories, the stress-vulnerabilty model is more generic, since a variety of factors can be subsumed under "vulnerabilities" (even including acquired vulnerabilities beyond genetics and influences during pregnancy, e.g., concussions, malnutrition in early childhood). The same is true for the term *stress*, which can include negative events (e.g., a breakup, losing a job, failing an exam) but also potentially positive events (e.g., childbirth, wedding, job promotion) or severe trauma (e.g., rape, life-threatening accident, war).

6.8 The Potential Role of Humanistic Psychology for Psychiatry

One of the main questions of psychology has always related to how we can lead satisfied lives. A behaviorist would claim that the fulfillment of physiological needs with food or sleep would lead to satisfaction. Cognitive behaviorists had challenged this view, but humanistic psychologists came up with alternative ideas of how inner fulfillment can be reached. Abraham Maslow, sometimes called the father of humanistic psychology, believed that each person and each experience is unique, and psychologists should focus on this uniqueness instead of relying on universal treatment strategies applied to everyone. He employed personal observations to formulate a concept named *The Hierarchy of Needs* [53, 54]. The original model contains five stages, which later have been expanded to eight [55]. These eight stages must be fulfilled in ascending order starting with four basic deficiency needs and followed by four more complex growth needs (Figure 6.1). The first stage relates to physiological needs, such as fresh air, food, enough sleep, and warmth. If these physiological needs are met, people long for safety – for example, they strive for a safe home, a secure job, and health. Then, the need to be close to others (love and belongingness) and the need for achievement and recognition by others become relevant. At a higher level, the needs are cognitive (desire to know and understand), aesthetic (wish for beauty and symmetry), self-actualization (need for self-fulfillment), and, finally, self-transcendence (desire to connect to something higher than ourselves and to move beyond the self). At this highest stage, individuals realize their greatest potential and their purpose in life and try to behave and act accordingly. Maslow [53] acknowledges that the need for self-actualization varies between individuals. One might try to become the ideal mother, whereas another person strives for athletic records or technical masterpieces.

There are several additional psychological approaches based on humanistic ideas. Foremost among them is the person-centered therapy by Carl Rogers [56]. His nondirective therapy approach focuses on human growth and individual potential and abilities. Second, there is the recovery approach that was originally developed for patients with severe schizophrenia [57] but has since been adapted for other psychiatric conditions, such as bipolar disorder [58]. It does not aim at full symptom reduction but encourages

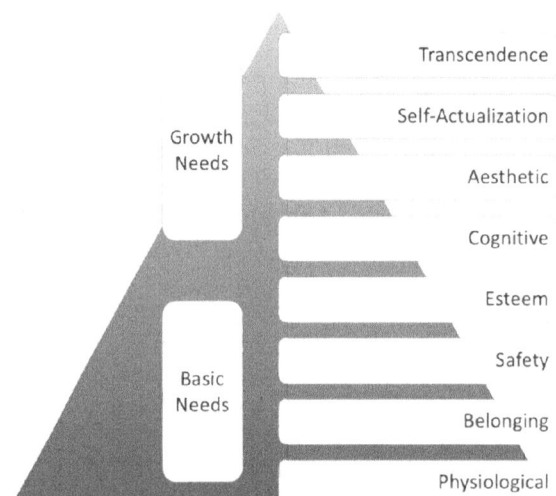

Figure 6.1 The Hierarchy of Needs model by Abraham Maslow.

Transcendence

Self-Actualization

Growth Needs

Aesthetic

Cognitive

Esteem

Safety

Basic Needs

Belonging

Physiological

people with severe mental diseases to express their individual goals and manage their symptoms, and it emphasizes resilience and personal responsibility [59, 60]. In addition, there are pragmatic programs such as the harm reduction approach that includes different strategies designed to reduce the negative consequences of addictive behavior. Taking into account the individual situation of the patient, this approach might prefer moderate substance use abstinence [61]. Also, positive psychology [62], defined as the study of what makes life most worth living and focusing on individual and social well-being, has its roots in humanistic psychology. Finally, on a more practical perspective, the humanistic idea that everybody is unique relates to the modern concept of personalized medicine that is presently discussed for psychiatric disorders [63].

How could these humanistic ideas be of value for mental health professionals? Unfortunately, nondirective humanistic psychotherapies in which patients set the pace are in sharp contrast to the strict economic and time constraints mental health professional face in various psychiatric settings today. However, there is evidence that humanistic psychotherapies are equally effective compared to other non-cognitive-behavioral therapies [64]. Finally, humanistic models provide guidance on basic principles of how best to approach our patients and colleagues.

References

1. A. M. Colman. *A Dictionary of Psychology*. Oxford University Press; 2015.

2. D. K. Lapsley, P. C. Stey. Id, ego, and superego. In Ramachandran V. S., ed. *Encyclopedia of Human Behavior*. Academic Press; 2012: 393–399.

3. N. Rennison. *Freud and Psychoanalysis: Everything You Need to Know about Id,* *Ego, Super-ego and More*. Oldcastle Books; 2015.

4. P. Cramer. Understanding defense mechanisms. *Psychodyn Psychiatry*. 2015;43:523.

5. O. F. Kernberg, M. A. Selzer, H. W. Koenigsberg, et al. *Psychodynamic Psychotherapy of Borderline Patients*. Basic Books; 1989.

6. J. P. Robledo, I. Cross, L. Boada-Bayona, et al. Back to basics: a re-evaluation of the

relevance of imprinting in the genesis of Bowlby's attachment theory. *Front Psychol.* 2022;13:1033746.

7.   P. R. Shaver, M. Mikulincer. Attachment-related psychodynamics. *Attach Hum Dev.* 2002;4:133–161.

8.   P. Ravitz, P. Watson, A. Lawson, et al. Interpersonal psychotherapy: a scoping review and historical perspective (1974-2017). *Harv Rev Psychiatry.* 2019;27:165–180.

9.   M. M. Weissman. Interpersonal psychotherapy: history and future. *Am J Psychother.* 2020;73:3–7.

10. R. E. Clark. The classical origins of Pavlov's conditioning. *Integr Psychol Behav Sci.* 2004;39:279–294.

11. I. P. Pavlov. *Conditioned Reflexes.* Oxford University Press; 1927.

12. B. Harris. Whatever happened to little Albert? *Am Psychol.* 1979;34:151.

13. B. F. Skinner. *Science and Human Behavior.* Simon and Schuster; 1965.

14. P. M. Lewinsohn. A behavioural approach to depression. In Freedman R. J., Katz M., eds. *The Psychology of Depression.* Wiley; 1974:157–174.

15. C. R. Martell, S. Dimidjian, R. Herman-Dunn. *Behavioral Activation for Depression: A Clinician's Guide.* Guilford Press; 2021.

16. P. Cuijpers, A. van Straten, E. H. Warmerdam. Behavioral treatment of depression: a meta-analysis of activity scheduling. *Clin Psychol Rev.* 2007;27:318–326.

17. M. K. Nock, M. J. Prinstein. A functional approach to the assessment of self-mutilative behavior. *J Consult Clin Psychol.* 2004;72:885–890.

18. M. C. Skewes, V. M. Gonzalez. The biopsychosocial model of addiction. In Miller, P., ed. *Principles of Addiction.* Elsevier; 2013:61–70.

19. A. T. Beck. *Depression: Clinical Experimental and Theoretical Aspects.* Harper & Row; 1967.

20. A. T. Beck. The current state of cognitive therapy: a 40-year retrospective. *Arch Gen Psychiatry.* 2005;62:953–959.

21. M. E. Seligman, S. F. Maier, J. H. Geer. Alleviation of learned helplessness in the dog. *J Abnorm Psychol.* 1968;73:256–262.

22. L. Y. Abramson, G. I. Metalsky, L. B. Alloy. Hopelessness depression: a theory-based subtype of depression. *Psychol Rev.* 1989;96:358.

23. L. Y. Abramson, M. E. Seligman, J. D. Teasdale. Hopelessness depression: a theory-based subtype of depression. *J Abnorm Psychol.* 1978;87:49.

24. K. E. Hawton, P. M. Salkovskis, J. E. Kirk, et al. *Cognitive Behaviour Therapy for Psychiatric Problems: A Practical Guide.* Oxford University Press; 1989.

25. O. D. Howes, R. M. Murray. Schizophrenia: an integrated sociodevelopmental-cognitive model. *Lancet.* 2014:383:1677–1687.

26. P. A. Garety, E. Kuipers, D. Fowler, et al. A cognitive model of the positive symptoms of psychosis. *Psychol Med.* 2001;31:189–195.

27. A. Bandura. *Social Learning Theory.* Prentice Hall; 1977.

28. A. Bandura, D. Ross, S. A. Ross. Transmission of aggression through the imitation of aggressive models. *J Abnorm Soc Psychol.* 1961;63:575–582.

29. A. Bandura, R. H. Walters. *Social Learning and Personality Development.* Holt Rinehart and Winston; 1963.

30. A. Bandura. *Social Foundations of Thought and Action: A Social Cognitive Theory.* Prentice-Hall; 1986.

31. A. Bandura. Social cognitive theory of mass communication. *Media Psychology.* 2001;3:265–299.

32. A. Bandura. The social and policy impact of social cognitive theory. In Mark, M., Donaldson S., Campbell B., eds. *Social Psychology and Evaluation.* Guilford Press; 2011:33–70.

33. A. Luszczynska, R. Schwarzer. Changing behavior using social cognitive theory.

In Hagger M. S., Cameron L. D., Hamilton K., et al., eds. *The Handbook of Behavior Change.* Cambridge University Press; 2020:32–45.

34. M. J. Gullo, Z. E. Papinczak, G. F. Freeney, et al. Precision mental health care for cannabis use disorder: utility of a biosocial cognitive theory to inform treatment. *Front Psychiatry.* 2021;12:1010.

35. D. J. Devoe, K. S. Cadenhead, B. Cornblatt, et al. Negative symptoms: associations with defeatist beliefs, self-efficacy, and maladaptive schemas in youth and young adults at-risk for psychosis. *Behav Cogn Psychother.* 2022;50:298–311.

36. B. Moeini, S. Bashirian, A. R. Soltanian, et al. Examining the effectiveness of a web-based intervention for depressive symptoms in female adolescents: applying social cognitive theory. *J Res Health Sci.* 2019;19:e00454.

37. J. Kabat-Zinn. Mindfulness-based stress reduction (MBSR). *Constr Hum Sci.* 2003;8:73.

38. M. M. Linehan. *Cognitive-behavioral treatment of borderline personality disorder.* Guilford Press; 1993.

39. B. Khoury, M. Sharma S. E. Rush, et al. Mindfulness-based stress reduction for healthy individuals: a meta-analysis. *J Psychosom Res.* 2015;78:519–528.

40. O. D. Kothgassner, A. Goreis, K. Robinson, et al. Efficacy of dialectical behavior therapy for adolescent self-harm and suicidal ideation: a systematic review and meta-analysis. *Psychol Med.* 2021;51:1057–1067.

41. X. Sun, C. Zhu, S. H. W. So. Dysfunctional metacognition across psychopathologies: a meta-analytic review. *Eur Psychiatry.* 2017;45:139–153.

42. S. C. Hayes, K. D. Strosahl, K. G. Wilson. *Acceptance and Commitment Therapy.* Guilford Press; 1999.

43. J. D. Teasdale, R. G. Moore, H. Hayhurst, et al. Metacognitive awareness and prevention of relapse in depression: empirical evidence. *J Consult Clin Psychol.* 2002;70:275–287.

44. C. Papageorgiou, A. Wells. An empirical test of a clinical metacognitive model of rumination and depression. *Cog Ther Res.* 2003;27:261–273.

45. C. Papageorgiou, A. Wells. *Depressive Rumination: Nature, Theory and Treatment.* Wiley; 2004.

46. A. Wells. *Metacognitive Therapy for Anxiety and Depression.* Guilford; 2009.

47. S. Nolen-Hoeksema, The role of rumination in depressive disorders and mixed anxiety/depressive symptoms. *J Abnorm Psychol.* 2000;109:504–511.

48. A. Wells. *Emotional Disorders and Metacognition: Innovative Cognitive Therapy.* Wiley; 2000.

49. L. Winter, J. Gottschalk, J. Nielsen, et al. A comparison of metacognitive therapy in current versus persistent depressive disorder: a pilot outpatient study. *Front Psychol.* 2019;10:1714.

50. J. Zubin, B. Spring. Vulnerability: a new view of schizophrenia. *J Abnorm Psychol.* 1977;86:103–126

51. S. F. Taylor, T. B. Grove, V. L. Ellingrod, et al. The fragile brain: stress vulnerability, negative affect and GABAergic neurocircuits in psychosis. *Schizophr Bull.* 2019;45:1170–1183.

52. C. Goh, M. Agius. The stress-vulnerability model how does stress impact on mental illness at the level of the brain and what are the consequences? *Psychiatr Danub.* 2010;22:198–202.

53. A. H. Maslow. A theory of human motivation. *Psychol Rev.* 1943;50:370–396.

54. A. H. Maslow. *Motivation and Personality.* Harper and Row; 1954.

55. A. H. Maslow. *Motivation and Personality.* 2nd ed. Harper & Row; 1970.

56. C. R. Rogers. *On Becoming a Person: A Therapist's View of Psychotherapy.* Houghton Mifflin Harcourt; 1995.

57. K. T. Mueser, P. S. Meyer, D. L. Penn, et al. The illness management and recovery program: rationale, development, and preliminary findings. *Schizophr Bull.* 2006;32:S32–S43.

58. G. Murray, N. D. Leitan, N. Thomas, et al. Towards recovery-oriented psychosocial interventions for bipolar disorder: quality of life outcomes, stage-sensitive treatments, and mindfulness mechanisms. *Clin Psychol Rev.* 2017;52:148–163.

59. S. Sharfstein. Recovery model will strengthen psychiatrist-patient relationship. *Psychiatric News.* 2005;40:3.

60. R. Warner. Recovery from schizophrenia and the recovery model. *Curr Opin Psychiatry.* 2009;22:374–380.

61. G. A. Marlatt. Harm reduction: come as you are. *Addict Behav.* 1996;21:779–788.

62. M. E. Seligman, M. Csikszentmihalyi. Positive psychology: an introduction. *Am Psychol.* 2000;55:5–14.

63. I. K. Wium-Andersen, M. Vinberg, L. V. Kessing, et al. Personalized medicine in psychiatry. *Nord J Pychiatry.* 2017;71:12–19.

64. R. Elliott, J. Watson, L. Timulak, et al. Research on humanistic-experiential psychotherapies: updated review. In Barkham M., Lutz W., Castonguay L. G., eds. *Bergin and Garfield's Handbook of Psychotherapy and Behavior Change: 50th Anniversary Edition.* John Wiley & Sons; 2021:421–467.

General Aspects of Psychopharmacology

Grace S. Pham and Sanjay J. Mathew

7.1 Introduction

Psychopharmacology is the study of how drugs affect the brain and body and impact emotion, behavior, and psychiatric symptoms. The use of drugs to treat mental illness dates back to ancient times, as a variety of herbs with psychoactive properties were given to patients suffering from grief in Greek and Roman times [1]. In the early 20th century, psychiatrists began using barbiturates (e.g., Veronal, Verpnal, Medinal) to treat mental disorders, but these were often addictive and had severe side effects [2]. In the 1950s, the discovery of chlorpromazine, the first antipsychotic drug, marked a major breakthrough in the treatment of mental illness [3]. This discovery led to the development of other classes of psychotropic drugs, including antidepressants, anxiolytics, and mood stabilizers. As contemporary psychiatry practice has gradually prioritized reciprocity (i.e., shared decision-making) over paternalism, so too have general practicing best practices increasingly emphasized collaboration and patient education [4]. In this chapter, we will review general aspects integral to the use of psychotropic medications in psychiatric practice.

7.2 Pharmacokinetics and Pharmacodynamics

An understanding of pharmacokinetics and pharmacodynamics is essential in prescribing and managing medications. Pharmacokinetics refers to how the body processes drugs, while pharmacodynamics relates to how drugs affect the body. Pharmacokinetics consists of four primary stages: absorption, distribution, metabolism, and elimination [5]. When a medication is taken, its absorption into the bloodstream is influenced by the drug's chemical properties, its formulation, and the route of administration. Once in the bloodstream, the medication is distributed throughout the body, where it may interact with target tissues and organs. The extent of distribution is influenced by factors such as the drug's chemical properties and the patient's physiological characteristics, such as body composition and hydration status [5]. After distribution, the medication must be metabolized by the liver into an excretable form, and this process is influenced by genetic factors and the patient's liver function. Finally, the rate of elimination of the medication through urine or feces is influenced by several factors, including kidney function and the drug's chemical properties [5].

Pharmacodynamics, on the other hand, refers to how drugs interact with the body's cells and tissues. The primary target of psychiatric medications is the central nervous system, where psychotropic medications work by altering the levels or activity of neurotransmitters [6]. By understanding how medications are absorbed, distributed, metabolized, and eliminated, one can make informed decisions about medication selection and dosing [7]. Similarly, by understanding how medications interact with the body, one can predict potential side effects, tailor medication choices to individual patients, and make adjustments to dosing and treatment regimens as needed.

7.3 Selecting Medications

When selecting medications, one must consider the patient's diagnosis, medical history, current symptoms, potential side effects, and medication interactions [8]. The patient's diagnosis should first be ascertained through thorough evaluation. Different psychiatric disorders require different types of medications, as major depressive disorder is typically treated with antidepressant medications, while bipolar disorder may require mood stabilizers or antipsychotic medications [9]. The patient's medical history, including any preexisting medical conditions or allergies, must then be considered [10]. Certain medications may be contraindicated or require dose adjustments in patients with liver or kidney disease, for example. Additionally, some patients may be allergic to certain medications or have a history of adverse reactions to particular drugs. The patient's current symptoms and severity of illness must also be considered when selecting medications [11]. Potential side effects of medications must also be considered in the medication selection process. One must balance the potential benefits of a medication with its potential side effects. For example, some antidepressant medications may cause sexual dysfunction, weight gain, or sedation, which can be problematic for some patients [12]. Medication interactions must also be considered when selecting medications. Some medications may interact with each other, leading to increased or decreased levels of the drug in the body or potential adverse effects, as seen in carbamazepine and valproic acid [13]. Additionally, patients may be taking other medications for nonpsychiatric conditions, and one must be aware of potential drug interactions with psychiatric medications.

Ultimately, the medication selection process involves a careful consideration of the patient's diagnosis, medical history, current symptoms, potential side effects, and medication interactions. Regular monitoring and adjustments to medication dosing and treatment regimens are often necessary to ensure optimal treatment outcomes.

7.4 Comorbidities and Medication Selection

Comorbid psychiatric conditions are common in patients with mental health disorders, and often affect the choice of medication for treatment [14]. It is important to be aware of comorbidities when selecting medications to ensure safe and effective treatment in light of potential medication interactions. For example, patients with depression may also have a comorbid anxiety or bipolar disorder [14, 15]. In such cases, a medication that is effective for depression may not be effective for anxiety or bipolar disorder. In addition, certain medications may interact with other medications the patient is taking for other medical conditions, such as hypertension or diabetes [16]. Another important factor to consider is the potential for adverse effects. Some medications may exacerbate certain medical conditions, and it is important to avoid prescribing medications that could cause harm. For example, patients with bipolar disorder who also have renal or hepatic dysfunction may not be able to tolerate certain mood stabilizers, such as lithium or valproic acid, respectively [17].

Patients with comorbid conditions may also require careful monitoring. For example, patients with depression and comorbid substance use disorders may be at increased risk for nonadherence to treatment, and may require more frequent monitoring of medication adherence [18]. Patients with comorbid anxiety and cardiovascular disease may require more frequent monitoring of blood pressure and heart rate [19].

When selecting medications for patients with comorbidities, psychiatrists should also consider nonpharmacological interventions, such as psychotherapy or lifestyle modifications [20]. Comorbidities may require a multidisciplinary approach, such as collaborating with other health care professionals to develop a comprehensive treatment plan [21].

7.5 Initiating Medications

Before initiating a medication, one must first consider the patient's medical history, current medications, potential side effects, and optimal dosing regimens in order to select an appropriate medication [11]. Another consideration is the patient's current medications, as medication interactions may lead to adverse effects or decreased effectiveness of the medications [22]. One must also consider potential side effects of the medication when initiating a new drug. Common side effects may include dizziness, dry mouth, nausea, or constipation. However, some medications may cause more serious side effects, such as weight gain, sexual dysfunction, or increased risk of suicidal thoughts or behaviors [23]. It is imperative to inform patients about potential side effects and work with them to manage any symptoms that may arise.

Optimal dosing regimens must also be considered when initiating a new medication. The initial dose of a medication may vary depending on the patient's age, weight, medical history, and other factors. Additionally, some medications may require a loading dose to reach therapeutic levels more quickly [24]. Regular monitoring of the patient's symptoms and side effects is critical during the initiation of medications, so that dosing adjustments can be made in a timely fashion in order to achieve optimal outcomes. The frequency of monitoring may vary depending on the medication, the patient's response, and other factors.

7.6 Switching Medications

Switching medications is a common practice in psychopharmacology, especially when a patient is not responding adequately to an initial treatment or is experiencing significant side effects [25]. However, switching medications can be complex and requires careful consideration of several factors, including the patient's current medication regimen, medical history, and treatment goals. The new medication should be compatible with any current medications, and the timing of the switch should be carefully planned. In some cases, a washout period may be necessary to avoid adverse interactions between medications [26]. The patient's medical history is another important consideration when switching medications, as patients with certain medical conditions, such as liver or kidney disease, may require lower doses or may need to avoid certain medications altogether [17]. Additionally, patients with a history of adverse reactions to certain medications may need to avoid those medications when switching.

The new medication should be chosen based on the patient's symptoms and the desired treatment outcomes. For example, a patient with depression who is not responding to an SSRI may benefit from switching to a different class of antidepressant medication, such as an SNRI or a tricyclic antidepressant [27]. Equivalency charts may assist in determining what dose conversions to utilize, like in the instance of switching antipsychotics [28]. An alternative formulation or mode of administration may be helpful when one of the desired outcomes is improved adherence, such as switching from oral antipsychotics to long-acting injectables [29]. It is important to consider the potential side effects of the new medication and monitor the patient for any adverse effects. Side effects may include dizziness, nausea, headache, or changes in mood or behavior. Patients should be educated regarded potential side effects and feel empowered to report symptoms that may arise. The dosing regimen and titration of the new medication must also be carefully considered when switching medications and should be tailored to the patient's lifestyle and needs.

Finally, regular monitoring is critical when switching medications. One must monitor the patient's response to the new medication and adjust the dose or regimen as needed to ensure optimal treatment outcomes. The frequency of monitoring (which may include blood levels) may vary depending on the medication, the patient's response, and other factors.

7.7 Augmentation Strategies

Augmentation strategies are often employed when initial treatments for mental health conditions, such as depression or anxiety, are not effective or only partially effective. Augmentation refers to the addition of a second medication, usually to an existing medication regimen, to enhance the therapeutic effects of the primary medication [30]. Augmentation strategies may also be used to address persistent symptoms or side effects of the primary medication. There are several classes of medications that may be used in augmentation strategies, including antipsychotics, mood stabilizers, and other classes of antidepressants [31]. The choice of augmentation agent will depend on the individual patient's symptoms, medication history, and medical history.

Antipsychotics are often used as augmentation for depression that is unresponsive to traditional antidepressant medications. They may be used at a low dose and can help enhance the therapeutic effects of the antidepressant medication. Commonly used antipsychotics in augmentation therapy include aripiprazole, quetiapine, and olanzapine [32]. More recently, brexpiprazole and cariprazine have received FDA approval as an adjunctive treatment in MDD [33]. Mood stabilizers, such as lithium [34] or valproic acid [35], may also be used as an augmentation strategy for depression or other mood disorders. Mood stabilizers can help stabilize mood and prevent relapse in patients who have not responded well to traditional antidepressants [36]. Other classes of antidepressants may also be used in augmentation strategies. For example, adding a medication that increases the activity of the neurotransmitter norepinephrine, such as bupropion or desipramine, may enhance the therapeutic effects of a traditional SSRI antidepressant [37].

In addition to medication augmentation, other nonpharmacological interventions may be used to enhance the effects of traditional medications. For example, cognitive behavioral therapy (CBT) or other forms of psychotherapy may be used in conjunction with medication to help patients develop coping skills and improve their ability to manage symptoms [38].

Of note, augmentation strategies may increase the risk of adverse effects, and regular monitoring of the patient is necessary to ensure optimal treatment outcomes. Patient education is also important to ensure that they understand the rationale behind the augmentation strategy and to help manage any concerns or questions they may have.

7.8 Tapering and Discontinuation

Tapering refers to the gradual reduction of medication dosage over time, while discontinuation refers to the complete cessation of a medication. The goal of tapering and discontinuation is to minimize the risk of withdrawal symptoms and prevent relapse [39]. Abrupt discontinuation of psychiatric medications can lead to withdrawal symptoms, which can range from mild to severe depending on the medication and the patient's individual characteristics [40]. Common withdrawal symptoms can include nausea, headaches, dizziness, irritability, insomnia, and anxiety. In some cases, withdrawal symptoms can be severe, such as in the case of benzodiazepines or other sedatives [41].

The process of tapering medications must be tailored to each individual patient, taking into account their specific medication regimen, medical history, and individual characteristics. The patient's response to tapering must be monitored closely and adjustments made as needed. The tapering schedule will depend on the specific medication and the duration of treatment, as well as the patient's individual characteristics [42]. The decision to discontinue medication must be made carefully, weighing the potential risks and benefits of continuing treatment versus the risks and benefits of discontinuation [43]. In some cases, medication may need to be continued indefinitely, as in the case of chronic psychiatric conditions [44].

There are several factors that should be considered when making the decision to discontinue medication, including the duration and severity of symptoms, the potential risks of medication use, the patient's response to previous attempts at discontinuation, and the presence of other medical or psychiatric conditions [45]. In general, it is recommended that psychiatric medications be discontinued gradually, over a period of weeks or months [46]. It is important to monitor the patient's response to the tapering process and to adjust the tapering schedule as needed to minimize the risk of withdrawal symptoms and prevent relapse. Patients should be educated about the tapering and discontinuation process, including the potential risks and benefits, and the importance of closely following the prescribed tapering schedule [47]. Regular follow-ups with the patient are important throughout the tapering and discontinuation process, to monitor the patient's response and to provide support and guidance as needed.

7.9 Managing Side Effects

Most psychotropic medications can cause a range of adverse effects, some of which may be minor and tolerable while others can be severe and interfere with treatment compliance or quality of life. Managing medication side effects is an important part of psychiatric treatment and requires careful consideration of the medication's mechanism of action, the patient's individual risk factors, and the impact of side effects on the patient's overall well-being [48].

It is important to regularly monitor patients for potential side effects, especially during the first few weeks of medication treatment. Patients should be encouraged to report any symptoms that they experience, even if they seem mild or unrelated to the medication. It is important to understand how a medication affects the brain and the nervous system, and how this can lead to side effects. For example, antidepressants that primary target serotonin receptors can cause side effects such as sexual dysfunction, gastrointestinal symptoms, and changes in appetite and weight [12]. Every patient is unique, and their individual risk factors (age, gender, genetics, medical history, lifestyle factors, and co-occurring psychiatric or medical conditions) can influence the likelihood and severity of medication side effects. For example, older patients may be more prone to cognitive side effects from antipsychotics [7], while patients with a history of substance use disorder may be more susceptible to abuse or dependence of certain medications [49].

If side effects are interfering with treatment, adjusting the medication dosage or timing may be necessary. This may involve decreasing the dose or splitting the daily dose into smaller doses taken throughout the day [50]. For example, patients who experience sedation from antidepressants may benefit from taking the medication at night instead of in the morning [51]. In some cases, adding an adjunctive medication to the treatment regimen may help manage side effects; for example, adding diphenhydramine, benztropine, deutetrabenazine, valbenazine, etc. for extrapyramidal symptoms caused by antipsychotics [52]. If side effects persist despite dose adjustments and adjunctive treatments, switching to a different medication with a different mechanism of action or side effect profile may be necessary. As mentioned earlier, switching medications should be done carefully and under close supervision, as there may be risks associated with abrupt discontinuation of the current medication or the initiation of a new medication.

Finally, it is important to educate patients about the potential side effects of their medications and to provide support and guidance for managing them. Patients should be encouraged to ask questions and to report any concerns that they have. They should also be provided with resources and tools for managing side effects, such as lifestyle recommendations, over-the-counter treatments, and self-monitoring tools [53].

7.10 Monitoring and Assessing Medication Efficacy

Monitoring and assessing medication efficacy involves tracking the patient's symptoms and the response to medication over time [54]. There are several factors that should be considered when monitoring and assessing medication efficacy, including the severity and duration of symptoms, the potential for medication interactions and side effects, and the patient's response to previous medication treatments [55].

One key tool is the use of rating scales, measures that can be used to evaluate the severity of symptoms, track changes in symptom severity over time, and assess the impact of treatment. The Hamilton Rating Scale for Depression is a research tool for assessing the severity of depression symptoms [56]. Other rating scales used in psychopharmacology clinical trials include the Young Mania Rating Scale for bipolar disorder [57] and the Positive and Negative Symptom Scale for schizophrenia [58]. In addition to rating scales, other measures that can be used to assess medication efficacy include patient self-report measures (including the Patient Health Questionnaire 9 [PHQ-9], General Anxiety Disorder 7 [GAD-7], and Post-Traumatic Stress Disorder Checklist for DSM-5 [PCL-5]), clinician observation, and physiological measures such as heart rate and blood pressure [59]. These measures can be used in combination with rating scales to provide a more complete picture of the patient's overall response to treatment.

Regular follow-up appointments are essential for monitoring medication efficacy. During these appointments, one can evaluate the patient's symptoms and side effects, adjust medication doses or formulations as needed, and assess the patient's overall response to treatment [60]. The frequency of follow-up appointments will depend on the specific medication and the severity of the patient's condition. Patients should be encouraged to report any changes in symptoms or side effects as soon as they occur. This can facilitate timely adjustments to the treatment plan to optimize medication efficacy and minimize the risk of side effects.

7.11 Polypharmacy

In the field of psychiatry, polypharmacy is a common practice due to the high prevalence of comorbid mental and physical health conditions, as well as the complexity of psychiatric disorders [61]. However, the use of multiple medications also increases the risk of adverse drug reactions, drug–drug interactions, and medication nonadherence, which can result in poor treatment outcomes. One should carefully consider the risks and benefits of polypharmacy when selecting medications. When treating a patient with multiple comorbidities, it may be necessary to prescribe multiple medications to address each condition adequately. However, when possible, one should try to limit the number of medications prescribed to avoid potential interactions and side effects [62].

A thorough review of the patient's medication regimen is imperative in identifying potential drug–drug interactions and adverse effects [62]. One should assess the patient's medication history, including prescription, over-the-counter medications, and dietary supplements. Prioritizing medications helps focus on the most essential medications, reducing the risk of adverse drug interactions [61, 63]. One should consider the medication's effectiveness and side effects and the patient's preferences when making decisions. Collaborative care involves coordinating with the patient, their primary care physician, and other specialists. It can help avoid duplicative treatments and improve communication, which leads to better outcomes [64]. Medication nonadherence is a significant problem in psychiatry and can lead to poor treatment outcomes [65]. To reduce nonadherence, one should involve the patient in the decision-making process, educate them about the medication's purpose and potential side effects, and monitor them for adherence. Lastly, monitoring patients for adverse effects of medications by using vital signs, laboratory values, and eliciting any signs or symptom can prevent the worsening of the side effects and improve patient outcomes [66]. Periodic evaluation of medication efficacy and side effects can help avoid unnecessary medications and ensure that the treatment plan is still appropriate.

7.12 Additional Safety Considerations

Safety is a crucial consideration in the use of psychotropic medications, which have the potential to cause adverse effects. Side effects, medical comorbidities, and polypharmacy, as discussed in the preceding sections, are important to keep in mind in ensuring the safety of a psychotropic regimen. Other best practices pertinent to safety include gradual titration of medications, special considerations for pregnant and breastfeeding women, acute suicidality caused by psychotropic medications, and assessing medication adherence.

Psychotropic medications often need to be titrated up to a therapeutic dose gradually. This allows patients to acclimate to the medication and reduces the risk of adverse effects. Close monitoring during the titration phase is necessary to ensure that the medication is effective and safe for the patient [67].

Pregnant and breastfeeding women require special considerations when it comes to the use of psychotropic medications. Some medications can be harmful to the developing fetus or the breastfeeding infant [68]. One should carefully weigh the potential benefits and risks of medication use during pregnancy and breastfeeding and consult with the patient's obstetrician or pediatrician as necessary [68].

Some psychotropic medications, particularly antidepressants, can increase the risk of suicidal ideation or behavior [69]. One should monitor patients closely for signs of suicidal ideation or behavior, particularly during the early stages of treatment when the risk is highest.

Lastly, medication adherence is critical to the effectiveness and safety of psychotropic medications. It is important to work with patients to ensure that they understand the importance of taking their medications as prescribed and to address any barriers to adherence that a patient may be experiencing [70].

7.13 Pharmacogenetics

The use of pharmacogenetics in psychiatry can help identify genetic variations that affect an individual's response to psychotropic medications. By understanding an individual's genetic makeup, one can determine the optimal dose and type of medication, as well as identify potential risks for adverse effects [71]. This approach can improve the safety and effectiveness of treatment as well as reduce the likelihood of trial-and-error prescribing. There are several genes that have been identified as relevant to psychotropic medication response. For example, genetic variations in the cytochrome P450 enzymes, which are responsible for metabolizing many medications, can affect how quickly or slowly a medication is broken down and eliminated from the body [72]. Variations in these enzymes can lead to either reduced or increased medication effectiveness and/or side effects. Additionally, genetic variations in transporters that affect the reuptake of neurotransmitters, such as the serotonin transporter gene, can affect an individual's response to antidepressants. For example, individuals with a variation in the serotonin transporter gene may be more likely to respond to SSRIs than to other antidepressants [73].

While pharmacogenetic testing has the potential to improve medication selection, it is important to note that it is not yet widely used in clinical practice, and its precise role in clinical management is still unclear [74]. Challenges include the cost and availability of testing as well as the need for education and training on how to interpret and apply the results.

7.14 Conclusion and Future Directions

Psychopharmacology is a constantly evolving field that is shaped by new research, advances in technology, and changes in clinical practice. As such, it is important to stay up to date with the latest developments and to be aware of the future directions of the field.

As discussed earlier, advances in genomics and other fields are making it possible to develop medications that are more targeted and effective for specific patients. By understanding a patient's genetic profile, psychiatrists may one day choose medications that are more likely to be effective and avoid those that are likely to cause side effects or be ineffective [75].

New discoveries in the pathophysiology of mental illness may uncover additional psychopharmacologic options. Inflammation has been linked to a number of mental health disorders, including depression and anxiety [76]. Recent research has focused on developing medications that target inflammatory pathways in the body, with the aim of reducing inflammation and improving symptoms of mental illness. Some of the medications being studied include anti-inflammatory agents such as aspirin [77] and omega-3 fatty acids [78]. The gut and brain are connected via a bidirectional communication system known as the gut-brain axis. Recent research has shown that the gut microbiome, the collection of microorganisms that live in the gut, can have a significant impact on mental health [79]. This has led to the development of new medications that target the gut microbiome, as well as the use of probiotics and prebiotics to improve mental health outcomes [80].

Psychedelic drugs like psilocybin and MDMA are being studied for their potential to treat mental health disorders, including depression, anxiety, and PTSD [81]. Research has shown that these drugs can have a powerful therapeutic effect, and they are being studied in clinical trials as potential treatments for a range of mental health disorders. While the use of these drugs is still highly controversial, they may play a significant role in the future of psychopharmacology.

Drug repurposing involves the use of existing medications for new indications. This can involve testing medications that are already approved for one use in a different population or for a different condition. Drug repurposing can be a cost-effective and time-efficient way to develop new treatments for mental health disorders, and is an area of growing interest in psychopharmacology [82].

In summary, psychopharmacology and clinical practice are guided by evidence-based medicine as well as individual patient circumstances. It is important to establish rapport with patients and tailor medication regimens to their diagnoses, past experiences, and medical and psychiatric comorbidities, and to monitor for drug efficacy and side effects over time. New advances in psychopharmacology may provide alternative treatment options as well as improve efficiency in medication selection and management.

References

1. Braslow, J. T. & Marder, S. R. History of psychopharmacology. *Annu Rev Clin Psychol* 15, 25–50 (2019).

2. Geels, F. W., Pieters, T. & Snelders, S. Cultural enthusiasm, resistance and the societal embedding of new technologies: psychotropic drugs in the 20th century. *Technol Anal Strateg Manag* 19, 145–165 (2007).

3. Baumeister, A. A. The chlorpromazine enigma. *J Hist Neurosci* 22, 14–29 (2013).

4. Pelto-Piri, V., Engström, K. & Engström, I. *Paternalism, autonomy and reciprocity: ethical perspectives in encounters with patients in psychiatric in-patient care.* http://www.biomedcentral.com/1472-6939/14/49 (2013).

5. Fan, J. & De Lannoy, I. A. M. Pharmacokinetics. *Biochem Pharmacol* 87, 93–120 (2014).

6. Zarkowski, P. A. Relative prevalence of 10 types of pharmacodynamic interactions in psychiatric treatment. *Int J Psychiatry Med* 55, 82–104 (2020).

7. Catterson, M. L., Preskorn, S. H. & Martin, R. L. Pharmacodynamic and pharmacokinetic considerations in geriatric psychopharmacology. *Geriatric Psychiatry* 20, 205–218 (1997).

8. Vieweg, W. V. R., Levy, J. R., Fredrickson, S. K., et al. Psychotropic drug considerations in depressed patients with metabolic disturbances. *Am J Med* 121 647–655. Preprint at https://doi.org/10.1016/j.amjmed.2007.08.043 (2008).

9. Dwight-Johnson, M., Lagomasino, I. T. & Simpson, G. M. Underuse of evidence-based pharmacotherapies for affective disorders. *Psychiatric Serv* 54, 1076–1078 (2003).

10. Miller, B. J., Paschall III, C. B. & Svendsen, D. P. Mortality and medical comorbidity among patients with serious mental illness. *Psychiatric Serv* 57, 1482–1487 (2006).

11. Howland, R. H. Questions to ask when selecting medication. *J Psychosoc Nurs Ment Health Serv* **50**, 13–15 (2012).

12. Posternak, M. A. & Zimmerman, M. The effectiveness of switching antidepressants during remission: a case series of depressed patients who experienced intolerable side effects. *J Affect Dis* 69 www.elsevier.com/locate/jad (2002).

13. Bourgeois, B. F. Pharmacologic interactions between valproate and other drugs. *Am J Med* **84**, 29–33 (1988).

14. Silva Neves, F., Fernandes Malloy-Diniz, L. & Corrêa, H. Suicidal behavior in bipolar disorder: what is the influence of psychiatric comorbidities? *J Clin Psychiatry* **70**, 13–18 (2009).

15. Almeida, O. P., Draper, B., Pirkis, J., et al. Anxiety, depression, and comorbid anxiety and depression: risk factors and outcome over two years. *Int Psychogeriatr* **24**, 1622–1632 (2012).

16. Ratliff, S. & Mezuk, B. Depressive symptoms, psychiatric medication use, and risk of type 2 diabetes: results from the Health and Retirement Study. *Gen Hosp Psychiatry* **37**, 420–426 (2015).

17. Hayes, J. F., Marston, L., Walters, K., et al. Adverse renal, endocrine, hepatic, and metabolic events during maintenance mood stabilizer treatment for bipolar disorder: a population-based cohort study. *PLoS Med* **13**, e1002058 (2016).

18. Lingam, R. & Scott, J. Treatment non-adherence in affective disorders. *Acta Psychiatrica Scandinavica* **105**, 164–172 Preprint at https://doi.org/10.1034/j .1600-0447.2002.1r084.x (2002).

19. Cosh, S. M., Pinto, R., Denson, L. & Tully, P. J. Understandings and experiences of adherence to secondary prevention for patients with cardiovascular disease and comorbid depression or anxiety. *Psychol Health Med* **28**, 1479–1486 (2022). doi:10 .1080/13548506.2022.2060515.

20. Frost, R., Bauernfreund, Y. & Walters, K. Non-pharmacological interventions for depression/anxiety in older adults with physical comorbidities affecting functioning: systematic review and meta-analysis. *Intern Psychogeriatrics* **31**, 1121–1136 Preprint at https://doi.org/10 .1017/S1041610218001564 (2019).

21. Andersson, A. C., Ainalem, I., Berg, A. & Janlov, A. C. Challenges to improve inter-professional care and service collaboration for people living with psychiatric disabilities in ordinary housing. *Qual Manag Health Care* **25**, 44–52 (2016).

22. Wolff, J., Reißner, P., Hefner, G., et al. Pharmacotherapy, drug-drug interactions and potentially inappropriate medication in depressive disorders. *PLoS ONE* **16**, e0255192 (2021).

23. Demyttenaere, K. & Jaspers, L. Review: bupropion and SSRI-induced side effects. *J Psychopharmacology* **22**, 792–804 (2008).

24. Hirschfeld, R. M. A., Allen, M. H., Mcevoy, J. P., Keck, P. E. & Russell, J. M. Safety and tolerability of oral loading divalproex sodium in acutely manic bipolar patients. *J Clin Psychiatry* **60**(12), 815–818 (1999).

25. Essock, S. M., Covell, N. H., Davis, S. M., et al. Effectiveness of switching antipsychotic medications. *Am J Psychiatry* **163**, 2090–2095 (2006).

26. Yates, S. J., Ahuja, N., Gartside, S. E. & McAllister-Williams, R. H. Serotonin syndrome following introduction of venlafaxine following withdrawal of phenelzine: implications for drug washout periods. *Therap Adv Psychopharmacology* **1**, 125–127 Preprint at https://doi.org/10.1177/ 2045125311413497 (2011).

27. Connolly, K. R. & Thase, M. E. If at first you don't succeed: a review of the evidence for antidepressant augmentation, combination and switching strategies. *Drugs* **71**, 43–64 (2011).

28. Andreasen, N. C., Pressler, M., Nopoulos, P., Miller, D. & Ho, B. C. Antipsychotic dose equivalents and dose-years: a standardized method for comparing exposure to different drugs. *Biol Psychiatry* **67**, 255–262 (2010).

29. Sajatovic, M., Levin, J., Ramirez, L. F., et al. Prospective trial of customized adherence enhancement plus long-acting injectable antipsychotic medication in homeless or recently homeless individuals with schizophrenia or schizoaffective disorder. *J Clin Psychiatry* **74**, 1249–1255 (2013).

30. Wainwright, L. Underutilised augmentation strategies for mood disorders. *Austral N Z J Psychiatry* **54**, 1039 Preprint at https://doi.org/10.1177/0004867420924106 (2020).

31. Mojtabai, R., Amin-Esmaeili, M., Spivak, S. & Olfson, M. Remission and treatment augmentation of depression in the United States. *J Clin Psychiatry* **82**, 21m13988 (2021).

32. Wright, B. M., Eiland, E. H. & Lorenz, R. Augmentation with atypical antipsychotics for depression: a review of evidence-based support from the medical literature. *Pharmacotherapy* **33**, 344–359 Preprint at https://doi.org/10.1002/phar.1204 (2013).

33. Vasudev, A. , Chaudhari, S., Sethi, R., et al. A review of the pharmacological and clinical profile of newer atypical antipsychotics as treatments for bipolar disorder: considerations for use in older patients. *Drugs Aging* **35**, 887–895 Preprint at https://doi.org/10.1007/s40266-018-0579-6 (2018).

34. Adli, M., Hollinde, D. L., Stamm, T., et al. Response to lithium augmentation in depression is associated with the glycogen synthase kinase 3-beta-50T/C single nucleotide polymorphism. *Biol Psychiatry* **62**, 1295–1302 (2007).

35. Ghabrash, M. F., Comai, S., Tabaka, J., et al. Valproate augmentation in a subgroup of patients with treatment-resistant unipolar depression. *World J Biol Psychiatry* **17**, 165–170 (2016).

36. Hantouche, E. G., Akiskal, H. S., Lancrenon, S. & Chatenêt-Duchêne, L. Mood stabilizer augmentation in apparently 'unipolar' MDD: predictors of response in the naturalistic French national EPIDEP study. *J Affect Disord* **84**, 243–249 (2005).

37. Marshall, R. D., Johannet, C. M., Collins, P. Y., et al. Bupropion and sertraline combination treatment in refractory depression. *J Psychopharmacol* **9**, 284–286 (1995).

38. Wiles, N., Thomas, L., Abel, A., et al. Cognitive behavioural therapy as an adjunct to pharmacotherapy for primary care based patients with treatment resistant depression: results of the CoBalT randomised controlled trial. *Lancet* **381**, 375–384 (2013).

39. Van Geffen, E. C. G., Hugtenburg, J. G., Heerdink, E. R., Van Hulten, R. P. & Egberts, A. C. G. Discontinuation symptoms in users of selective serotonin reuptake inhibitors in clinical practice: tapering versus abrupt discontinuation. *Eur J Clin Pharmacol* **61**, 303–307 (2005).

40. Tint, A., Haddad, P. M. & Anderson, I. M. The effect of rate of antidepressant tapering on the incidence of discontinuation symptoms: a randomised study. *J Psychopharmacol* **22**, 330–332 (2008).

41. Guaiana, G. & Barbui, C. Discontinuing benzodiazepines: best practices. *Epidemiol Psychiatr Sci* **25**, 214–216 (2016).

42. Horowitz, M. A., Moncrieff, J., de Haan, L., et al. Tapering antipsychotic medication: practical considerations. *Psychol Med* **52**, 32–35 Preprint at https://doi.org/10.1017/S0033291721003299 (2022).

43. Ostrow, L., Jessell, L., Hurd, M., Darrow, S. M. & Cohen, D. Discontinuing psychiatric medications: a survey of long-term users. *Psychiatric Serv* **68**, 1232–1238 (2017).

44. Harrow, M., Jobe, T. H. & Faull, R. N. Do all schizophrenia patients need antipsychotic treatment continuously throughout their lifetime? A 20-year longitudinal study. *Psychol Med* **42**, 2145–2155 (2012).

45. Cosci, F. & Chouinard, G. Acute and persistent withdrawal syndromes following discontinuation of psychotropic medications. *Psychotherapy Psychosomatics* **89**, 283–306 Preprint at

https://doi.org/10.1159/000506868 (2020).

46. Tondo, L. & Baldessarini, R. J. Discontinuing psychotropic drug treatment. *BJPsych Open* **6**(2), e24 (2020).

47. Groot, P. C. & van Os, J. How user knowledge of psychotropic drug withdrawal resulted in the development of person-specific tapering medication. *Ther Adv Psychopharmacol* **10**, 204512532093245 (2020).

48. Malik, S. Understanding, assessing, and managing the side effects of psychotropic medications. *Psychiatric Annals* **51**, 399–400 Preprint at https://doi.org/10.3928/00485713-20210806-02 (2021).

49. Jones, J. D., Mogali, S. & Comer, S. D. Polydrug abuse: a review of opioid and benzodiazepine combination use. *Drug Alcohol Dependence* **125**, 8–18 Preprint at https://doi.org/10.1016/j.drugalcdep.2012.07.004 (2012).

50. Weissman, E. M. & Dellenbaugh, C. Impact of splitting risperidone tablets on medication adherence and on clinical outcomes for patients with schizophrenia. *Psychiatric Serv* **58**, 201–206 (2007).

51. Mayers, A. G. & Baldwin, D. S. Antidepressants and their effect on sleep. *Hum Psychopharmacol* **20**, 533–559 Preprint at https://doi.org/10.1002/hup.726 (2005).

52. Stahl, S. M., Sy, S. & Maguire, G. A. How and when to treat the most common adverse effects of antipsychotics: expert review from research to clinical practice. *Acta Psychiatrica Scandinavica* **143**, 172–180 Preprint at https://doi.org/10.1111/acps.13266 (2021).

53. Ashoorian, D., Davidson, R., Rock, D., Dragovic, M. & Clifford, R. A clinical communication tool for the assessment of psychotropic medication side effects. *Psychiatry Res* **230**, 643–657 (2015).

54. Rush, A. J. Isn't it about time to employ measurement-based care in practice? *Am J Psychiatry* **172**, 934–936 Preprint at https://doi.org/10.1176/appi.ajp.2015.15070928 (2015).

55. Fournier, J. C., DeRubeis, R. J., Hollon, S. D., et al. Differential change in specific depressive symptoms during antidepressant medication or cognitive therapy. *Behav Res Ther* **51**, 392–398 (2013).

56. Kieslich da Silva, A., Reche, M., Lima, A. F. D. S., et al. Assessment of the psychometric properties of the 17- and 6-item Hamilton Depression Rating Scales in major depressive disorder, bipolar depression and bipolar depression with mixed features. *J Psychiatr Res* **108**, 84–89 (2019).

57. Prisciandaro, J. J. & Tolliver, B. K. An item response theory evaluation of the Young mania rating scale and the Montgomery-Asberg depression rating scale in the systematic treatment enhancement program for bipolar disorder (STEP-BD). *J Affect Disord* **205**, 73–80 (2016).

58. Khan, A., Lindenmayer, J. P., Opler, M., et al. A new integrated negative symptom structure of the positive and negative syndrome scale (PANSS) in schizophrenia using item response analysis. *Schizophr Res* **150**, 185–196 (2013).

59. Blenkiron, P. & Goldsmith, L. Patient-reported outcome measures in community mental health teams: pragmatic evaluation of PHQ-9, GAD-7 and SWEMWBS. *B J Psych Bull* **43**, 221–227 (2019).

60. John Rush, A., Trivedi, M. H., Wisniewski, S. R., et al. Acute and longer-term outcomes in depressed outpatients requiring one or several treatment steps: a STAR*D report. *Am J Psychiatry* **163** www.star-d.org (2006).

61. Möller, H. J., Seemüller, F., Schennach-Wolff, R., et al. History, background, concepts and current use of comedication and polypharmacy in psychiatry. *Intern J Neuropsychopharmacol* **17**, 983–996 Preprint at https://doi.org/10.1017/S1461145713000837 (2014).

62. Kukreja, S., Kalra, G., Shah, N. & Shrivastava, A. Polypharmacy in psychiatry: a review. *Mens Sana*

Monographs **11**, 82–99 Preprint at https://doi.org/10.4103/0973-1229.104497 (2013).

63. Delara, M., Murray, L., Jafari, B., Banji, A., Goodarzi, Z., et al. Prevalence and factors associated with polypharmacy: a systematic review and meta-analysis. *BMC Geriatrics* **22**(1) 601 (2022).

64. Barkil-Oteo, A. Collaborative care for depression in primary care: how psychiatry could 'troubleshoot' current treatments and practices. *Yale J Biol Med* **86**, 139–146 (2013).

65. Cutler, R. L., Fernandez-Llimos, F., Frommer, M., Benrimoj, C. & Garcia-Cardenas, V. Economic impact of medication non-adherence by disease groups: a systematic review. *BMJ Open* **8**, e016982. Preprint at https://doi.org/10.1136/bmjopen-2017-016982 (2018).

66. Coates, M., Spanos, M., Parmar, P., Chandrasekhar, T. & Sikich, L. A Review of methods for monitoring adverse events in pediatric psychopharmacology clinical trials. *Drug Safety* **41**, 465–471 Preprint at https://doi.org/10.1007/s40264–017-0633-z (2018).

67. Caffrey, A. R. & Borrelli, E. P. The art and science of drug titration. *Ther Adv Drug Safety* **11** , 2042098620958910. Preprint at https://doi.org/10.1177/2042098620958910 (2020).

68. Payne, J. L. Psychopharmacology in pregnancy and breastfeeding. *Med Clin North Am* **103**, 629–650 Preprint at https://doi.org/10.1016/j.mcna.2019.02.009 (2019).

69. Bauer, M. S., Wisniewski, S. R., Marangell, L. B., et al. Are antidepressants associated with new-onset suicidality in bipolar disorder? A prospective study of participants in the systematic treatment enhancement program for bipolar disorder (STEP-BD): antidepressants and suicidality in bipolar disorder. *J Clin Psychiatry* **67**, 48–55 (2006).

70. Deane, F. P., McAlpine, E., Byrne, M. K., Davis, E. L. & Mortimer, C. Are carer attitudes toward medications related to self-reported medication adherence amongst people with mental illness? *Psychiatry Res* **260**, 158–163 (2018).

71. Bousman, C., Al Maruf, A. & Muller, D. J. Towards the integration of pharmacogenetics in psychiatry: a minimum, evidence-based genetic testing panel. *Curr Opin Psychiatry* **32**, 7–15 Preprint at https://doi.org/10.1097/YCO.0000000000000465 (2019).

72. Mostafa, S., Polasek, T. M., Bousman, C. A., et al. Pharmacogenomics in psychiatry: the challenge of cytochrome P450 enzyme phenoconversion and solutions to assist precision dosing. *Pharmacogenomics* **23**, 857–867 Preprint at https://doi.org/10.2217/pgs-2022-0104 (2022).

73. Niitsu, T., Fabbri, C., Bentini, F. & Serretti, A. Pharmacogenetics in major depression: a comprehensive meta-analysis. *Prog Neuropsychopharmacol Biol Psychiatry* **45**, 183–194 (2013).

74. Stingl, J. C. Mindful pharmacogenetics: drug dosing for mental health. *Am J Psychiatry* **175**, 395–397 Preprint at https://doi.org/10.1176/appi.ajp.2018.18020134 (2018).

75. Stein, M. B. & Smoller, J. W. Precision psychiatry: will genomic medicine lead the way? *JAMA Psychiatry* **75**, 663–664 Preprint at https://doi.org/10.1001/jamapsychiatry.2018.0375 (2018).

76. Morris, A. A., Zhao, L., Ahmed, Y., et al. Association between depression and inflammation-differences by race and sex: the META-health study. *Psychosom Med* **73**, 462–468 (2011).

77. Berk, M., Woods, R. L., Nelson, M. R., et al. Effect of aspirin vs placebo on the prevention of depression in older people: a randomized clinical trial. *JAMA Psychiatry* **77**, 1012–1020 (2020).

78. Carney, R. M., Freedland, K. E., Rubin, E. H., et al. *Omega-3 augmentation of sertraline in treatment of depression in patients with coronary heart disease: a randomized controlled trial.* https://jamanetwork.com (2009).

79. Jang, S. H., Woo, Y. S., Lee, S. Y. & Bahk, W. M. The brain–gut–microbiome axis in

psychiatry. *Int J Molecul Sci* 21, 1–17 Preprint at https://doi.org/10.3390/ijms21197122 (2020).

80. Liu, R. T., Walsh, R. F. L. & Sheehan, A. E. Prebiotics and probiotics for depression and anxiety: a systematic review and meta-analysis of controlled clinical trials. *Neurosci Biobehavior Rev* 102, 13–23 Preprint at https://doi.org/10.1016/j.neubiorev.2019.03.023 (2019).

81. Davis, A. K., Barrett, F. S., May, D. G. Effects of psilocybin-assisted therapy on major depressive disorder: a randomized clinical trial. *JAMA Psychiatry* 78, 481–489 (2021).

82. Truong, T. T. T., Panizzutti, B., Kim, J. H. & Walder, K. Repurposing drugs via network analysis: opportunities for psychiatric disorders. *Pharmaceutics* 14, 1464. Preprint at https://doi.org/10.3390/pharmaceutics14071464 (2022).

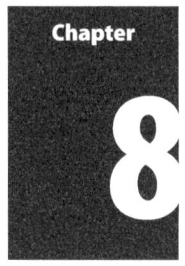
Neurostimulation Treatments

Luis A. Wische-Fernandez and Salih Selek

8.1 Introduction

Psychiatry has incorporated at different times seemingly disparate models that explain illness. Psychoanalytic theory was followed by molecular, genetic, and neurotransmitter-based conceptualizations. The latter model led to effective pharmacologic treatment. However, this global, nonspecific approach can also come with untoward effects on the function of the brain and/or body, such as antipsychotic-associated prolactinemia or the decreased libido seen with some antidepressants, to name a few.

Functional imaging has more recently elucidated the role of whole brain networks as they relate to psychiatric illness. One way to modulate these networks or circuits is by stimulating the brain with the direct application of electricity or its induction through magnetic fields. The resultant plastic changes appear to outlive the initial stimulus and may affect discrete networks.

This chapter will focus on electroconvulsive therapy (ECT) and will describe modalities such as transcranial magnetic stimulation (TMS), vagus nerve stimulation (VNS), deep brain stimulation (DBS), and magnetic seizure therapy (MST).

8.2 Electroconvulsive Therapy

8.2.1 History

Medicinal, artificially induced seizures had their beginnings in the work of Lazlo Meduna, a neuropathologist from the early 20th century. His studies of postmortem brains showed illness-specific variations in glial counts. Higher numbers were seen in patients having suffered from epilepsy while the opposite occurred in schizophrenia. At the time it appeared that the two conditions were somewhat mutually exclusive. Meduna hypothesized that psychosis could improve through seizure-mediated increases of glia. To test this, he sought chemicals with epileptogenic potential and found some degree of success in using intramuscular camphor. He later switched to pentyenetetrazol, which he found tended to induce seizures more quickly, offering greater comfort to the patient. By 1934, Meduna had effectively reversed catatonia in several individuals using chemically induced seizures and went on to publish his findings in 1937 [1].

Ugo Cerletti and his student Lucio Bini conducted experiments with animals using electricity as the epileptogenic stimulus. Their work extended to involve successful human trials in 1938 [2]. Soon their method of induction replaced chemical means in part due to the side effects of the latter (prior to onset of seizure patients would experience discomfort that they would later recall). The popularity of ECT soared as evidence mounted regarding its effectiveness in treating a large swath of mental illness. The field of brain stimulation was born.

Through the 1940s, the use of ECT became widespread and waned somewhat by 1950 with the introduction of chlorpromazine. Nevertheless, ECT survived as a treatment modality and continued to evolve likely due to its unmatched efficacy.

Its peculiar side effect profile did limit its appeal, though, especially when compared to pharmacotherapy. Patients could experience shattered teeth, broken bones, and postictal confusion lasting up to half a day. Over the years, however, elegant refinements brought about comfort and safety through the introduction of a bite block, anesthesia, muscle paralyzing agents, and a physiologically compatible version of the stimulus. These advances led to the minimization of side effects associated with ECT treatment and its consolidation as a safe and effective intervention when well indicated, despite the fact that misconceptions about its use remain common.

8.2.2 Minimization of Cognitive Side Effects

Early ECT caused retrograde autobiographical memory loss, anterograde amnesia, and severe post-treatment confusion. These have been greatly minimized through the focalization of the stimulus and the maximization of stimulus efficiency.

With regards to the modifiable variables in ECT practice, electrode placement disproportionately drives cognitive side effects. Bilateral (BL) treatments, while highly effective, pass energy through the dominant hemisphere, hippocampus, and other midline structures. One eliminates the involvement of these brain areas by delivering a unilateral (UL) stimulus to the nondominant hemisphere. To produce a sufficiently robust seizure with a similar efficacy to that of BL, the UL stimulus requires a charge of six times the patient's seizure threshold (ST) [3].

One can further minimize cognitive effects by modulating the stimulus itself. Older machines produced sine waves no different than those obtained from a wall socket. The majority of their energy would fall on neurons already in the refractory state. This meant that unnecessarily high doses of electricity resulted in a relatively low yield. Higher energy caused greater side effects. In contrast, modern machines deliver block-like pulses that can be narrowed to the range of 0.5–1.5 ms (brief pulse) or < 0.5 ms (ultra-brief pulse). The narrower these become, the less energy is required to cause a seizure (efficiency increases). Although there's a relative lowering of the ST, the charge density also decreases, eliciting seizures that are less robust. This is the reason why ultra-brief pulses are ineffective when delivered bilaterally and why they have to be given at six times ST when given through UL electrode placement [4].

8.2.3 Mechanism of Action

While the mechanism of action of ECT remains to be elucidated, evidence hints at the role of its inhibitory and anticonvulsant properties. Systems in the body adapt to a myriad of environmental, metabolic, and trophic pressures. Just as hypertension causes left ventricular hypertrophy in the heart, the repeated application of seizures causes an upregulation of inhibitory mechanisms in the brain. Multiple observations support this hypothesis. For one, as the treatment series progresses, the expression of seizures lessens, and the ST rises. Additionally, studies looking at the effects of barely suprathreshold stimuli showed that the resultant seizures lacked antidepressant properties. Although seizures were induced, their magnitude was insufficient in causing a significant counterresponse on the part of the brain. Giving a series of these led to an efficacy similar to that of sham treatment. Localization also matters. Strong antiepileptic mechanisms specifically at the frontal poles appear to be involved in achieving a response [4].

Additionally, ECT leads to increases in brain-derived neurotrophic factor (BDNF), neurogenesis, and volume increases in the hippocampus [5, 6]. Incidentally, nascent cells resemble inhibitory interneurons. On a macro level, ECT normalizes the default mode network's overactivity, a feature associated with introspection and rumination in depression [7].

8.2.4 Pre-ECT Medical Evaluation

The physician performing the pretreatment physical should be educated regarding ECT-specific physiological responses. The application of a stimulus to the head can lead to brief bradycardia and asystole (usually < 6 seconds in duration). This occurs as a result of direct parasympathetic effects exerted through vagal stimulation. As the seizure entrains and fully generalizes, the opposite occurs. A sympathetic response results in marked tachycardia and hypertension. In addition, ECT can cause transient intracranial and intraocular pressures.

For these reasons, all the physicians involved will consider the patient's cardiac fitness, presence of implantable cardioverter defibrillators, hypertension, congestive heart failure, significant valvular disease, recent pneumonia, glaucoma, and space-occupying lesions. A basic workup includes an EKG, CBC, and CMP.

In certain states, patients will undergo mandatory testing for the activity of pseudo cholinesterase, a liver enzyme responsible for cleaving succinylcholine, a muscle paralyzer administered during ECT anesthesia. Those with impaired function can remain paralyzed for several hours and will require sedation and mechanical ventilation [8]. In these instances, rocuronium can serve as a safe alternative.

No absolute contraindications exist with regards to ECT. However, treatment is generally avoided in patients with space-occupying lesions that cause increased intracranial pressure [9].

8.2.5 ECT Session: Sequence of Events

Prior to arrival, the patient should be kept on "nothing by mouth" (NPO) status for at least 6 hours prior to treatment. If on insulin, they should be advised to postpone doses until after treatment completion as to avoid hypoglycemia.

On arrival, nursing starts an intravenous access (IV), attaches electrocardiogram (EKG) leads, and dons pulse oximetry and an automated blood pressure cuff. The elect roencephalography (EEG) leads are then placed over the forehead and behind the ear at the mastoid process. Pre-cleaning these areas with alcohol prep-pads eliminates skin oils, improves contact, and prevents EEG artifact secondary to movement. This aids in determining the cessation of the seizure.

The pre-procedure time-out can include patient identifiers, planned electrode placement, list of pre-medications, and the planned induction agent. This practice, in the author's opinion, offers the psychiatrist the ability to correlate the effect of anesthesia's medications on seizure expression.

Pre-treatment medications allow for the manipulation of individual patient variables affected by ECT. For example, in a hypertensive individual, low doses of a short-acting calcium channel blocker such as nifedipine can mitigate post-treatment rises in blood pressure without altering the seizure. Beta blockers show efficacy but have the unwanted effect of blunting seizure expression and compounding stimulus-associated bradycardia and asystole. The latter phenomena result with greater frequency in RUL electrode placement and when giving subthreshold stimuli as part of determining ST [10]. Anticholinergics such as glycopyrrolate or atropine mitigate these vagally driven effects while decreasing airway secretions, but at the cost of potentiating postictal tachycardia [11].

Muscle soreness results from succinylcholine-associated fasciculations. A tension headache can also occur due to the direct stimulation at the neuromuscular junction of facial and forehead muscles. Ketorolac, at the dose of 15 mg IV, given before or after the ECT-induced seizure can address those issues [12].

Once fully sedated after infusion of the anesthetic, the patient receives succinylcholine, a depolarizing paralytic agent. As mentioned earlier, rocuronium serves as an alternative in very rare situations of pseudocholinesterase deficiency [13]. Full muscle relaxation allows for manual mask bagging. High-frequency bag ventilation maximizes oxygen saturation prior to the period of high neuronal metabolic demand. It also facilitates the induction of the seizure by causing hypocapnia [14].

Post-treatment medication addresses the immediate sequelae of treatment. Seizures of limited expression (low-amplitude delta waves and weak postictal suppression) pose a challenge when determining seizure duration. As a means of preventing possible ictal activity from reaching the 5-minute mark (defined then as status epilepticus), a request for 1–2 mg IV of midazolam can be called out before the 2-minute mark. This allows sufficient time for preparation, administration, circulation, and diffusion of the medication across the blood–brain barrier. After cessation of a seizure, postictal delirium can occur, which can be treated with a short-acting benzodiazepine or an additional dose of the chosen induction agent. If the patient remains significantly hypertensive and tachycardic, a low dose of labetalol or esmolol can be given IV. The latter, being selective, avoids the risk of symptom exacerbation in patients with asthma.

8.2.6 Seizure Quality in Relation to Efficacy

For many years, duration served as the only measure by which to judge the quality of a seizure. Two additional EEG features appear to correlate with efficacy. One is the amplitude of the delta waves, and the other is postictal suppression, or the abruptness with which the brain enacts full electrical silence [15]. The first represents seizure intensity, while the degree of flatlining reflects the brain's inhibitory counterresponse. However, correlation does not equal causation, and some interpret the above measures as a possible reflection of physiological differences of those individuals that respond to ECT. These parameters can also be used to guide the stepwise increase of stimulus intensity as the ST rises. This is important given that barely suprathreshold seizures are ineffective while highly suprathreshold ones result in unnecessary side effects.

8.2.7 Effect of Anesthetic on Seizure Quality

The effects of anesthetic agents range from antiepileptic properties to sympathomimetic effects, which, in turn, influence the quality of the seizure. Propofol, a short-acting anesthetic, exerts a dampening effect on seizure expression. These effects present more prominently when involving right UL ECT treatment, as patients require more sessions and higher stimulus intensities. Propofol delays the response to ECT [16].

Ketamine, when used as an anesthetic for ECT, does not confer additional anti-depressant benefits [17]. It does, however, lead to increases in seizure expression. Because of this, it is often combined with either propofol or methohexital in patients with a peculiarly high ST. Its use as monotherapy leads to dissociative effects, a longer time to postictal recovery, and higher dropout rates [18].

8.2.8 Concurrent Pharmacotherapy

Two camps exist when it comes to the use of psychotropics during an index course of ECT. One believes in discontinuing medications due to their potential of causing side effects, while the other sees the possibility of a synergistic effect. Tricyclic antidepressants appear to exert a protective effect with regards to cognitive side effects, perhaps through noradrenergic processes. The use of nortriptyline appears to confer an increase in remission of about ~15%. A similar agent, Venlafaxine, improves outcomes to a lesser degree while possibly causing an nonsignificant worsening in side effects [19].

As this is a seizure-based treatment, as a general rule, benzodiazepines and anticonvulsants (for mood stabilization) should be avoided. The latter, however, should be continued if used as a treatment for epilepsy.

8.2.9 Maintenance Treatment

Despite the exceptional rates of response and remission provided by ECT treatment, those results are often short-lived. Among patients treated for depression with ECT, a large portion of remitters will relapse within 6 months of conclusion of the treatment [20]. The use of maintenance ECT treatments at regular intervals appears to augment the effects of psychotropic treatment and decrease the risk of relapse [17].

8.3 Transcranial Magnetic Stimulation

Transcranial magnetic stimulation (TMS) first received approval as a treatment for resistant depression during the 2000s. This modality creates an electrical current over the chosen area of the brain through magnetic induction. It has been widely practiced since 2007 and is currently being reimbursed by many medical insurance carriers. The treatment entails giving a series of 25–30 daily treatments lasting less than 1 hour each. Like ECT, TMS is noninvasive and involves fewer restrictions on treatment days. The classic region of interest in treating depression is the left dorsolateral prefrontal cortex. Due to its convenience and wide availability, TMS is becoming the first choice when it comes to neurostimulation. Current research is focused on the modulation of stimulus patterns and its application to different brain regions of interest.

8.4 Vagus Nerve Stimulation

In the mid-2000s, the US Food and Drug Administration approved a low-amplitude vagus nerve stimulator to address treatment-resistant depression. Unlike other techniques, this does require a surgical intervention. Short-term studies failed to show positive outcomes. However, a subsequent retrospective study noted the occurrence of a response in some patients after 6 months. Interest in VNS has been revived as newer long-term studies surface.

8.5 Deep Brain Stimulation

Deep brain stimulation, as the name implies, involves the placement of electrodes deep in the brain parenchyma. The technique has been used for approximately two decades in the treatment of neurological disorders such as Parkinson's disease. Currently, it is still an experimental treatment when it comes to the treatment of depression.

8.6 Magnetic Seizure Therapy

Magnetic seizure therapy combines the features of ECT and TMS. Like the former, it induces a seizure. Instead of using the direct application of current, it creates a seizure focus through powerful magnetic induction. Currently the treatment course is similar to that of ECT. It is still in trial phases, however.

There are several other neurostimulation methods undergoing trials. They have yet to be proven to be effective. Nonetheless, over the history of psychiatry, there has never been such an interest in neurostimulation as a treatment modality in psychiatry, and a new psychiatric subspecialty, *interventional psychiatry*, is currently in its dawn.

References

1. Fink M. The intimate relationship between catatonia and convulsive therapy. *J ECT*. 2010;26(4):243–245

2. Cerletti U. Old and new information about electroshock. *Am J Psychiatry*. 1950;(107):87–94.

3. Sackeim HA, Prudic J, Devanand DP, Nobler MS, Lisanby SH, Peyser S, et al. A prospective, randomized, double-blind comparison of bilateral and right unilateral electroconvulsive therapy at different stimulus intensities. *Arch Gen Psychiatry*. 2000;57(5):425–434.

4. Sackeim HA. Convulsant and anticonvulsant properties of electroconvulsive therapy: towards a focal form of brain stimulation. *Clin Neurosci Res*. 2004;4(1-2):39–57.

5. Perera TD, Dwork AJ, Keegan KA, Thirumangalakudi L, Lipira CM, Joyce N, et al. Necessity of hippocampal neurogenesis for the therapeutic action of antidepressants in adult nonhuman primates. *PLoS ONE*. 2011;6(4):e17600.

6. Nordanskog P, Dahlstrand U, Larsson MR, Larsson EM, Knutsson L, Johanson A. Increase in hippocampal volume after electroconvulsive therapy in patients with depression: a volumetric magnetic resonance imaging study. *J ECT*. 2010;26(1):62–67.

7. Dichter GS, Gibbs D, Smoski MJ. A systematic review of relations between resting-state functional-MRI and treatment response in major depressive disorder. *J Affect Disord*. 2015;172:8–17.

8. Soliday FK, Conley YP, Henker R. Pseudocholinesterase deficiency: a comprehensive review of genetic, acquired, and drug influences. *AANA J*. 2010;78(4):313–320.

9. Taylor S. Electroconvulsive therapy: a review of history, patient selection, technique, and medication management. *South Med J*. 2007;100(5):494–498.

10. Hartnett S, Rex S, Sienaert P. Asystole during electroconvulsive therapy: does electrode placement matter? A systematic review. *J ECT*. 2023;39(1):3–9.

11. Rasmussen P, Andersson JE, Koch P, Secher NH, Quistorff B. Glycopyrrolate prevents extreme bradycardia and cerebral deoxygenation during electroconvulsive therapy. *J ECT*. 2007;23(3):147–152.

12. Rasmussen K. A randomized controlled trial of ketorolac for prevention of headache related to electroconvulsive therapy. *Pain Stud Treatm*. 2013;1(2):5–8.

13. Yuksel E, Sergin D, Tanatti B, Alper I. Rocuronium-sugammadex use in electroconvulsive therapy of patients with pseudocholinesterase enzyme deficiency. *J Clin Anesth.* 2013;25(8):680–681.

14. Aksay SS, Bumb JM, Janke C, Hoyer C, Kranaster L, Sartorius A. New evidence for seizure quality improvement by hyperoxia and mild hypocapnia. *J ECT.* 2014;30(4):287–291.

15. Azuma H, Fujita A, Sato K, Arahata K, Otsuki K, Hori M, et al. Postictal suppression correlates with therapeutic efficacy for depression in bilateral sine and pulse wave electroconvulsive therapy. *Psychiatry Clin Neurosci.* 2007;61(2):168–173.

16. Vaidya PV, Anderson EL, Bobb A, Pulia K, Jayaram G, Reti I. A within-subject comparison of propofol and methohexital anesthesia for electroconvulsive therapy. *J ECT.* 2012;28(1):14–19.

17. Hausmann A, Post T, Post F, Dehning J, Kemmler G, Grunze H. Efficacy of continuation/maintenance electroconvulsive therapy in the treatment of patients with mood disorders: a retrospective analysis. *J ECT.* 2019;35(2):122–126.

18. Yen T, Khafaja M, Lam N, Crumbacher J, Schrader R, Rask J, et al. Post-electroconvulsive therapy recovery and reorientation time with methohexital and ketamine: a randomized, longitudinal, crossover design trial. *J ECT.* 2015;31(1):20–25.

19. Sackeim HA, Dillingham EM, Prudic J, Cooper T, McCall WV, Rosenquist P, et al. Effect of concomitant pharmacotherapy on electroconvulsive therapy outcomes: short-term efficacy and adverse effects. *Arch Gen Psychiatry.* 2009;66(7):729–737.

20. Sackeim HA, Haskett RF, Mulsant BH, Thase ME, Mann JJ, Pettinati HM, et al. Continuation pharmacotherapy in the prevention of relapse following electroconvulsive therapy: a randomized controlled trial. *JAMA.* 2001;285(10):1299–1307.

Ethico-legal Considerations in Psychiatry

Edward Poa

9.1 Overview: Basic Principles

Four ethical principles underly most of the ethical and legal issues that arise in psychiatry, as in all of medicine. They are autonomy, beneficence, nonmaleficence, and justice [1]. Many of the ethical considerations in psychiatry arise from the balance between two of these: the autonomy of the patient and the beneficence of the clinician.

The ethical principle of autonomy is the concept that individuals possess the right to self-determination, deciding what will happen to their bodies. Justice Benjamin Cardozo, who would later become a Supreme Court Justice, wrote in a legal opinion, "Every human being of adult years and sound mind has a right to determine what shall be done with his own body" [2]. Each individual is presumed to possess the ability to make their own medical decisions unless they are found to lack the capacity to do so. A unique consideration in psychiatry is that the patient's decisions, driven by their thoughts and emotions, may be affected by the symptoms of their mental illness.

Beneficence is the physician's obligation to work for the benefit of the patient. A physician has a fiduciary duty to their patient – to put the best interests of the patient above other interests, including the physician's financial or other interests in the course of treatment. Of course, the actual preferences of the patient may differ from their best interests.

Nonmaleficence is the principle of doing no harm. This is perhaps most easily illustrated by the American Medical Association's prohibition against physicians participating in executions and the American Psychiatric Association's prohibition against psychiatrists participating in torture [3, 4]. While these examples are straightforward, this principle needs to be balanced against others in situations where pain/hurt is caused to a patient but in the service of a greater benefit (e.g., surgery to excise a malignant tumor, medication side effects from an antibiotic). The weighing of the benefits and harms can be challenging when considering treatments with significant side effects or relatively lower chances of success.

Justice is the principle of fairness and equity for all individuals. This is the foundation of making emergency and basic medical care available for all as well as how to allocate limited medical resources such as organ transplants. It is also a factor in instances such as triage, when limited resources are focused on those individuals with the greatest likelihood of benefit or those who would suffer most from a delay of care.

Besides the above four ethical principles, there are two other concepts that often come into play in emergency psychiatry: *parens patriae* and police power [5]. *Parens patriae* is the concept that the government, as a "parent" of the people, has a responsibility to care for its vulnerable citizens who need protection. This underlying principle is used for hospitalizing an individual when they have a debilitating condition that could lead to grave harm if left untreated (e.g., an individual with florid psychotic symptoms with no concern for food, drink, or shelter from the elements). Such a hospitalization may occur against the individual's wishes if they are found to lack capacity to recognize their situation and the potential consequences of such. Police power is the concept that the state has a responsibility for preventing an individual from harming another. Police power arises as a factor when an individual is deemed to be an imminent threat to a third party, perhaps through an expressed intent of violence or murder. Some jurisdictions mandate or permit a clinician to break confidentiality in order to warn or protect the third party, while other jurisdictions do not permit it.

9.2 Confidentiality

The confidentiality and security of personal health information are crucial in all of medicine due to its private and sensitive nature. In psychiatry, confidentiality takes on even greater importance; the nature of the information disclosed to psychiatrists may include personal secrets, traumas, feelings about others, fears, and so on. The patient takes the risk to share this sensitive information in case it can be helpful in their treatment, and they do so because they have a reasonable expectation that it will be kept confidential.

In some cases, a psychiatrist may be evaluating an individual for an administrative or legal purpose (e.g., work evaluation, different types of competency evaluations), in which case there may not be confidentiality. It is critical that the psychiatrist fully discloses the evaluation's purpose and lack of confidentiality to the evaluee, and that the evaluee is able to give informed consent to proceed [6].

Due to the nature of the work, some unique nuances of confidentiality exist in psychiatry. Records pertaining to the diagnosis and treatment of substance use disorders enjoy an even greater level of protection than that already afforded to their personal health information in their medical records [7]. When authorizing the release of their medical records, patients can decide whether or not to release substance use disorder–related information as distinct from other records. This helps combat the stigma and repercussions of such information becoming public, and to encourage individuals to seek help for such disorders. An exception exists, however: A clinician may have to report to licensing boards if they are treating a health care provider in whom an ongoing substance use disorder or other psychiatric condition is jeopardizing the safety of patients.

Exceptions to confidentiality also exist for the patient's benefit, in that information can be released without express consent. These can include the release of protected health information to third-party payors for payment or to other clinicians for continuity of care. Other exceptions can also occur when an individual is incapacitated or in emergency circumstances [8].

Another exception to confidentiality can exist when a patient is deemed to be a threat to a third party. Different states vary widely in what may be required, permitted, or allowed in such a circumstance. Some states require a clinician to warn or protect a third party when their patient has expressed a credible threat against an identifiable person and possesses the ability to carry it out [9]. These are sometimes referred to as "Tarasoff" laws based on the original landmark case from California that established a duty to warn, and later to protect, third parties. State laws may stipulate if this is accomplished by directly warning the identifiable person or notifying law enforcement. Alternatively, the psychiatrist may also discharge the duty by hospitalizing the patient (as a means of preventing the patient access to the third party). Hospitalization is probably the most frequent response to such instances, as it allows for maintenance of safety, an opportunity to treat any condition that could be resulting in the violent intent, and perhaps avoidance of the need to break confidentiality. There may no longer be a need to warn the third person or law enforcement if the hospitalization and treatment result in the cessation of the violent intent.

Other states have "permissive" statutes that do not require but do allow a clinician to warn others in instances of threats to third parties. This can be further complicated when a state permits the breaking of confidentiality in these situations but does not explicitly grant immunity from a civil action or complaint for doing so. In those jurisdictions, the clinician will have to make a decision to break confidentiality and warn or to maintain confidentiality and not disclose. If breaking confidentiality, their patient could still bring action against them for breach of confidentiality (if the state has not expressly grant immunity for breaking confidentiality). If confidentiality is maintained, a potential injured third party could also sue the clinician. Still other states have no established duty or permission to disclose, thereby placing the clinician at risk if they choose to do so. It is therefore critical that psychiatrists know the laws in their state, as that should guide their actions in such situations.

Confidentiality may also be broken to prevent a patient from harming themselves. This might take the form of informing police so that they can perform a check on an outpatient who has given an indication of suicidal intent or providing information when petitioning the courts for involuntary hospitalization or treatment [10].

As for all physicians, psychiatrists are mandated reporters of suspected child abuse/neglect as well as vulnerable adult abuse/neglect/exploitation. Information that leads to this suspicion may arise in a psychiatric history whereas it may not in a routine medical history. The patient may be the possible victim or perpetrator of the possible abuse, neglect, or exploitation. A report can potentially create tensions or ruptures in the patient–physician relationship, as well as tensions in the relationship between the physician and their patient's caregivers (parents, adult children, siblings, etc.). While it is not entirely preventive of a therapeutic rupture, it can sometimes help to inform the affected individuals when a mandated report needs to be made, explaining that it must be done even if the clinician is not certain that abuse or neglect occurred [11]. This can at least avoid the additional anger that may occur if the affected individuals learn of the report later from other sources and come to believe that the clinician intentionally withheld the fact of the report from them.

9.3 Informed Consent and Decision-Making

Informed consent for treatment is critical in the process of caring for patients. Three critical components are necessary for an individual to give informed consent for care. The first is that the patient have available the necessary information about the current situation and options. The second is the capacity of the patient to give informed consent. The third is voluntariness [12].

To make a knowing, or intelligent, decision, a patient must have the necessary information about their medical situation and the options available, including the pertinent risks, benefits, and other consequences of each option. Two standards exist for what information needs to be provided to the patient [13]. The first is the "reasonable professional standard," which is the information that would be provided by a reasonable professional under the same or similar circumstances. The second is the more patient-centered "reasonable patient standard," which is the information a reasonable or average patient would need in a similar circumstance. A further extension of this patient-centered approach is also to provide any additional information that each particular patient would want to know in making a decision. For example, if a physician knows that their patient finds information about cardiac side effects to be highly important because they lost a parent to an arrhythmia, they will provide details about even very rare cardiac side effects of an intervention that they might not review with any other "reasonable patient."

Once information has been provided, the patient must then possess the capacity to utilize the information and give informed consent. The criteria for assessing their ability to do so, elucidated by Appelbaum and Grisso, consists of four abilities: (1) an understanding of the situation and relevant information, (2) an appreciation of the situation and its consequences, (3) a rational decision-making process, and (4) communication of a choice [14].

The first two criteria flow directly from their ability to understand the information that has been provided by their clinicians (based on the reasonable professional or reasonable patient standard). The degree that an individual needs to understand the information may vary based on the benefit-to-risk ratio of the proposed intervention. A procedure with a high amount of benefit to possible risk (such as a simple blood draw for routine laboratories) usually does not require an extensive explanation or a highly sophisticated understanding of the process by the patient. Conversely, an intervention with a low ratio of benefit to possible risk (such as a research study from which the patient will not directly benefit, or an experimental chemotherapy drug with significant side effects) requires greater explanation and a higher degree of understanding from the patient.

The third criterion is the patient's ability to use a rational decision-making process in their decision. This does not require flawless logic or judgment but instead allows for the wide variability of personal preferences, feelings, opinions, experience, and thoughts that individuals may bring to their health care decisions. Patients may have personal preferences and experiences that cause them to weigh options very differently than a physician might, but these do not make their decision-making process irrational. A rational decision-making process does not require the patient to use a decision-making process similar to the one the clinician would have used. Delusional or frankly illogical rationale, perhaps resulting from a condition such as psychosis or a neurocognitive disorder, is usually the threshold at which an individual is found to lack the capacity to give informed consent.

The final criteria of communication of the choice includes the consistent and reliable ability of the individual to express their decision. The classic example used to illustrate this last element would be a patient with locked-in syndrome; they can understand and reason logically but are unable to communicate their decision and therefore would lack the capacity to give informed consent.

An underlying factor to all these components is memory; one must possess adequate memory to be able retain the information about the situation, options, and consequences, to then use that information in forming a decision, and then communicate it consistently. An individual who is unable to remember information reliably may use rational processes in coming to a decision but utilize different information each time due to memory loss. They might provide a different decision each time they are asked to give informed consent. Such an individual would lack the capacity to give informed consent, and whatever decisions they gave could not be relied upon by the treating clinicians.

Finally, voluntariness is the ability to make a free choice without being subjected to coercion. Examples of coercion or lack of voluntariness include the recruitment of prisoners for research studies or overwhelming financial compensation for tissue or organ donation. It also means that the clinician providing the explanation of the proposed intervention may provide their opinion and recommendations, but they should refrain from attempting to sway decisions with personal appeals or threats of consequences if the "wrong" decision is made.

When an individual lacks the capacity to give informed consent, decisions need to be made by a surrogate decision-maker. Depending on the jurisdiction and circumstance, the surrogate decision-maker may be a family member, medical staff, or an administrative/judicial process. Also, they may use different approaches to making such decisions, based on the local laws. This can include using the substituted judgment standard (what the individual would have wanted if they possessed capacity, based on their expressed preferences) or the best interests standard (which option would likely lead to the greatest benefit when weighed against risks) [15].

The balance of individual autonomy and clinician beneficence plays out most dramatically when a patient is experiencing a psychiatric emergency resulting in imminent danger (suicidality, homicidality, florid psychosis) and lacks capacity to give informed consent for hospitalization or treatment. At this point, the scale favors beneficence over patient autonomy, resulting in an involuntary admission to the hospital in order to protect the patient.

There can be a distinction between involuntary hospitalization (which usually provides safety in that it prevents physical harm to the patient but may not actually treat the precipitating condition) and involuntary treatment (which can be more invasive whether in the form of medications or therapy but is much more likely to improve the clinical status of the patient). Individuals who are involuntarily hospitalized (as well as voluntarily hospitalized) have a right to treatment so that they have the means to improve so that they can be released from the hospital [16]. Similarly, individuals who are involuntarily hospitalized may also have the right the refuse treatment. Depending on the jurisdiction, the process for involuntarily treating a patient may be a separate process than the one for involuntarily hospitalizing the patient.

Informed consent is one of the areas where psychiatry and the rest of medicine have some divergence. When an individual lacking capacity is treated in an emergency setting, both medicine and psychiatry have mechanisms for providing life-saving treatment. For emergency psychiatric conditions, involuntary hospitalization occurs as described above. For medical or surgical conditions, the life-saving procedure is initiated based on the assumption that the patient would have consented if they were able to.

In a non-emergency medical setting, individuals lacking capacity to give informed consent can have a surrogate decision-maker assigned to assist in making decisions (if one hasn't been designated by the patient previously). The surrogate decision-maker is assigned based on the local laws, and it is often a relatively fast and smooth process (and may occur in the context of the clinical interaction). However, in the non-emergency psychiatric setting, there is often no clear or efficient process of assigning a surrogate decision-maker. Some jurisdictions allow for the individual themselves to name a legally authorized representative or to assign someone from a rank order list of usual interested parties (e.g., partners, parents, siblings, children). In many other states the only available routes might be a designated medical power of attorney or guardianship.

When an individual may have a condition that does not necessarily cause them to require emergency treatment, but instead prevents them from making decisions in their own interest, the balance between autonomy and beneficence again arises. Here, the local government will step in via a guardianship or similar process, by which another person is appointed to make decisions for the individual in their own best interests. This may apply to all decisions or only to personal (such as housing and marriage) or financial decisions.

The different approach between the two situations can be traced to abuses of the psychiatric field and patients. Individuals have been abused or exploited by their family members using psychiatric hospitalization and removal of decision-making power. Political dissidents have been labeled mentally ill and forcibly medicated to both invalidate their concerns and silence them. The First Amendment guarantee of freedom of speech has been interpreted as freedom of thought, as one cannot generate free speech without free thought. As such, society is cautious about imposing psychiatric treatment on an individual unless safety is involved, in order to avoid the slippery slope of treatment for nonconformist or unpopular beliefs.

Informed consent may not be required in certain situations. Besides emergency treatment, therapeutic waiver and therapeutic privilege are two other exceptions [17]. Therapeutic waiver is when a patient waives their right to informed consent and instead defers to the judgment of another individual, sometimes the physician. Therapeutic privilege is when the physician deems that the consent process (usually due to the information provided) would harm the patient or worsen their clinical situation. This is a very rarely used exception and should be approached cautiously and with consultation.

9.4 Dual Relationships

Psychiatrists, like all physicians, have a fiduciary duty to their patients in that they must put the interests of their patient above other interests in the clinical relationship. This reflects the profound power differential between patients and physicians as well as the trust that people need to be able to place in their health care providers. In the case of psychiatrists, this is especially true because the patient often discloses highly personal information that can make them vulnerable to anyone who has access to it. For this reason, dual relationships (where the patient and psychiatrist have another relationship in addition to the clinical relationship) are either highly discouraged or forbidden [18].

Some jurisdictions explicitly forbid sexual relationships between mental health clinicians and their patients or former patients, with serious penalties (including loss of license) as a consequence. Many of these jurisdictions also mandate that health care providers make a report if they have knowledge of a sexual relationship between a mental health clinician and a patient.

Nonsexual relationships such as business relationships or friendships are also highly discouraged. The one-sided power differential and intimate knowledge the psychiatrist may possess about their patient increase the risk of manipulation or coercion. A patient may also feel unable to disagree or break off the nontreatment relationship for fear of losing an essential treatment relationship. The patient may also have difficulty understanding that their psychiatrist's obligation to act in their best interests only applies in their clinical relationship and not in their other interactions.

References

1. B. Varkey. Principles of clinical ethics and their application to practice. *Med Princ Pract.* 2021;30:17–28.

2. Schoendorff v. Society of New York Hosp (1914) 105 N.E. 92, 93.

3. American Medical Association. AMA principles of medical ethics. 2001. https:// code-medical-ethics.ama-assn.org/ principles/ (accessed February 2, 2023).

4. American Psychiatric Association. The principles of medical ethics with annotations especially applicable to psychiatry. 2013. https://www.psychiatry .org/File%20Library/Psychiatrists/ Practice/Ethics/principles-medical-ethics .pdf (accessed January 30, 2023).

5. B. Hamm. Ethical practice in emergency psychiatry: common dilemmas and virtue-informed navigation. *Psychiatr Clin N Am.* 2021;44:627–640.

6. American Psychiatric Association. The principles of medical ethics with annotations especially applicable to psychiatry. 2013. https://www.psychiatry .org/File%20Library/Psychiatrists/ Practice/Ethics/principles-medical-ethics .pdf (accessed January 30, 2023).

7. M. H. Gendel. Forensic and medical legal issues in addiction psychiatry. *Psychiatr Clin N Am.* 2004;27(4):611–626.

8. J. H. Khan. Confidentiality and capacity. *Emerg Med Clin North Am.* 2020;38 (2):283–296.

9. J. L. Knoll. The psychiatrist's duty to protect. *CNS Spectr.* 2015;20(3):215–222.

10. American Psychiatric Association. The principles of medical ethics with annotations especially applicable to psychiatry. 2013. https://www.psychiatry .org/File%20Library/Psychiatrists/ Practice/Ethics/principles-medical-ethics .pdf (accessed January 30, 2023).

11. J. H. Khan. Confidentiality and capacity. *Emerg Med Clin North Am.* 2020;38 (2):283–296.

12. R. R. Tampi, J. Young, S. Balachandran, et al. Ethical, legal and forensic issues in geriatric psychiatry. *Curr Psychiatry Rep.* 2018;20(1):1.

13. R. W. Brendel and R. Schouten. Legal concerns in psychosomatic medicine. *Psychiatr Clin N Am.* 2007;30(4):663–676.

14. P. S. Appelbaum and T. Grisso. Assessing patients' capacities to consent to treatment. *N Engl J Med.* 1988;319 (25):1635–1638.

15. J. G. Wong, I. C. H. Clare, M. J. Gunn and A. J. Holland. Capacity to make healthcare decisions: its importance in clinical practice. *Psychol Med.* 1999;29 (2):437–446.

16. B. Ostermeyer, A. M. Shoaib and S. Deshpande. Legal and ethical challenges, part 1: general population. *Psychiatr Clin N Am.* 2017;40:541–553.

17. R. W. Brendel and R. Schouten. Legal concerns in psychosomatic medicine. *Psychiatr Clin N Am.* 2007;30 (4):663–676.

18. American Psychiatric Association. The principles of medical ethics with annotations especially applicable to psychiatry. 2013. https://www.psychiatry .org/File%20Library/Psychiatrists/ Practice/Ethics/principles-medical-ethics .pdf (accessed January 30, 2023).

Transcultural Aspects of Mental Health Care

Syed Shahzeb Ayaz and Ali Abbas Asghar-Ali

10.1 Culture

Culture is the distinctive customs, values, norms, beliefs, knowledge, art, and language of a society or community [1]. The richness of culture promotes a sense of collective belongingness, which influences the way individuals may express themselves, communicate with others, and hold expectations.

Culture may also be defined as "All the learned behaviors, beliefs, norms, and values held by a group of people and passed down from one generation to the other as a mechanism of preserving the group" [2]. It is imperative to acknowledge that culture is not a static construct but rather necessitates adaptation as communities evolve.

Historical context can help us better understand the ever-evolving nature of culture. The suffrage movement expanded voting rights for women in the United States. This represented a substantial change in US culture, leading to a shift in the involvement of women in governance in ways that were not part of the culture previously. Similarly, first-generation immigrant Americans demonstrate the dilemma of conforming to perceived static cultural values. It is not uncommon for members in this generation to experience pressures on their cultural identity as they try to maintain traditions and customs from their country of origin while also acclimating to the new environment and culture.

The United States is becoming more diverse than ever before [3]. As one of the most populous countries in the world, it is necessary for the United States to dedicate attention and resources to understand and address the needs of the intersecting cultural identities of the individuals in the country.

Culture influences how individuals interpret and respond to their symptoms and illness [4]. The scientific literature confirms that illness and distress are shaped by cultural contexts [5]. This chapter focuses on the relationship between culture and psychiatry and ways in which clinicians can implement culturally informed approaches to tailor their treatment planning. Additionally, facilitators and barriers to implementation of culturally informed care in the clinical setting will be addressed.

10.2 Transcultural Psychiatry

The term *transcultural psychiatry* was first used by Dr. Eric D. Wittkower to focus his studies that "go beyond the boundaries of any culture and, indeed, focus on differences observed in many cultures" [7]. Wittkower established the first university transcultural psychiatry unit at McGill University and thereafter established the newsletter, *Transcultural Research in Mental Health Problems*, which in 1997 was renamed *Transcultural Psychiatry* [6].

The field of cultural psychiatry emerged to address three main concerns: questions about how psychopathology and healing practices could be understood from a universal or relative perspective; how best to provide psychiatric care to diverse populations; and appreciation of psychiatric theoretical underpinnings and practice perspectives as outcomes of specific cultural events and their relationship to globalization [7]. Early studies of psychiatric conditions assumed that Western psychiatric diagnoses could be applied globally. However, this was not reflective of regions outside North America and Western Europe. In fact, 90% of *the Diagnostic and Statistical Manual (DSM)*, Fourth Edition categories were culturally bound to Euro-American societies; yet the label "culture-bound syndrome" was to be used for other, "exotic" regions [8]. Eventually, advances in medical anthropology replaced culture-bound syndrome with cultural syndromes, cultural idioms of distress, causal explanations, and folk diagnostic categories.

As described by the World Psychiatric Association Transcultural Psychiatry Section, transcultural psychiatry hopes to achieve five main objectives [9]:

- Exploration of the similarities and differences in the manifestations of mental illness in different cultures;
- Identification of cultural factors that predispose people to mental illness and promote mental health;
- Assessment of the effect of identified cultural factors on the frequency and nature of mental illness;
- Study of the form of treatment practiced or preferred in different cultural settings;
- Comparison of different attitudes toward the mentally ill in different cultures.

As noted above, the term *culture-bound syndrome* had limitations, which were addressed in the *DSM–5 Text Revision (DSM-5-TR)* [10] with the use of the broader term, *cultural concepts of distress*. This new term encompasses the different ways that individuals may represent their experiences and their understanding of emotional distress and behavioral problems. Furthermore, the *DSM-5-TR* describes three components within cultural concepts of distress. The first, cultural idioms of distress, refers to the ways in which individuals express feelings and emotions across cultures. They may be phrased as metaphors, sayings, or idioms that reflect cultural values but cannot be linked to a syndrome or a disorder. For example, "feeling blue" reflects emotions of sadness or depression but is insufficient to meet the criteria for major depressive disorder. The second component is cultural explanations. These are labels and attributions about how individuals experience their symptoms and how they expect to respond to treatment. For instance, some cultural perspectives may lead a person to be more likely to address depression as a clinical illness warranting treatment, while other cultural perspectives may view depression as a personal failing. Cultural perspectives often lead to definitions of "normal" and "abnormal" mood. The third component of cultural concepts of distress is cultural syndromes. These are described as a set of symptoms and attributions that co-occur among individuals of cultural groups that are associated with distress or dysfunction. Thus, within the cultural group, the symptoms of distress are recognized as consistent or familiar experiences.

Cultural concepts of distress stem from folk or professional diagnostic systems for mental and emotional distress, and they also reflect the influence of biomedical concepts. They have four key features in relation to the *DSM-5 TR*:

- Cultural concepts of distress and *DSM* diagnostic categories do not necessarily correlate on a one-to-one basis – that is, there is not a specific cultural concept of distress that leads to a specific illness, and vice versa.
- Cultural concepts of distress may be useful when considering symptomatology that may not meet criteria of a mental disorder and apply to a broad range of symptom and functional severity.
- In common parlance, a single cultural term may often represent more than one type of cultural concept of distress.
- Cultural concepts of distress may change over time in response to changes in the local and global environment.

An understanding of cultural concepts of distress enhances identification of an individual's concerns; avoids misdiagnosis; obtains accurate clinical information; guides clinical research; clarifies cultural epidemiology; and improves clinical rapport, engagement, and therapeutic efficacy.

10.3 Practicing Transcultural Psychiatry

Several tools have been developed to assist clinicians in incorporating the objectives of transcultural psychiatry in their practice. This section highlights a few such tools and provides guidance on how they may be used in clinical care.

10.3.1 Cultural Formulation Interview

The first transcultural psychiatry tool is the cultural formulation interview (CFI), which is featured in the *DSM-5 TR*. It is a semistructured interview that enables exploration of the cultural context of the experiences of an individual with mental health concerns. The CFI provides a person-centered approach to assess how individuals, as well as their social network, conceptualize, experience, and respond to their illness.

The core CFI is composed of 16 questions, which also have been reformulated for use with an informant. Additionally, there are 12 supplementary modules that augment the CFI.

The core CFI (16 questions) is divided into four domains. The first, **cultural definition of the problem**, aims to understand how individuals view and understand their distress, how they frame their distress for others in their social network, and how they prioritize their concerns. The second, **cultural perceptions of cause, context, and support**, helps determine what individuals identify as the cause of their distress, how others in their social network view the cause for their distress, what support is available to them, and how their social environment and cultural identity affect them. The third, **cultural factors affecting self-coping and past help-seeking**, focuses on how individuals cope with their distress, the sources of help they may have sought, and their usefulness and barriers experienced while seeking help. The final domain, **cultural factors affecting current help-seeking**, explores what individuals perceive as potential sources of help that they deem to be appropriate or that members of their social network have suggested and identifies individuals' concerns about the clinician–patient relationship.

The CFI Informant Version reframes the core CFI so that the clinician can address the same areas covered in the core CFI with a member of an individual's support network, such as a friend or family member who has knowledge of the individual's circumstances and cultural values. The Informant Version may be used to augment information gathered from the individual or serve as the primary interview in circumstances in which the individual is unable to participate in the interview.

Among the 12 supplementary modules, 8 are designed to explore the domains of the core CFI in greater depth. Three modules focus on the specific needs of children and adolescents, older adults, and immigrants and refugees. Lastly, one module is designed specifically to ascertain the perspectives and experiences of a caregiver.

Three other noteworthy cultural assessment tools include the Culture, Respect, Assess/Affirm, Sensitivity, Self-Awareness (CRASH), the HUMBLE (Humble in the assumptions one makes; Understanding one's own background and culture; Motivating oneself in further learning about the individual's cultural background; Beginning to incorporate the attained knowledge into practice; Life-Long Learning; and Emphasizing respect in one's interactions) and the LEARN (Listen; Explain; Acknowledge; Recommend; Negotiate). These tools are best applied with cultural humility in mind. Cultural humility is a process of committing to an ongoing relationship with patients, communities, and colleagues that requires humility as individuals continually engage in reflective practices and self-critique [11].

10.3.2 Crash

CRASH provides key components for clinicians to consider in their approach to clinical interactions. As its first step, clinicians are reminded to "consider culture" in the care of an individual. It is important to remember that the degree of affiliation that an individual may have with a specific aspect of their cultural identity is influenced by intersecting aspects of their identity, such as their age, gender, sexual orientation, and degree of acculturation.

Clinical Vignette: A pregnant woman who identifies as a practicing Muslim requested a female obstetrician at her first appointment. Since then, she has been cared for by a female obstetrician. On the day of her scheduled delivery, a male obstetrician introduced himself as the physician for the day. When the patient and her husband expressed concern, the treatment team noted that they were not aware of a gender preference, and that "there is nothing that we can do about it now." This led to distress and an uncomfortable experience for the patient.

Evaluation: In this case, the health care team failed to acknowledge a previously expressed need by the patient; they did not assess the significance of the patient's request and did not offer options for how culturally consistent care could have been provided. Given the Islamic ethics concerning cross-gender interaction and emphasis on modesty, a practicing Muslim woman may be uncomfortable being examined by a male physician [12].

The second component of the CRASH model emphasizes the need for clinicians to "show respect" in their clinical interaction. As the authors explain, "understanding that demonstrations of respect are more important than gestures of affection or shallow intimacy and finding ways to learn how to demonstrate respect in various cultural contexts" [13]. Examples of how to express respect include the following:

- "I want to make sure I treat you respectfully. How are you accustomed to being greeted by a physician in the community in which you grew up?"
- "What can I do to make you feel respected in this office?"
- "Are there things that we do that make you feel disrespected?"

It is important for clinicians to draw from their personal experience with different cultures, genders, occupations, generations, and so forth to employ the most "respectful" approach. It is advisable to begin conversations using formal salutations and the last name of the patient. Thereafter, assessing for the preferred name and pronouns can help place the patient at ease and represent a respectful approach.

The third component of CRASH is "Assess," which asserts the importance of collecting a person's cultural history along with the medical and family history. Some questions for this assessment include:

- "Please tell me about your family background."
- "Could you share a little about your family's heritage?"
- "Are there cultural issues that are important to consider in our work together?"

The goal for assessment is to avoid cultural assumptions and assess individual identities, health preferences, beliefs, understanding of health conditions, language proficiency, acculturation level, and health literacy.

The next component of the CRASH model is to "Affirm" the differences between the clinician and the patient. It recognizes the possibility of bias in relation to cultural beliefs, values, and behaviors. As a result of unfamiliarity, clinicians may be more inclined to make assumptions. However, it is necessary for clinicians to set aside their beliefs and grant the patient the role of an expert in their experience.

The next component of CRASH is "Self-Awareness," which urges clinicians to develop an awareness of their own cultural values and assumptions. Importantly, self-awareness requires that clinicians develop a better understanding of themselves and perform ongoing exploration of patterns of behaviors that may be unconsciously mediated. Examination of these behaviors, their impact on equitable care, and corrective action are necessary in practicing self-awareness.

The fifth component in CRASH is "Show Sensitivity." Clinicians are well served by developing empathy, which allows them to be more sensitive to patients' point of view and anticipate their needs.

The last element of CRASH is "Humility," which encourages clinicians to approach clinical interactions from a position of humility. While clinicians may be asked to expand their cultural knowledge and self-awareness, it is expected that they cannot be "experts" in every person's culture. This acceptance of being a "novice" in the patient's cultural experience and identity is a form of humility. Additionally, it is necessary for clinicians to commit to a lifetime of reflection and self-critique while learning from their patients' lived experiences.

10.3.3 HUMBLE

Humility is central in the HUMBLE model of cultural humility, designed to inform and guide clinicians and their organizations in practicing cultural humility.

Illustration: A 72-year-old male veteran attended his primary care appointment at his local community clinic. Although the clinician specializes in working with individuals in the veteran's age range, he has not previously worked with veterans. During the clinical interaction, the clinician sought to learn more about the individual's experience as a veteran and how it differed from nonveteran experiences. He made sure to demonstrate respect through words, affirmations, and behavior and was successful in building rapport with the patient. Following the appointment, the clinician jotted down apparent themes in the veteran's narrative and found it important to educate himself on health care needs and disparities among male veterans to allow better care of the individual and other veterans in his practice.

The HUMBLE model emphasizes the importance of acknowledging personal biases and replacing them with receptivity toward the personal journey of individuals. Through this, clinicians can foster a relationship of trust and respect with their patient. In practicing humility, clinicians and their teams can promote an inclusive environment with mutual understanding and effective communication.

10.3.4 LEARN

The LEARN model of cultural communication is another framework to assist clinicians and their team in addressing cross-cultural interactions with patients. The first step, Listen, requires clinicians to actively listen to the patient's concerns and perspectives while ensuring they are empathic, and to avoid indulging in their assumptions and judgments. The second step, Explain, involves providing clear explanations of medical concepts and procedures in a manner that is understandable by the patient. Acknowledge requires recognizing and respecting cultural differences that may influence the patient and clinician's relationship and inform value-driven care. The fourth step, Recommend, involves making recommendations for treatment that take the patient's cultural background and preferences into consideration. Lastly, Negotiate involves working collaboratively with the patient in developing a plan that is considerate, accommodating, and feasible in light of cultural values and preferences.

Illustration: A mental health clinician is caring for a 53-year-old woman who has recently moved to the United States from a West African country to live with her son after her husband's death. Her son made the appointment and brought her to the clinic because of his concerns that his mother was exhibiting depressive symptoms. He was also worried that she may have been struggling to adjust to the new environment and family structure. She has been hesitant to seek treatment due to cultural beliefs about mental health. The clinician thoroughly listens to the patient's concerns and experiences both from herself and, with her permission, from her son. The clinician pays special attention to the cultural understanding and the patient and son's expectations. They take time to explain that symptoms of depression can impact the day-to-day life of individuals, which can create additional challenges when adjusting to a new life. The clinician appreciates that it is necessary to understand the cultural perspectives to accurately develop a formulation. While doing so, the clinician acknowledges the patient's cultural beliefs regarding mental health and how they may be influencing her decision in seeking treatment while destigmatizing mental health treatment and underscoring its importance in overall well-being. The clinician makes treatment recommendations while keeping the multiple dimensions in mind. Finally, with the patient's and son's input and understanding, they develop a treatment plan that is acceptable, consistent with cultural practices, and feasible to implement.

As illustrated in this example, the LEARN model allows clinicians and their teams to improve communication with patients from diverse cultural backgrounds, build rapport and trust, and establish more effective and person-centered care.

10.4 Implementation Barriers

There is a growing call for transcultural care in the provision of mental health care [14]. Nonetheless, clinicians may face barriers that prevent them from widely implementing transcultural psychiatry. One such barrier is language. Approximately 47% of immigrants in the United States are not proficient in English [15]. Unsurprisingly, language barriers can lead to miscommunication between clinicians and their patients. Language barriers can reduce both clinician and patient satisfaction with the interaction while also decreasing patient safety and the overall quality of care delivered. While interpreter services are critical in such circumstances, they add cost to care and increase the length of treatment encounters [16]. Additionally, even in the presence of an interpreter, the depth and rapport of the conversation can get lost in the interpretation process, resulting in diminishing effects on quality of care and patient satisfaction [17]. Thus, while a transcultural approach is critical to incorporating culture in the understanding of a person, language barriers may provide additional challenges to the therapeutic alliance.

Cultural humility in the practice of transcultural psychiatry requires not only acceptance of the perspective but also training. Unfortunately, trainings related to cultural psychiatry are not widely available or implemented, which is a barrier to the adoption of the desired practices [18, 19]. As established previously, culture is an evolving phenomenon through the exposure to institutions, mainstream media, and technology. It is, however, worthwhile to consider a cautionary note when devising a training to address transcultural interactions. Trainings may embed stereotypical representations of clinicians and patients that may reinforce stereotyping and amplify the "us" versus "them" dynamic. This could lead to implicit discrimination by clinicians toward individuals whom they serve.

Another barrier to applying cultural humility in clinical practice is time constraints. To understand the diverse cultural backgrounds and health care needs of their patients, clinicians need to first dedicate time to learning the concepts and practices. Attitudinal changes are also needed. Often, clinical sessions are not structured to allow a thorough discussion of culturally relevant information, which may lead clinicians to rely on assumptions or on superficial understanding of the information and circumstances [20, 21]. To minimize the risk of defaulting to heuristics, clinicians need to be deliberate in how they choose to incorporate transcultural practices. We recommend that clinicians familiarize themselves with the different models described in this chapter to adopt processes and approaches that work best for their setting. With time constraints, it is also important to consider how the entire clinical team can contribute to working from a culturally informed position. This may require training of nonclinical staff and education of patients. For example, patients can be invited to consider, even before their visit, personal values and cultural factors that they may want to address at their visit.

10.5 Conclusion

Transcultural psychiatry was conceptualized more than 50 years ago and emphasizes the appreciation of culture in the delivery of health care. Clinicians have several tools to implement to improve their provision of culturally responsive care with humility.

References

1. *APA Dictionary of Psychology.* American Psychological Association, 2023. Available at https://dictionary.apa.org/. Last accessed April 7, 2023.

2. P. A. Hays. Addressing the complexities of culture and gender in counseling. *J Couns Dev.* 1996;74(4):332–338.

3. J. B. Wright, D. Wolfe, P.Krishnakumar, C., et al. Census release shows America is

more diverse and more multiracial than ever. CNN Politics [Internet]. CNN. 2021. Available from: https://www.cnn.com/2021/08/12/politics/us-census-2020-data/index.html. Last accessed April 11, 2023.

4. R. Lewis-Fernández, ed. *DSM-5 Handbook on the Cultural Formulation Interview*. American Psychiatric Publications; 2016.

5. R. D. Alarcón, C. C. Bell, L. J. Kirmayer LJ, et al. Beyond the funhouse mirrors: research agenda on culture and psychiatric diagnosis. In *A Research Agenda for DSM-V*. American Psychiatric Association; 2002:219–281.

6. E. Delille. Eric Wittkower, and the foundation of Montréal's Transcultural Psychiatry Research Unit after World War II. *Hist Psychiatry*. 2018;29(3):282–296.

7. K. Bhui, D. Bhhugra. *Textbook of Cultural Psychiatry* (2nd ed.). Cambridge University Press; 2018.

8. A. Kleinman. Triumph or pyrrhic victory? The inclusion of culture in *DSM-IV*. *Harv Rev Psychiatry*. 1997;4(6):343–344.

9. Transcultural Psychiatry. World Psychiatric Association – Transcultural Psychiatry Section. https://www.wpa-tps.org/about-wpa-tps/transcultural-psychiatry/. Accessed April 6, 2023.

10. American Psychiatric Association. *Diagnostic and Statistical Manual of Mental disorders* (5th ed., text rev.). 2022. https://doi.org/10.1176/appi.books.9780890425787.

11. K. A. Yeager, S. Bauer-Wu. Cultural humility: essential foundation for clinical researchers. *Appl Nurs Res*. 2013;26(4):251–256.

12. A. I. Padela, P. R. del Pozo. Muslim patients and cross-gender interactions in medicine: an Islamic bioethical perspective *J Med Ethics*. 2011;37:40–44.

13. G. Rust, K. Kondwani, R. Martinez, et al. A crash-course in cultural competence. *Ethn Dis*. 2006;16(2 Suppl 3):S29–S36.

14. L. Wylie, R. Van Meyel, H. Harder, et al. Assessing trauma in a transcultural context: challenges in mental health care with immigrants and refugees. *Public Health Rev*. 2018;39(1):22.

15. A. Budiman. *Key findings about U.S. immigrants*. Pew Research Center, August 20, 2020. https://www.pewresearch.org/fact-tank/2020/08/20/key-findings-about-u-s-immigrants. Accessed April 9, 2023.

16. H. Al Shamsi, A. G. Almutairi, S. Al Mashrafi, T. Al Kalbani. Implications of language barriers for healthcare: a systematic review. *Oman Medl J*. 2020;35(2):e122.

17. P. K. Goenka. Lost in translation: impact of language barriers on children's healthcare. *Currt Opin Pediatr*. 2016;28(5):659–666.

18. H.-M. Lekas, K. Pahl, C. Fuller Lewis. Rethinking cultural competence: shifting to cultural humility. *Health Serv Insights*. 2020; 13:1178632920970580.

19. R. A. Taylor, M. V. Alfred. Nurses' perceptions of the organizational supports needed for the delivery of culturally competent care. *West J Nurs Res*. 2010;32(5):591–609.

20. S. Boi. Nurses' experiences in caring for patients from different cultural backgrounds. *NT Research*. 2000;5(5):382–389.

21. S. R. Kirkham. Nurses' descriptions of caring for culturally diverse clients. *Clin Nurs Res*. 1998;7(2):125–146.

Chapter 11

Child and Adolescent Psychiatry

Cristian Patrick Zeni and Priscilla Granja Machado

11.1 Introduction

Child and adolescent psychiatry (CAP) is a complex and challenging subspecialty in psychiatry. The different dynamic issues displayed by patients and their families, the impact of patient's different developmental levels and their cultural backgrounds, the often challenging ethical issues faced, and the prominent impact of environmental factors on patient's mental health are among the characteristics that make it fascinating.

Following the organization of pediatrics as a separate health care discipline at the beginning of the 19th century, child and adolescent mental health care mostly developed at the beginning of the 20th century, with very few reports of mental illness in youth before 1900 [1]. Behavioral and emotional disorders were considered nonexistent in children because they were thought to be not mature enough to develop those conditions. CAP grew along, and never fully separated from, its partner fields of pediatrics, neurology, education, and psychology. Concomitant to advances in medicine, the study of biological factors (genetics, neuroimaging) has flourished in the late 20th and early 21st centuries, where a significant amount of research has provided a better understanding of brain functioning and development, evidence-based therapies (biological and psychosocial), and the integration of the different factors involved in the pathophysiology of mental disorders.

In this chapter, we will present a brief overview of development, and specific aspects of the assessment, diagnosis, and treatment, of children and adolescents.

11.2 Development

Childhood is where the most intense development takes place [2]. There are many ways to classify it, and the main convention is to divide childhood into infancy, preschool years, middle childhood years, and adolescence.

The study of development is usually divided in physical, social, cognitive, communication, and emotional development, and the average milestones have been extensively studied. A comprehensive milestone checklist can be found on the CDC website (www .cdc.gov/ncbddd/actearly/milestones/index.html), and an application for monitoring development is available at www.cdc.gov/ncbddd/actearly/milestones-app.html [3].

We encourage the reader to review the existing developmental theories (Freud's psychosexual, Erikson's psychosocial, Skinner behavioral, Piaget's cognitive, Bowlby's attachment, Bandura's social learning, and Vygotsky's sociocultural). It is a common understanding that children are not "small adults," and that different stimuli will have more or less impact depending on the timing of those stimuli, due to developmental variations. In addition, advances in neurobiological studies (neuroimaging, pre-birth) of the last few decades have shed light on new areas of research. The complexity revealed by the current findings allows a better understanding of the numerous possibilities of variation in human emotional and behavioral development, and the deviations we call mental disorders.

11.3 Assessment

The only currently available tool for the assessment of infant, children, and adolescents is the clinical interview [4, 5]. There are no specific biological markers (blood, imaging, tests) to establish a psychiatric diagnosis. Some instruments, questionnaires, neuro-psychological assessments, and labs can help exclude, or confirm the clinical hypothesis.

Every step of the assessment should be conveyed to the patient and guardians. It is important to clarify expectations, state limits of confidentiality, obtain consent/assent to contact third parties, and review guardianship paperwork.

Some parts are uniquely used in this population, such as school reports and information from other family members. These sources of information can provide valuable insight about how the environment influences behaviors. Also, disruptive or externalizing symptoms (hyperactivity, aggression) are usually better reported by observers, such as caregivers or teachers. On the other hand, the child is usually the best source of information for internalizing symptoms, such as sadness or nervousness. Some diagnoses require the behavior to be observed in multiple settings in order not to attribute to a mental disorder what can be a relational problem.

Behaviors should be evaluated considering what is in a developmentally appropriate range (normal) for specific ages. Attention span, for example, should increase from childhood to adolescence.

The psychiatrist should respect cultural beliefs and traditions of each family and consider that family origin or immigration status may contribute to patient presentation. In some cultures, depression may be seen as weakness or a curse, and expressing emotions may be poorly tolerated in others.

It is important to promote a moment (usually without the guardians) when the patient can safely talk about substance use and physical/emotional/sexual abuse. Patients will be understandably very guarded to talk about these issues in the presence of others. Depending on the findings, local authorities may need to be contacted. Please make sure to be educated in the local legal practices regarding communication of risk and protection of children and adolescents rights.

11.3.1 Specific Aspects of Clinical Interview

- **Children** – parents/caregivers should be seen without the child in a first moment. This allows parents to express their concerns, share their feelings, evaluate family dynamics, and start a collaboration with the psychiatrist. The psychiatrist can also educate the parents on how to approach the child about the interview, in a language that they can understand (e.g., to a "feelings doctor"), and explain that they are safe to say anything that they think or feel in confidence.
- **Adolescents** – due to the increasing autonomy and resistance in this age range, the adolescent should be seen without the parents initially. The principles of privacy and

confidentiality must be discussed at the beginning of the interview, especially when approaching topics such as trauma and drug use.
- **Infants** – infants should always be seen with the caregivers, and particular interest and attention are dedicated to the dyadic/triadic interactions.

Children of different ages require different interview approaches. Infants will always be observed with the caregiver in various situations, such as playing, feeding, and so on. The psychiatrist will often play or draw with preschool children. Not all children and adolescents will be able to talk directly/openly about symptoms/feelings. The sole use of verbal language should be expected as patients reach adolescence.

11.3.2 Content of the Interview

The content mostly will not differ from that utilized while interviewing adults but will be adapted to the patient's level of communication. As a summary, the patient and caregiver should be inquired about the present complaint from their perspective; the thorough history of the complaint; a review of psychiatric symptoms including suicidality; past and current treatments and their effects; family psychiatric and medical history; developmental aspects; an evaluation of social aspects including family composition, school and afterschool activities, hobbies, and friends; and a description of a typical day of the patient.

11.3.3 Use of Rating Scales/Questionnaires

Rating scales/questionnaires are ancillary to the clinical interview and do not replace a thorough assessment. Screening questionnaires can help identify youth at risk for developmental delays (like the Denver Developmental Screening Test), emotional/behavioral problems (Child Behavior Checklist), or environmental risk factors (Stressful Life Events Schedule). Diagnostic questionnaires/interviews can generate/strengthen diagnostic impressions. Those are particularly important in research studies, like the Kiddie Schedule for Affective Disorders and Schizophrenia (K-SADS). Rating scales allow the objective quantification and monitoring of changes during treatment. Examples of those are the Kutcher Adolescent Depression Scale and the Affective Reactivity Index (irritability).

11.3.4 Referrals

The assessment of some conditions will require the participation of specific professionals, especially pediatricians and pediatric neurologists. Psychologists can assess the patient using standardized, valid, and reliable instruments to measure intelligence or identify specific learning disabilities.

11.3.5 Labs/Imaging

Labs may be required to rule out medical conditions causing emotional or behavioral problems. The assessment of metabolic activity is also important before starting several medications due to their potential impact on endocrinologic, hepatic, renal, and hematologic systems. Other exams may be indicated according to presentation (electroencephalogram for patients with suspected epilepsy), brain imaging studies (e.g., magnetic resonance imaging, polysomnography), or lumbar punctures.

11.3.6 Diagnosis

The two most popular classification system are the Diagnostic and Statistical Manual of Mental Disorders, Fifth edition (DSM-5) [6] and the International Classification of Diseases (ICD-11) [7]. These were not created specifically for children and adolescents. There are specific manuals for diagnosis of infants and preschool-age children (DC:0–5) [8] and for patient with intellectual disabilities (Diagnostic Manual – Intellectual Disability: A Clinical Guide for Diagnosis – DM-ID 2) [9].

We do not recommend the sole use of a manual when generating a diagnosis or treating youth. A comprehensive case evaluation is preferred, such as the 4P Factor Model, which is based on the biopsychosocial model [10]. In this model, a case conceptualization includes predisposing, precipitating, perpetuating, and protective factors. As per DSM-5, for example, a fictional 12-year-old boy could be diagnosed with conduct disorder. Using the biopsychosocial model, the formulation could be: "J is a 12yo boy presenting with increasing behavioral problems including stealing, lying, bullying peers, showing no remorse for his actions. Predisposing factors for his conduct problems are a family history of substance use and emotional neglect, and very low birthweight. Precipitating factor is the imprisonment of his adoptive father, and the perpetuating factor is negative peer influence. As protective factors, patient likes playing soccer, and has health insurance."

The following are some of the main aspects of the most common mental disorders that can have their onset in childhood.

Intellectual disability disorder (IDD) is a neurodevelopmental disorder that begins in childhood, characterized by limitations in both intelligence and adaptive skills with varying severity. The cause of IDD and the severity of impairment affect when and how a child presents difficulties. The overall goals of management of intellectual disability are to lessen the effects of disability and improve functioning, and to promote optimal functioning in the child's different settings. Interventions should begin early and be individualized, continuous, and multidisciplinary.

Autism spectrum disorders (ASD) are neurodevelopmental disabilities that affect multiple areas of development, especially relationally. Clinical manifestations are usually identified around the second year of life but may clearly manifest in older patients when social demands increase.

Elimination disorders include enuresis and encopresis. Primary enuresis (diurnal or nocturnal) refers to episodes of urinary incontinence in children who are ≥5 years of age, and usually resolves spontaneously in most patients. Enuresis is involuntary, so punishing the child will not help and can be counterproductive. The child pediatrician should be involved in the assessment. Secondary enuresis is usually associated with trauma or other medical/environmental conditions leading to a regressive state, and raises suspicion for abuse (especially sexual). Encopresis (functional fecal incontinence) refers to the inability to control the discharge of bowel contents after the acquisition of toileting skills. There is a strong association with psychosocial triggers and family dysfunction.

Attention deficit hyperactivity disorder (ADHD) is a behavioral condition with persistent and pervasive core symptoms of inattention, hyperactivity, and impulsivity. Evaluation for ADHD is usually indicated by the school and should be initiated in children ≥4 years of age who have persistent symptoms or poor school performance.

Although the combined subtype is the most common, hyperactivity/impulsivity are more frequent in boys, and female patients more often present inattention, forgetfulness, and learning difficulties.

Learning disorders (LDs) are a set of cognitive difficulties that result in academic achievement at a level less than expected for the individual's intellectual performance. Risk factors include family history of LD, poverty, prematurity, developmental and mental health conditions, prenatal alcohol exposure, neurologic conditions, and chromosomal disorders. The specific types are reading disability (dyslexia), written expression (dysgraphia), and mathematical (dyscalculia). Neurodevelopmental disorders are typically comorbid.

Oppositional defiant disorder (ODD) typically begins in preschool years. The prominent feature is a persistent pattern of angry or irritable mood, argumentative or defiant behavior, and vindictiveness. Symptoms must occur in multiple environments. The symptoms lead to conflicts with adults (family, teachers, and/or peers). Individuals with the more defiant behavior aspects tend to have comorbid attentional problems, substance use, and/or conduct disorder.

Conduct disorder (CD) consists of a pattern of behaviors and actions that harm the well-being of others and violate rules and societal norms. More frequent in boys, in the United States its prevalence ranges from 2% to 10%. Parental substance use, poor supervision, domestic violence, and low socioeconomic status are associated with CD. Only around one-third of the children will continue to present those symptoms later in life.

Anxiety: worries and fears are a natural and adaptive part of childhood development and important for good coping and survival. Anxiety disorders are the most common psychiatric disorders with onset in childhood, and frequently cooccur with other psychiatric disorders. Childhood anxiety disorders are associated with educational underachievement, increased risk for depression, substance use disorder, and suicide. Examples of anxiety disorders more common in children are separation anxiety, specific phobias, social phobia, and selective mutism.

Obsessive-compulsive disorder (OCD) : Some rituals, such as lining up objects and counting multiple times, may be normal during development. The rigid pattern, and the time spent on compulsive behaviors and thoughts associated with them will define the presence of OCD. It is important to differentiate OCD from separation anxiety or ASDs. OCD tends to start in childhood and adolescence, having a bymodal onset distribution.

Post-traumatic stress disorder (PTSD) is a condition characterized by flashbacks, nightmares, and severe anxiety, as well as uncontrollable thoughts about the traumatic event. Maltreatment (physical/emotional neglect/abuse and sexual abuse) and disasters, may trigger those symptoms, which can sometimes cause a significant change in usual behavior and even be observed in a child's play. It may be hard for children to disclose traumatic situations, and a trauma-informed approach is recommended.

Depressive disorders are less common in children, and become more common during adolescence (around 8%, more prevalent in females). Symptoms are the same as in adults, with the addition that the mood can be irritable instead of sad. Suicidality is particularly concerning during adolescent years and should be closely monitored.

Bipolar disorder in children and adolescents is characterized by recurrent episodes of increased energy and elevated mood (mania or hypomania) and depressive episodes. Bipolar disorder severely affects the normal development and psychosocial functioning of the youth and is associated with high rates of suicidality (around 45%).

Disruptive mood dysregulation disorder (DMDD) is a diagnosis added to DSM-5 in an attempt to reclassify the diagnosis of children and adolescents who could be misdiagnosed with bipolar disorder and receive treatment with antipsychotics. Youth with DMDD present chronic sad/irritable mood and severe, disproportional to cause, long, and frequent anger outbursts. So far, it is very hard to distinguish DMDD from ODD or ADHD with irritability, and most of those patients still receive antipsychotics.

Psychosis/schizophrenia: since childhood schizophrenia is rare (0.4%), the acute onset of psychosis in a child or adolescent must prompt consideration of other medical etiologies before attributing behavior to a primary psychosis diagnosis, especially in those with no family history of psychotic disorders. Children who have altered mental status without evidence of drug intoxication warrant a diligent evaluation with auxiliary studies based on clinical presentation.

Eating disorders: most body image distortions and eating disorders have an onset during adolescence, and anorexia nervosa, bulimia nervosa, and binge eating disorder are the most common ones. Youth with eating disorders need an interdisciplinary team. Family therapy is crucial for recovery.

Sleep disorders: The average normal sleep time ranges in infants from 12 to 16 hours/day and decreases gradually so that adolescents sleep from 8 to 10 hours a day. Sleepwalking and parasomnias are common in children and are usually transient and benign. In some cases they can impair academic function and daytime behavior. Polysomnography should not be routinely indicated for children.

Gender dysphoria: children generally are assigned a gender at birth based on genital anatomy or chromosomes. Some youth may have a gender identity that is not congruent with their assigned gender at birth. When there is distress with that discrepancy, the condition is called gender dysphoria. Suicide attempt rates in this population are as high as 36%, more than seven times that of the general population.

Substance use disorder (SUD): although experimentation with recreational drugs may be common during adolescence, there is a significant prevalence of SUD. Initiation and early patterns of use are strongly influenced by social and familial environmental factors, while later levels of use are strongly influenced by genetic factors. SUDs are associated with a number of negative consequences among youth, including accidents, death, health effects, crime, unplanned pregnancy, and lower achievement. Substance use should be always brought up during adolescent routine evaluations.

Personality disorders diagnoses are not unanimous among child and adolescent psychiatrists, due to ongoing development and the strong environmental element in youth emotional and behavioral problems.

Organic disorders: Physical illnesses can cause behavioral and emotional changes. Acute or chronic intoxications, metabolic problems, and infections that affect the central nervous system (encephalitis, meningitis) can cause delirium, loss of conscience, agitation, and anxiety, among other symptoms. Acute changes in behavior in a previously typically developing child indicate the need for a thorough clinical investigation, and the same should be done in atypical presentations of psychiatric problems.

11.4 Treatment

The treatment of children and adolescents with mental, emotional, and behavioral problems should receive the same attention as their assessment. Collaboration with the family and a multidisciplinary team including several professions (psychologists, social workers, occupational, physical and speech therapists, educators, and dietitians) are key to promoting better outcomes.

Once a diagnostic conclusion is made, it is important to help parents process and understand the findings and their meaning. The psychiatrist needs to have the flexibility to be supportive while also making sure the patient receives the appropriate care. Many psychiatric disorders present with a chronic course, which require the professional to develop a long-term partnership for a successful treatment.

Genetics is a factor that may be perceptible in the evaluation and treatment processes, as many parents will have experienced mental disorders themselves. Considering their struggles will provide information for the clinician and signal to parents/caregivers that the clinician will be sensitive to family issues. Legal situations (divorce agreements, guardianships, etc.), educational level of the parents, socioeconomic status (for example, private insurance), and cultural aspects must also be considered when discussing the diagnostic impressions with the families.

11.4.1 Pharmacological Treatment

The cornerstone of psychiatric management, psychotropics have a major role in the treatment of children and adolescents [11]. Youth cannot and should not be prescribed the same medications and in the same doses as adults, due to pharmacokinetic differences. Furthermore, some neurotransmitter pathways are not yet established as in adult life, which will make some medications ineffective in youth [12].

Before prescribing medication for children, one should consider if improvement is possible with more conservative approaches. When balancing risk and benefit, the psychiatrist needs to include the impact on self-esteem and the potential psychological dependence. In many anxiety disorders and mild depression, an initial psychopharmacological approach should only be tried when psychotherapy is not available or significant suffering or impairment is present. Depriving the youth of trying to improve using their cognitive, emotional, and social support may have a detrimental effect on their self-esteem and defer the appropriate measures to be implemented. Of course, this is not the case where the use psychopharmacological agents is mandatory, such as in mania or psychosis.

Regarding general rules when prescribing, starting with low doses is recommended in youth. Titration should continue until (1) satisfactory decrease in symptoms is achieved; (2) superior limit of therapeutic range is reached; (3) impairing side effects manifest; (4) or a plateau in target symptoms, or worsening with an increased dose, occurs.

Table 11.1 presents the most commonly used psychopharmacological agents for youth. Not all are FDA approved, but their inclusion in the table is supported by a series of cases or open trials.

11.4.2 Psychosocial Approaches

Psychotherapy is an interpersonal treatment based on psychological principles [13]. It should be planned individually, seeking to help patient and their families cope or manage symptoms/impairments of a psychiatric/organic disorder or adverse circumstances. Psychotherapy can be provided individually and in groups.

Table 11.1 Pharmacological agents for the treatment of children and adolescents

Class	Name	Indication	Dose	Side Effects
Typical antipsychotics (First generation)	Haloperidol	Agitation/aggression/psychosis	Children: 1–4 mg/day Adolescents: 2–10 mg/day	EPS, sedation
	Chlorpromazine	Agitation/aggression/psychosis	Children: 150–200 mg/day Adolescents: 225–375 mg/day	Sedation, orthostatic hypotension, weight gain
Atypical antipsychotics (Second generation)	Risperidone	Agitation/aggression/psychosis* Bipolar Mania/Mixed* Irritability in autism* Aggression in Conduct Disorder	Children: 1–2 mg/day Adolescents: 2.5–4 mg/day	Weight gain, hyperprolactinemia
	Clozapine	Treatment resistant mania or psychosis	Children: 100–350 mg/day Adolescents: 225–450 mg/day	Agranulocytosis, sedation, weight gain, constipation, enuresis, seizures
	Quetiapine	Bipolar mania* Bipolar depression	Children: 150–400 mg/day Adolescents: 250–550 mg/day	Weight gain, sedation
	Paliperidone	Bipolar mania/mixed* Psychosis*	Children/Adolescents: 3–6 mg/day	Weight gain, hyperprolactinemia
	Olanzapine	Bipolar mania/mixed* Psychosis*	Children: 5–10 mg/day Adolescents: 10–15 mg/day	Weight gain, sedation, hyperglycemia, dyslipidemia
	Lurasidone	Psychosis* Bipolar depression*	20–80 mg/day	Nausea, drowsiness
	Asenapine	Bipolar mania/mixed* Psychosis*	10–17a: 2.5–10 mg/day	Weight gain
	Ziprasidone	Bipolar mania/mixed Psychosis*	Children: 40–100 mg/day Adolescents: 80–140 mg/day	EKG abnormalities (prolonged QTc), sedation
	Aripiprazole	Bipolar mania/mixed* Psychosis* Irritability in autism*	Children: 5–15 mg/day Adolescents: 10–20 mg/day	Somnolence, tremor, EPS

Table 11.1 (cont.)

Class	Name	Indication	Dose	Side Effects
Antidepressants SSRIs SSRIs	Fluoxetine	Depression* Anxiety* Bulimia	Children: 10–40 mg/day Adolescents: 10–80mg/day	Headaches, gastrointestinal distress, diarrhea, sexual dysfunction, weight gain
	Paroxetine	Not indicated due in youth due to documented increase in suicidality		
	Sertraline	Depression Anxiety	50–200 mg/day	Headaches, gastrointestinal distress, diarrhea, sexual dysfunction
	Citalopram	Depression Anxiety	10–40 mg/day	Headaches, gastrointestinal distress, diarrhea, sexual dysfunction, weight gain, EKG abnormalities
	Escitalopram	Depression* Anxiety*	2.5–20 mg/day	Headaches, gastrointestinal distress, somnolence, diarrhea, sexual dysfunction, weight gain
	Fluvoxamine	Depression OCD*	25–300 mg/day	Dry mouth, dizziness, sexual dysfunction
Tricyclics	Imipramine	ADHD Enuresis	Up to 2.5 mg/kg/day)	Dry mouth, dizziness, sexual dysfunction, EKG abnormalities
	Clomipramine	OCD*	Up to 3–5 mg/kg/day	Dry mouth, dizziness, urinary retention, sexual dysfunction, EKG abnormalities
Other antidepressants	Bupropion	ADHD Depression	3–6 mg/kg/day	Headache, insomnia, hypomania, dry mouth, blurred vision, sudoresis, tremors
	Venlafaxine	Depression Anxiety ADHD	Children: 12.5–37.5 mg Adolescents: 25–225 mg	Headaches, GI distress, diarrhea, sexual dysfunction, weight gain

Drug	Indication	Dosing	Side effects
Trazodone	Insomnia	25–50mg/day	Sedation, hypotension
Mirtazapine	PTSD-related nightmares	15–45 mg/day	Sedation, weight gain, hypotension
Duloxetine	Generalized Anxiety Disorder*	30–60mg/day (max. 120 mg)	Sedation, decreased appetite, headaches, dry mouth
Atomoxetine	ADHD*	Start 0.5 mg/kg/day Max 1.2 mg/kg/day	Insomnia, dizziness, emotional lability, headaches, dry mouth, urinary retention, liver and pancreatic abnormalities
Mood stabilizers			
Lithium	Bipolar Mania*, Mixed*, Depression Aggression in Conduct Disorder	Start 300 mg/daily Increase 150/300 mg, monitoring serum levels	Sedation, somnolence, fatigue, tremors, gastrointestinal distress, hypothyroidism, kidney dysfunction, enuresis, SIADH, intoxication
Valproic acid Valproate Divalproate	Bipolar Mania/Mixed Aggression	Children: 1000–1200 mg/day Adolescents: 1000–2500 mg/day Start 125/250 mg/day and increase 125/250 mg, monitoring serum levels	Sedation, somnolence, fatigue, tremors, GI distress, hypothyroidism, weight gain, PCOS, liver, pancreatic, and hematologic abnormalities
Carbamazepine	Bipolar Mania	Children: 200–600 mg Adolescents: 300–1200 mg	Sedation, somnolence, fatigue, tremors, double vision, menstrual alterations, liver and hematologic disturbances, hyponatremia.
Oxcarbazepine	Not indicated in youth. Only randomized clinical trial in bipolar mania did not show difference from placebo.		
Topiramate	Bipolar Mania	< 12yo: 5–9 mg/kg/day > 12yo: 100–200 mg/day	Sedation, somnolence, fatigue, weight loss, memory impairment

Table 11.1 (cont.)

Class	Name	Indication	Dose	Side Effects
Stimulants	Methylphenidates	ADHD	5–60 mg/day (0.3–1 mg/kg/day)	Appetite decrease, insomnia, restlessness, irritability, headaches, rebound hyperactivity, mania, psychosis, growth delay
	Amphetamines	ADHD	5–40 mg/day (around 60% of the dose of methylphenidates)	
Other agents	Clonidine	ADHD	3–10 µg/kg/day (0.05–0.4 mg/day)	Sedation, headache, dry mouth, rebound hypertension
Anti-hypertensives	Guanfacine	ADHD	0.5–3 mg/day	

ADHD, Attention-deficit/hyperactivity disorder; EKG, electrocardiogram; EPS, extrapyramidal symptoms; OCD, obsessive-compulsive disorder; PCOS, polycystic ovary syndrome; PTSD, post-traumatic stress disorder; SIADH, syndrome of inappropriate antidiuretic hormone secretion.

There are different types of psychotherapies, ranging from more simple approaches, such as psychoeducation or parent training that can be done in school settings, to complex and multi-level interventions such multisystemic family therapy. Psychotherapy can be highly specialized, like trauma-focused therapy or specific protocols for pediatric anxiety or OCD.

Evidence is available for the effectiveness of cognitive-behavioral therapy (for anxiety disorders, sleep disorders, eating disorders, PTSD, OCD), psychodynamic psychotherapy (for anxiety disorders, interpersonal conflict), motivational interviewing (for substance use), dialectical behavior therapy (for mood dysregulation), applied behavioral analysis (for autism), supportive psychotherapy, and family therapy. There are no compelling data that one major psychotherapy is superior to the others for treatment of pediatric depression; thus, the choice usually rests on availability and patient preference. Choosing a therapist should involve knowing their training and experience treating pediatric disorders, as well as how family members are included in the treatment process. Psychotherapy for youth is more effective when caregivers and other significant people in the child's environment are included to support and maintain treatment gains.

11.5 Final Remarks

Child and adolescent psychiatry has evolved greatly over the past century. It is now known that several mental disorders have their onset in childhood, so the work with this population has the potential of significantly influencing the developmental trajectories of children, adolescents, and their families, and improving outcomes. The importance of family, school, and environmental factors cannot be understated in the evaluation and treatment of youth. The same can be said about the participation of a myriad of professionals to ensure that all the needs of our patients are met. Few professions and specialties can be more challenging and rewarding, as our young patients can provide amazing insights and show so much resilience in the face of their struggles.

References

1. Rey J, Assumpção F, Bernad C, Çuhadaroğlu Ç, Evans B, Fung D, et al. *IACAPAP e-Textbook of Child and Adolescent Mental Health.* International Association for Child and Adolescent Psychiatry and Allied Professions; 2015.

2. Papalia DE, Martorell G. *Experience Human Development.* 15th ed. Mcgraw Hill Education; 2023.

3. U.S. Department of Health & Human Services. *Centers for Disease Control and Prevention.* U.S. Department of Health & Human Services; 2023. Available from: https://www.cdc.gov/.

4. Cepeda C, Gotanco L. *Psychiatric Interview of Children and Adolescents.* American Psychiatric Association Publishing; 2017.

5. Mcconaughy SH. *Clinical Interviews for Children and Adolescents: Assessment to Intervention.* The Guilford Press; 2013.

6. American Psychiatric Association. *Diagnostic and Statistical Manual of Mental Disorders.* 5th ed. American Psychiatric Publishing; 2013.

7. World Health Organisation. *ICD-11.* Who.int. 2019. Available from: https://icd.who.int/.

8. Zero to Three. *DC: 0–5: Diagnostic Classification of Mental Health and Developmental Disorders of Infancy and Early Childhood.* Zero to Three; 2016.

9. Fletcher RJ, Al E. *Diagnostic Manual – Intellectual Disability: A Textbook of Diagnosis of Mental Disorders in Persons with Intellectual Disability: DM-ID-2.* Nadd Press; 2016.

10. Engel G. The clinical application of the biopsychosocial model. *American Journal of Psychiatry.* 1980;137 (5):535–544.

11. Isolan L, Kieling C, Zeni CP, Conceicao TV, Pianca TG. Psicofarmacos na infancia e adolescencia. In Cordioli AV, Gallois CG, Passos IC, eds. *Psicofármacos: Consulta rápida.* 6th ed. Artmed; 2023.

12. Zeni CP, Isolan LR. Psicofarmacologia na infancia e adolescencia. In Halpern R, ed. *Manual de Pediatria do Desenvolvimento e Comportamento.* Manole; 2015.

13. Weersing V, Dirks M. Psychotherapy for Children and Adolescents: A Critical Overview. In Martin A, Volkmar F, Bloch M, eds. *Lewis's Child and Adolescent Psychiatry: a Comprehensive Textbook.* Wolters Kluwer; 2017.

Chapter 12

Principles of Geriatric Psychiatry

Antonio L. Teixeira and Jennifer R. Gatchel

12.1 Introduction

According to the 2021 American Community Survey, there were almost 56 million people aged 65 and over in the United States, comprising approximately 17% of the total population. In less than two decades, it is projected that older adults will outnumber children and adolescents for the first time in US history [1]. This demographic transformation characterized by a marked increase in the absolute number and proportion of older adults has already contributed to increased health care costs. Furthermore, given the shortage of geriatric psychiatrists, primary care physicians and general psychiatrists will increasingly be responsible for the diagnosis and management of older adults presenting with mental health problems.

With aging, people are prone to develop age-related (or degenerative) conditions potentially affecting all body systems. As a consequence, older adults have increased prevalence of physical comorbidities and disabilities. In addition, older adults go through changes in their social roles and networks. Many persons move from being an active player in the working force to retirement, impacting their finances and social status. Individuals may transition from living with a family and/or spouse to living alone, experiencing loss of family members, or assuming a caregiver role.

In this context of biological and psychosocial changes superimposed on any premorbid psychological vulnerability, older adults can develop psychiatric conditions for the first time. Although not officially recognized by the DSM-5 or ICD-11 as discrete entities, these late-life psychiatric disorders have unique biological, clinical and therapeutic features compared to presentations earlier in life [2]. Noteworthy, late-life psychiatric disorders may often be associated with dementia and other neurodegenerative diseases, and in many cases may be the initial presenting symptoms of such disorders. Clinicians must manage not only patients with these conditions but also aging patients with a chronic and/or a recurrent psychiatric disorder. In either case, they must acknowledge the specificities involved in the medical management of older adults, including polypharmacy, multiple physical morbidities, decreased functioning of body systems (e.g., impaired hearing, vision, renal and liver functions), concomitant pharmacokinetic changes, along with social (e.g., isolation) and economic (e.g., poverty) issues (Table 12.1).

In this chapter, we will discuss late-life psychiatric disorders, highlighting how they frequently overlap as well as the related therapeutic challenges. To emphasize the dynamic nature of psychiatric management of older adults and set a framework for the subsequent discussion, we will start with a clinical vignette.

Table 12.1 Aging-related biological, psychological, and social factors

Biological	Psychological	Social
Physiological aging of systems	Bereavement	Retirement/new social roles
Physical morbidity (e.g., diabetes, cardiovascular diseases)	Caregiving	Isolation
Neurodegenerative diseases	Loneliness	Impoverishment
Polypharmacy		

12.1.1 Clinical Vignette

An 85-year-old woman was referred to our geriatric clinic because of "neurotic excoriations." Since the year prior to consultation, she was very fixated on supposed changes in her face, especially in her eyebrows. She described "stitches, like fishing lines" getting out of her eyebrows, so she was frequently picking her face. She tried multiple treatments under the guidance of dermatologists without any effect. She was referred to a psychiatrist who prescribed an antipsychotic that she did not tolerate. Regarding her medical history, she had controlled high blood pressure and no past history of psychiatric disorders. Besides the fixation on her face skin, she acknowledged reduced energy, irritability, and memory problems, denying any functional impairment. She was the main caregiver of her husband who had moderate to advanced dementia. They lived alone in their own house. Her report was corroborated by her son. Her clinical examination was unremarkable except for superficial excoriating lesions in the eyebrows. She also displayed reduced performance in a cognitive screening test (23 out of 30 in the Montreal Cognitive Assessment, expected value ≥ 25, with marked recall impairment).

As diagnostic formulation, patient had late-life obsessive-compulsive spectrum disorder (skin picking disorder), subsyndromal depressive symptoms, and minor neurocognitive disorder. Working hypotheses and therapeutic plan were carefully discussed with patient and family, who agreed with them. Laboratory workup (complete blood cell count, comprehensive metabolic and thyroid panels) and brain MRI were requested, and the results were unrevealing. She was prescribed a selective serotonin reuptake inhibitor that significantly minimized the skin picking behavior. On longer-term follow-up, cognitive complaints and related functional impairments became more prominent, prompting the diagnosis of probable Alzheimer's disease.

Although this case might not be seen as a typical one because of the lack of multiple physical morbidities and polypharmacy, the patient presented with late-life psychiatric conditions: skin picking and depressive symptoms. She also had cognitive impairment (mild cognitive impairment, amnestic type) that evolved with functional decline and, as a consequence, the eventual diagnosis of major neurocognitive disorder due to Alzheimer's disease. In this context, the emerging behavioral problems could be regarded as prodrome of the neurodegenerative disease. Her major complaint was related to skin picking disorder, but she also exhibited depressive symptoms not fulfilling the diagnosis of a major depression episode. The prevalence of major depressive disorder is lower in older adults compared to younger adults, but milder forms of depression are common. The patient responded well to a selective serotonin reuptake inhibitor that can help with both obsessive-compulsive and depressive symptoms. It is worth mentioning that, besides tolerability issues, there are serious concerns with the use of antipsychotics in older adults with neurocognitive disorders, including the increased risk of mortality, cardiovascular events, cognitive decline, and falls.

12.2 Delirium and Dementia

A common conundrum in clinical practice is defining whether an older adult presenting with cognitive impairment has delirium, dementia, or both. Without clear evidence from medical records or reports from family or caregivers that the patient's presentation is consistent with his/her baseline functioning, it is good practice to assume delirium.

Delirium is a clinical syndrome characterized by acute changes (hours to days) in arousal (or level of consciousness) and cognition (inattention, disorientation, forgetfulness), a fluctuating course, and variable behavioral presentation (hypoactivity, hyperactivity, or mixed). By definition, delirium is caused by an underlying condition, such as a urinary tract infection, medications or drugs, dehydration and other metabolic disorders, or post-surgical or anesthetic procedures [3]. The role played by medications, notably psychoactive and anticholinergic drugs, must be highlighted, as they account for up to 40% of delirium cases. These causative (or precipitating) factors are more likely to determine delirium in vulnerable individuals, including those 70 years of age or older, with cognitive impairment and/or sensory (hearing, visual) disturbances. Accordingly, the prevalence of delirium is higher in older compared to younger adults, with an incidence reported up to 50% after major-risk surgeries (e.g., heart surgeries).

Delirium diagnosis can be overlooked, especially in outpatient practice scenarios and with a hypoactive presentation that is the most frequent one. Many clinicians consider patients with delirium as being agitated or hyperactive, but these represent less than one-third of the cases. Once suspected, delirium must prompt thorough clinical (including neurologic) examination and laboratory tests to identify potentially treatable or reversible causes. Nonpharmacologic approaches are the cornerstone of managing behavioral problems in delirium, but antipsychotics may be necessary to reduce agitation and distressing symptoms of altered perception and thought. Although antipsychotics (e.g., olanzapine and risperidone) are effective for these indications, they do not influence the duration or severity of delirium, the length of hospital stay, or mortality, corroborating the major role played by underlying causes [4].

Traditionally, delirium has been understood as a transient condition, but a growing body of evidence has challenged this view. For example, persistent delirium was evidenced in approximately one-third of the cases at 1 month post hospital discharge, and up to 20% after 6 months [5]. Delirium is also closely associated with neurodegenerative diseases, notably Lewy body dementia, and is recurrent in this context. Finally, delirium has been implicated in persistent functional decline, and frequently unveils undiagnosed dementia.

Dementia is an umbrella term that describes a range of conditions whose course is associated with progressive decline of one or more cognitive functions (i.e., attention, executive function, learning/memory, language, perceptual-motor, and social cognition) leading to functional impairment and loss of independence. Importantly, the loss of independence is the main feature differentiating dementia from mild cognitive impairment (MCI). Although approximately one-third of older adults age 85 or older have some type of dementia, dementia is not viewed as a natural consequence of the aging process. Neurodegenerative diseases are the most common causes of dementia, with Alzheimer's disease, frontotemporal dementia (FTD), and Lewy body dementia being the most clinically relevant instances. Among non-neurodegenerative causes of dementia, it is worth considering vascular, infectious (e.g., HIV-associated neurocognitive disorder, neurosyphilis), related to traumatic brain injury (e.g., chronic traumatic encephalopathy), and toxic/metabolic (e.g., alcohol-related dementia, secondary to folate and B12 deficiencies, hypothyroidism). Of note, DSM-5 introduced the term "neurocognitive disorder" to refer to the continuum of cognitive decline spanning from mild neurocognitive disorder (or MCI/preclinical dementia) to major neurocognitive disorder (or dementia). According to DSM-5, neurocognitive disorder would also be a preferable term for conditions affecting younger adults evolving with cognitive decline, such as the one secondary to traumatic brain injury.

Alzheimer's disease (AD) accounts for more than 50% of the cases of dementia worldwide. The typical amnestic form of AD usually involves a 70-year-old or older adult presenting with progressive (months to years) forgetfulness. Atypical AD presentations include frontal variant AD (resembling FTD with apathy and socially inappropriate and/or repetitive behaviors), posterior cortical atrophy (with visuo-perceptual problems), and logopenic variant of primary progressive aphasia (word-finding difficulty with slow speech but preserved comprehension of words and articulation of phonemes). In clinical practice, the diagnosis of AD has been essentially clinical (based on clinical history and neurocognitive testing) and restricted to the stage of dementia. However, with the increasing availability of AD biomarkers beyond research scenarios (e.g., cerebrospinal fluid levels of beta-amyloid 42, tau, phospho-tau; amyloid positron-emission tomography), the diagnosis of AD can be performed at the MCI or predementia stage [6]. This integrated clinical biomarker–based diagnostic approach is important for the development and validation of disease-modifying therapies, such as monoclonal antibodies targeting beta-amyloid. The current available therapeutic strategies (acetylcho linesterase inhibitors and memantine) seem to temporarily improve and/or stabilize cognitive deficits, also helping with the management of behavioral problems.

With disease progression, more than 90% of patients with AD will develop a series of psychiatric symptoms, also referred to as behavioral and psychological symptoms of dementia (BPSD), a.k.a. neuropsychiatric symptoms [7] (Table 12.2). BPSD are a frequent reason for geriatric psychiatry referral. Compared to the relatively steady decline in cognitive parameters, BPSD tend to have a more irregular or fluctuating course. These BPSD can be categorized into three dimensions or domains: (1) affective (anxiety, dysphoria/irritability, depression, apathy); (2) perception/thought (psychosis, i.e., hallucinations and/or delusions); and (3) activity (agitation, impulse dyscontrol, wandering, rummaging, aggression). While each of these domains can be pharmacologically targeted, nonpharmacological approaches (e.g., behavioral activation, physical activity) are considered first-line therapeutic interventions for BPSD [8]. Despite that, their real-world implementation can be challenging. Antidepressants, mainly selective serotonin reuptake inhibitors (SSRIs), such as citalopram and sertraline, have been used in the management of affective symptoms as well as to target psychosis and agitation. Atypical antipsychotics (aripiprazole, brexpiprazole, risperidone, olanzapine) have been

Table 12.2 Core and accessory behavioral features of neurodegenerative dementias

	Alzheimer's disease	Frontotemporal dementia (behavioral variant)	Lewy body dementia
Core		Disinhibition; Apathy; Lack of empathy; Hyperorality (food preference change, binge eating); Repetitive behaviors (from simple stereotyped to complex compulsive behaviors).	Fluctuating arousal (with inhibited and/or agitated behaviors); Vivid visual hallucinations; REM sleep behavior disorder (act out vivid dreams).
Accessory	Apathy; Anxiety; Depression; Sleep disorders; Delusions; Agitation.	Agitation; Irritability.	Hallucinations in other sensorial modalities; Delusions; Apathy; Anxiety; Depression.

used for psychosis and disruptive behaviors, such as agitation and aggression. However, antipsychotics have a black box warning because of the increased risk of all-cause mortality with their use in patients with dementia and BSPD. Besides mortality rate, antipsychotics can influence morbidity, increasing the risk of falls and cognitive impairment, and cause anticholinergic (e.g., xerostomia, constipation) and motor (e.g., parkinsonism) side effects, which are critical issues in older adults. Therefore, the use of antipsychotics for BPSD must be carefully weighted and discussed with patient and family/caregivers. Historically, there have not been any FDA-approved medications to treat BPSD in dementia and neurodegenerative diseases, and use of pharmacological approaches has been off-label. While this largely remains the case, very recently pimavanserin, a $5\text{-}HT_{2A}$ receptor selective inverse agonist, was approved to treat Parkinson's disease psychosis, and brexipiprazole to treat agitation associated with Alzheimer's disease type dementia.

Frontotemporal dementia (FTD) refers to a heterogenous group of neurodegenerative diseases characterized by atrophy of the frontal and/or temporal lobes. This heterogeneity reflects both neuropathology (accumulation of Tau, TDP-43, or FUS) and clinical presentation (behavioral variant, primary progressive aphasia, and related variants). The topic is very complex and continuously evolving [9]. Pertinent to the current discussion, FTD is the second most common cause of neurodegenerative dementia for people younger than age 65, with a prevalence close to AD at this age, and is characterized by prominent behavioral problems. Given their disinhibition and socially inappropriate behaviors that can be can be misinterpreted as hypomania/mania, patients with behavioral variant FTD are not infrequently diagnosed with bipolar disorder, even without past history of mood disorders. The emergence of late-life mania/hypomania must prompt the consideration of secondary causes, including neurodegenerative diseases.

12.3 Depression and Anxiety

Depression is a common psychiatric syndrome among older adults, especially in medical settings and long-term care facilities [10]. The prevalence of major depressive disorder (MDD) among community-dwelling older adults is estimated at 1–4%, a rate lower than the one reported in younger adults. However, milder forms of depression are more prevalent in older adults compared to younger counterparts. This observation suggests that the DSM diagnostic criteria for MDD do not necessarily capture the complexity and heterogeneity of geriatric depression. Beyond the inherent heterogeneity of DSM criteria for MDD – where more than 200 combinations of symptoms can lead to its diagnosis – geriatric depression encompasses different conditions with supposedly distinct pathogenesis. Depression in an older adult can be an episode of recurrent MDD with early onset, that is, MDD starting before 40–50 years old with a pathogenesis involving the interplay among multiple biological, including genetic, and psychosocial factors. Conversely, depression emerging later in life, frequently referred as late-life depression, has less emphasis on low mood but increased somatic and cognitive concerns [2] and may be related to neurodegenerative and/or cerebrovascular pathology. Indeed, late-life depression has been conceptualized as a risk factor for dementia and/or as a prodrome of neurodegenerative changes [11].

The focus on somatic symptoms rather than depressed mood (masked depression or depression *sine* depression) alongside the potential impact of physical comorbidity on appetite, sleep, and energy that affects vegetative symptoms of depression pose a challenge for the recognition and management of late-life depression. While the reliance on vegetative symptoms may cause depression overdiagnosis, the lack of mood change report can lead to a premature dismissal of the diagnosis. In this context, the clinical assessment should include careful delineation of past and current depressive symptoms, contributing biological (e.g., cardiovascular and cerebrovascular diseases) and psychosocial factors and suicide risk. Bereavement and limited social support, among other factors, play a role in the pathogenesis of depression. Besides instruments to identify and determine the severity of depression (e.g., Geriatric Depression Scale, self-report; Montgomery-Asberg Depression Rating Scale, clinician-administered), cognitive screening test (e.g., Montreal Cognitive Assessment, Mini-Mental State Exam), collateral/informant report, and physical and neurological exam must all be part of the assessment.

As for younger adults, late-life depression treatment involves psychosocial and somatic approaches [12]. The relevance of physical activity, restful sleep, and appropriate nutrition for prevention and treatment of depression in older adults cannot be overstated. Evidence-based psychotherapies, such as cognitive-behavioral, acceptance and commitment, interpersonal, and problem-solving, proved to be effective for older adults with depression. Although many older adults prefer this type of intervention and/or fear drug interactions because of polypharmacy, there are concerns with cognitive, sensory (e.g., hearing), and physical (e.g., mobility) impairments and implementation issues (e.g., access to therapists).

Pharmacological treatment with antidepressants (SSRIs and SNRIs are first-line strategies) is usually effective and well tolerated by older adults. General principles in geriatric psychopharmacology include (1) choosing a specific antidepressant taking into account its side effect profile, (2) starting at a low dose, (3) increasing slowly, and

(4) discontinuing if not tolerated or lack of response. Meaningful side effects in older adults include anticholinergic (urinary retention, constipation, cognitive dysfunction), antihistaminergic (drowsiness, dizziness), and antiadrenergic (postural hypotension) effects. Other specific late-life risks to be monitored include hyponatremia, gastrointestinal bleeding, bone loss, and falls. A baseline electrocardiogram should be considered given the potential effect of antidepressants, especially tricyclics and citalopram, on QT prolongation. The role of pharmacogenetic testing to guide antidepressant treatment among older adults remains to be determined but might be helpful for patients who experienced major side effects or had failed antidepressant trials [13].

While electroconvulsive therapy (ECT) has been the traditional treatment of choice for patients with severe depression with suicidality, there is a growing interest in new neuromodulation methods, mainly repetitive transcranial magnetic stimulation, for depression in older adults. Of relevance, this is a group at risk of developing treatment-resistant or difficult-to-treat depression, in which augmentation and/or combination interventions are required. Along with older age, duration and severity of depression, physical comorbidities, comorbid anxiety, and executive dysfunction are predictors of poor antidepressant outcome such as non-response or non-remission [14].

Anxiety and depressive disorders are frequently comorbid, partly because of overlapping symptoms (restlessness, irritability, impaired concentration, insomnia), partly reflecting the transdiagnostic nature of fear and/or worry, defining features of anxiety. Approximately 50% of older adults with MDD have an anxiety disorder diagnosis, mainly generalized anxiety disorder (GAD) that is characterized by excessive and/or persistent worry. This comorbidity increases negative outcomes, including lower response to antidepressant treatment, higher rate of treatment discontinuation, greater risk for chronicity, and possibly greater cognitive impairment. The antidepressants SSRIs and SNRIs are considered the first-line treatment for late-life anxiety disorders. However, as seen in other age groups, benzodiazepines are frequently used as a pharmacological strategy for anxiety. While efficacious in reducing anxiety, there are potentially serious risks in older adults, notably falls and cognitive impairment. Other pharmacological alternatives include buspirone and gabapentinoids (pregabalin and gabapentin).

Bipolar disorder must also be considered on the differential diagnosis when assessing a mood disorder in an older adult. Bipolar disorder is less prevalent among older adults than younger adults (0.1–1.0% of community-dwelling elders) but is more common among clinical populations of older adults (geriatric outpatient psychiatric clinics, inpatient units, and nursing homes). Older adults with bipolar disorder are a heterogeneous group and include those with early onset of illness, those with newly diagnosed mania who have a history of a mood disorder, those with initial presentation of a mood disorder in late life, as well as those in whom symptoms of mania are secondary to a medical or neurological cause that or may or may not be reversible (secondary mania). Recognition and diagnosis may be complicated by the multiple medical and psychiatric comorbidities that are common in older-age bipolar disorder (cardiovascular and metabolic diseases, substance use disorders, anxiety disorders, and neurocognitive disorders). Though details of the complexity of diagnosis and management of older-age bipolar disorder are beyond the scope of the current chapter, bipolar disorder should be included on the differential diagnosis when considering depression vs. delirium vs. dementia in older adults. Mood stabilizers (lithium, valproic acid, lamotrigine) are the mainstay of treatment and require judicious dosing and monitoring of drug–drug interactions, serum levels, clinical side effects, and signs of toxicity. Psychosocial interventions are additional important components of treatment that, when adapted for cognitive symptoms, may improve health and functioning.

12.4 Psychosis and Other Psychiatric Disorders

Psychosis, a psychopathological term describing the presence of delusions, hallucinations, and/or formal thought disorder, is relatively common in later life. It can present in different contexts, and around 60% of the cases are supposedly secondary to neurological (mainly dementias) or medical causes and/or due to the effects of medications or illicit drugs [15–16]. Primary causes of late-life psychosis include late-onset schizophrenia, delusional disorder, and mood disorders. A careful clinical history, including information from collateral sources, can help differentiate between primary and secondary causes. For example, insidious onset of symptoms may suggest a primary psychotic disorder, while acute or subacute might indicate a secondary cause, such as medication or illicit drug related. Visual hallucinations presenting independently of auditory hallucinations also suggest secondary causes, such as Lewy body dementia. After defining the nature of the psychotic presentation, prompt treatment or removal of secondary causes are warranted. Given safety issues, antipsychotics should be used among older adults at the lowest effective doses and for the shortest time period when possible.

Less than 25% of cases of schizophrenia start after age 40 years (late onset), with a very small proportion starting after age 60 (very late onset). Being female, from a lower socioeconomic status, and having family history of schizophrenia or paranoid or schizoid personality disorders are risk factors for very late-onset schizophrenia. Delusional disorders, marked by fixed delusions involving one or more subtypes like persecutory, jealous, erotomanic, and somatic, also affect more women than men, with sensory impairment (hearing, vision) playing a pathogenic role.

The case in the clinical vignette was previously diagnosed with a delusional disorder, somatic type, highlighting how challenging it is to disentangle somatic delusions from severe somatic obsessions. Of note, the onset of obsessive-compulsive and related spectrum disorders (body dysmorphic, hair pulling, skin picking, hoarding) in the elderly is rare and mostly related to secondary causes, such as dementia [17]. However, hoarding is more prevalent in older adults compared to younger adults, reflecting the chronic nature of the disorder that tends to increase its severity overtime. As for obsessive-compulsive and related spectrum disorders, the prevalence of eating disorders among older adults is significantly smaller than younger adults, and late onset is very rare [18].

The problematic use of illicit or prescribed substances is an underrecognized problem in older adults. Therefore, this hypothesis should be considered in the differential diagnosis of late-life psychiatric presentations. Despite the fact that substance use disorders are less common in older compared to younger adults, the overall prevalence in the elderly is rising, including related complications such as drug overdose deaths [19]. More than half of the overdose deaths were related to opioids, highlighting the need for caution with the prescription of benzodiazepines, non-benzodiazepine hypnotic or Z-drugs, and gabapentinoids because of the risk of increased sedation. Benzodiazepines and Z-drugs (e.g., eszopiclone, zolpidem) are effective for the treatment of insomnia, especially in the short term, but side effects must be taken into account in older adults, including the risk of falls, delirium, and cognitive decline. For the long-term treatment, sedative antidepressants (mirtazapine, trazodone) and orexin antagonists (suvorexant, lemborexant) may be pharmacological alternatives, but nonpharmacological interventions, including sleep hygiene and cognitive and behavioral therapies, are preferred [20].

12.5 Conclusion

In summary, there are several particularities in the diagnosis and management of older adults, reflecting aging-related biological and psychosocial changes. For instance, older adults usually have multiple physical and neurological comorbidities and are risk for polypharmacy. The three D's of geriatric psychiatry – delirium, dementia, and depression – are common conditions that can pose diagnostic and therapeutic challenges in older adults. Delirium is frequently overlooked, and its clinical suspicion must prompt immediate and comprehensive investigation of the underlying cause(s). Dementia involves a series of neurodegenerative diseases and other causes that evolve with cognitive decline and different patterns of behavioral symptoms. The current therapeutic approach is based on the symptomatic management of cognitive and behavioral problems, but there is the recent emergence of disease-modifying therapies (anti-beta-amyloid monoclonal antibodies) that will be available in the near future. In this context, the etiologic diagnosis of dementia is a fundamental step, and recent biomarker development is facilitating this in clinical settings. Late-life depression has unique features, including the focus on somatic complaints instead of mood changes. Furthermore, older age and related characteristics, such as physical comorbidities and cognitive dysfunction, are risk factors for poor treatment response. Antidepressants, mainly SSRIs and SNRIs, are well tolerated by older adults, albeit not without risk of side effects, while there are serious concerns with the use of antipsychotics. Neuromodulation methods have emerged as promising therapeutic tools in geriatric psychiatry.

References

1. J. Vespa, The U.S. Joins Other Countries with Large Aging Populations. (2021). https://www.census.gov/library/stories/2018/03/graying-america.html.

2. S. Husain-Krautter & J. M. Ellison, Late Life Depression: The Essentials and the Essential Distinctions. *Focus (Am Psychiatr Publ)*, **19** (2021) 282–293.

3. E. R. Marcantonio, Delirium in Hospitalized Older Adults. *N Engl J Med*, **377** (2017) 1456–1466.

4. K. J. Neufeld, J. Yue, T. N. Robinson, S. K. Inouye, & D. M. Needham, Antipsychotic Medication for Prevention and Treatment of Delirium in Hospitalized Adults: A Systematic Review and Meta-Analysis. *J Am Geriatr Soc*, **64** (2016) 705–714.

5. M. G. Cole, A. Ciampi, E. Belzile, & L. Zhong, Persistent Delirium in Older Hospital Patients: A Systematic Review of Frequency and Prognosis. *Age Ageing*, **38** (2009) 19–26.

6. P. Scheltens, B. De Strooper, M. Kivipelto, H. Holstege, G. Chetelat, C. E. Teunissen, J. Cummings, & W. M. van der Flier, Alzheimer's Disease. *Lancet*, **397** (2021) 1577–1590.

7. R. R. Tampi & D. V. Jeste, Dementia Is More Than Memory Loss: Neuropsychiatric Symptoms of Dementia and Their Nonpharmacological and Pharmacological Management. *Am J Psychiatry*, **179** (2022) 528–543.

8. H. C. Kales, L. N. Gitlin, & C. G. Lyketsos, Assessment and Management of

Behavioral and Psychological Symptoms of Dementia. *BMJ*, **350** (2015) h369.

9. K. C. Jones, Update on Major Neurocognitive Disorders. *Focus (Am Psychiatr Publ)*, **19** (2021) 271–281.

10. G. S. Alexopoulos, Mechanisms and Treatment of Late-Life Depression. *Transl Psychiatry*, **9** (2019) 188.

11. N. S. Dias, I. G. Barbosa, W. Kuang, & A. L. Teixeira, Depressive Disorders in the Elderly and Dementia: An Update. *Dement Neuropsychol*, **14** (2020) 1–6.

12. R. M. Kok & C. F. Reynolds 3rd, Management of Depression in Older Adults: A Review. *JAMA*, **317** (2017) 2114–2122.

13. V. S. Marshe, F. Islam, M. Maciukiewicz, C. Bousman, H. A. Eyre, H. Lavretsky, B. H. Mulsant, C. F. Reynolds 3rd, E. J. Lenze, & D. J. Muller, Pharmacogenetic Implications for Antidepressant Pharmacotherapy in Late-Life Depression: A Systematic Review of the Literature for Response, Pharmacokinetics and Adverse Drug Reactions. *Am J Geriatr Psychiatry*, **28** (2020) 609–629.

14. C. Tunvirachaisakul, R. L. Gould, M. C. Coulson, E. V. Ward, G. Reynolds, R. L. Gathercole, H. Grocott, T. Supasitthumrong, A. Tunvirachaisakul, K. Kimona, & R. J. Howard, Predictors of Treatment Outcome in Depression in Later Life: A Systematic Review and Meta-analysis. *J Affect Disord*, **227** (2018) 164–182.

15. R. R. Tampi, J. Young, R. Hoq, K. Resnick, & D. J. Tampi, Psychotic Disorders in Late Life: A Narrative Review. *Ther Adv Psychopharmacol*, **9** (2019) 2045125319882798.

16. M. M. Reinhardt & C. I. Cohen, Late-Life Psychosis: Diagnosis and Treatment. *Curr Psychiatry Rep*, **17** (2015) 1.

17. A. N. Jazi & A. A. Asghar-Ali, Obsessive-Compulsive Disorder in Older Adults: A Comprehensive Literature Review. *J Psychiatr Pract*, **26** (2020) 175–184.

18. M. Mulchandani, N. Shetty, A. Conrad, P. Muir, & B. Mah, Treatment of Eating Disorders in Older People: A Systematic Review. *Syst Rev*, **10** (2021) 275.

19. K. Humphreys & C. L. Shover, Twenty-Year Trends in Drug Overdose Fatalities among Older Adults in the US. *JAMA Psychiatry*, **80** (2023) 518–520.

20. L. Wang, Y. Pan, C. Ye, L. Guo, S. Luo, S. Dai, N. Chen, & E. Wang, A Network Meta-analysis of the Long- and Short-Term Efficacy of Sleep Medicines in Adults and Older Adults. *Neurosci Biobehav Rev*, **131** (2021) 489–496.

Reproductive Psychiatry

Julia N. Riddle, Margo Nathan, Riah Patterson, and Anne Ruminjo

13.1 Introduction

Reproductive psychiatry specializes in mental illness in patients with a female reproductive system during the years from menarche to menopause. This topic is vital for all psychiatric clinicians that treat patients during their reproductive years. Syndromes included in this subspecialty include perinatal mood and anxiety disorders (PMADs), postpartum psychosis (PPP), premenstrual dysphoric disorder (PMDD), premenstrual exacerbation of underlying illness (PME), and mood changes associated with perimenopause. Of note, some psychiatric phenomena, such as PPP, perinatal anxiety, and PME, are not currently represented in the DSM-5. Tables 13.1 and 13.2 provide an overview of the epidemiological, diagnostic, and therapeutic aspects of reproductive psychiatry.

13.2 Important Terms

- **Trimesters of Pregnancy**
  - ○ First: Conception to ~12 weeks' gestation
  - ○ Second: ~12–28 weeks' gestation
  - ○ Third: ~28 weeks' gestation to birth

- **Antepartum:** Conception to delivery
- **Postpartum (PP):** After delivery
- **Perinatal/Peripartum:** Antepartum and postpartum
- **Gestational Age:** Age of pregnancy in weeks since last menstrual period
- **Follicular Phase:** From menstruation to ovulation, first half of cycle
- **Luteal Phase:** From ovulation to menstruation, second half of cycle. This phase is also often called the premenstruum.
- **Perimenopause:** Menstrual cycles become irregular in length, severity, and character while still maintaining a cycle within a year. Onset is usually in the fourth decade.
- **Menopause:** One year without a menstrual cycle, average age is 51 years.

13.3 Pathophysiology

Like other psychiatric and medical illnesses, PMADs, PMDD, and other reproductive illnesses are multifactorial and not yet fully understood. In addition to the sociological, societal, and political stressors, myriad biological hypothesis have gained traction.

In addition to genetic risks, research into the role of hormones and the neuroendocrine system in PPD and PMDD has pointed to the role of both metabolites of

Table 13.1 Prevalence of disorders of interest in reproductive psychiatry

Disorder/Syndrome	Prevalence (%)*	Timing of Onset
Perinatal Depression	15–20	During pregnancy – 12 months postpartum
Perinatal Anxiety Disorders	12–20	During pregnancy – 12 months postpartum
Postpartum OCD	2–4**	Up to 12 months postpartum
Postpartum Psychosis	0.2	Usually with first weeks postpartum
Premenstrual Dysphoric Disorder	4–8	Reproductive Years***
Premenstrual Exacerbation of Illness	60+	Reproductive Years***
Perimenopausal Mood Symptoms	45–68	4th and 5th decade of life

* Prevalence rates vary across different studies.
** Up to 9% in some studies
*** Reproductive years are defined as menarche to menopause. Not perinatal/postpartum prevalence is a report of percentage with illness of those pregnant or after a life birth.
Source: Hutner et al. [1].

Table 13.2 Broad overview of screening tools to assist in clinical assessment and common treatments

Disorder/Syndrome	Screening Tools	Common Treatments
Perinatal Depression	EPDS, PHQ-9	Therapy, SSRI/SNRI, augmenting agents, ECT, Brexanolone
Perinatal Anxiety Disorders	PASS, GAD-7	Therapy, SSRI/SNRI, augmenting agents,
Postpartum OCD	OCI-R, POCS, Y-BOCS	CBT/ERP therapy, SSRI/SNRI, augmenting agents
Postpartum Psychosis	MDQ	Lithium, inpatient care, ECT, neuroleptics, benzodiazepines
Premenstrual Dysphoric Disorder	DRSP	SSRI, OCPs, augmenting agents
Premenstrual Exacerbation of Illness	DRSP	Treat underlying disorder
Perimenopausal Mood Symptoms	PHQ-9, GAD-7, GREENE	Therapy, SSRI/SNRI, stimulants, OCPs

DRSP, Daily Record of Severity of Problem [13]; EPDS, Edinburgh Postnatal Depression Scale [2, 3]; GAD-7, Generalized Anxiety Disorder-7 [7]; GREENE, Greene Climacteric Scale [14]; MDQ, Mood Disorder Questionnaire [11, 12]; OCI-R, Obsessive Compulsive Inventory – Revised [8]; PASS, Perinatal Anxiety Screening Scale [6]; POCS, Perinatal Obsessive-Compulsive Scale [10]; PHQ-9, Patient Health Questionnaire-9 [4, 5]; Y-BOCS, Yale-Brown Obsessive-Compulsive Scale [9].

progesterone and their receptors in the brain (specifically GABA). Research has homed in on the hormonal shifts in the luteal phase of menstruation and in the late pregnancy, delivery, and early postpartum. It is during this time that reproductive hormones (estrogen, progesterone, and many others) change dramatically either to shed uterine lining (menstrual bleeding) or prepare for delivery of a fetus/baby. While continued research is required, data thus far has supported that there is something unique about the hormonal shift in these transitions, rather than the exact levels, that impact a subset of vulnerable women.

13.4 Obtaining a Reproductive History

We recommend obtaining a reproductive history from all patients. For women, this includes menarche, physical and mood symptoms prior to menses, history of hormonal contraception and if they impact mood (positively or negatively), pregnancy history and outcomes (this includes infertility, losses, assisted fertility, as well as mood outcomes in pregnancy and postpartum).

13.5 Pregnancy: General Considerations

13.5.1 Resources for Clinicians

Many states have clinician-staffed phone lines for maternal mental health that can be accessed by any provider. Additionally, Postpartum Support International (PSI) has a provider line. These can be used by any clinician that wants peer-to-peer guidance and resources.

13.5.2 Broad Psychological and Physiological Considerations

Psychologically, the early stage of pregnancy is often focused on privacy, care for self, and concern about pregnancy loss. Mid-pregnancy, especially when movement becomes detectable, can be a time of anxiety and excitement around changing roles. The third trimester can bring about new worries in terms of delivery and care. These thoughts can all be within the range of normal.

Physiologically, a pregnancy body will substantially increase in the following: blood volume, renal excretion, glomerular filtration rate, and hepatic metabolism. These changes can lead to increased dilution, excretion, and metabolism of many of the psychiatric medication that we use for treatment.

13.5.3 Sleep

Pregnancy and early postpartum are marked by alterations in sleep. In some cases, newborns will not sleep for more than 45 minutes at a time. Many new parents are not prepared for this dramatic change, and for those at risk of mental illness, lack of sleep can be destabilizing. We recommend discussing sleep strategies with all pregnant patients and their families in the third trimester. The goal is to aim for 3–4 uninterrupted hours even in the first days after birth [15]. These discussions can include utilizing extra bedrooms, doing shift work, or recruiting support for watching the newborn so the parent can rest.

13.5.4 Infant Feeding: Breastfeeding, Supplementing, and Formula Feeding

It is important to understand the feeding goals of your patients prior to delivery. For some patients, the goal of breastfeeding may be complicated by low milk supply, newborn feeding issues, or severe pain with feeding. For some woman, these concerns can be very unnerving. It is important to have delicate, nonjudgmental conversation around infant feeding while also understanding how much of their time is spent on feeding efforts in lieu of sleep, eating, and/or caring for themselves. Supplementing with formula can, in certain circumstances, be part of a treatment plan to allow a patient to sleep.

13.5.5 Loss/Infertility

Pregnancy loss occurs in 25% of pregnancies. While the majority of women will experience grief, they are also at increased risk of mental illness in the year (or more) following loss. History of loss is an important part of any psychiatric history. Grief counseling, therapy, and symptom monitoring for the development of illness are important.

13.6 Perinatal Psychiatric Illnesses

13.6.1 Perinatal Depressive and Anxiety Disorders (PMADS)

Perinatal Depression

By the DSM-5 criteria, perinatal depression (PND) is a major depressive episode that occurs during pregnancy or within the first 4 weeks postpartum [16]. Many women's mood specialists extend the timeline to 1 year postpartum. PND should not be confused with the baby blues – an episode of a few days, soon after delivery, of increased tearfulness, sensitivity, and mood lability experienced by 80% of new mothers. Severe depression, neurovegetative symptoms, and suicidality are not part of the baby blues.

Diagnostic interview should include questions about thoughts of harm to child, any worries that lead to neglect of self or childcare, and direct discussion about infant sleep and feeding to best understand the unique stressors during this time period.

Diagnosis and treatment are critical and if delayed can result in poor maternal and infant outcomes. These may include poor bonding and attachment, increased substance use, suicide, infanticide, neglect, low birth weight, and prematurity [1, 17].

Perinatal Anxiety

Perinatal anxiety (not currently a DSM-5–recognized phenomenon) is an anxiety disorder that presents or is exacerbated in the perinatal period. In addition to a standard assessment of anxiety, the astute reproductive psychiatrist will assess anxiety and worry related to the perinatal period: a thorough sleep history (what is preventing sleep onset or getting into bed when the opportunity arises, such as Googling new questions, checking the baby for breathing, discussing myriad "what ifs"), characterize the types of worry, intrusive thoughts/images, and discussing symptoms with collateral informants. Infant feeding must also be nonjudgmentally discussed, as this can be highly distressing to the anxious patient. The treating clinician must also be careful not to ascribe all changes in sleep, worry, appetite, focus, and energy to the sentiment of "that's just pregnancy/postpartum."

The Perinatal Anxiety Screening Scale (PASS) is a useful screening to understand and track specific symptoms at intake and during treatment.

Risk Factors

Risk factors for PMADS include prior psychiatric illness, family history of PMADS, limited social support, history of interpersonal violence or abuse, unplanned and/or unwanted pregnancy, smoking, prior perinatal loss, and psychosocial stressors, particularly during pregnancy [1, 18]. Anxiety and depression are often comorbid, and antepartum anxiety is a risk factor for postpartum depression. Other risk factors include issues with breastfeeding, infant in an intensive care unit (NICU), preterm birth, and trauma delivery.

Treatment

See **Risk Discussions** for how to approach treatment decisions with patients.
Nonpharmacological treatment includes:

- Psychotherapy, hopefully with a perinatal specialist, particularly CBT and IPT
- Protecting sleep (see **Sleep** section)
- Yoga
- Mindfulness practices

Pharmacological Treatment as follows:

- Treat as you would other unipolar depression and anxiety with the following considerations:
  - Minimize the number of agents by optimizing one agent before adding the next.
  - Increase medications in the third trimester as clinically necessary in setting of increased GFR, renal clearance, hepatic metabolism, and blood volume.
  - Specifics in pregnancy below. For medications not covered, please consult online and locally provided tools.

- Brexanolone is the first FDA-approved medication specifically for moderate to severe postpartum depression. It is a 60-hour infusion of allopregnanolone that requires inpatient monitoring [19, 20]. Zuranolone, an oral formulation of the same steroid, is currently in the process of FDA approval.
- In severe cases, electroconvulsive therapy (ECT) is an effective option for perinatal depression.
- Repetitive transcranial magnetic stimulant (rTMS) shows promise in early studies of PPD [21].

13.6.2 Perinatal Obsessive-Compulsive Disorder

Perinatal OCD can occur as either a worsening of preexiting OCD or as new-onset illness. Some key features different from non-perinatal OCD:

- Common obsessions and compulsions include contamination (focused on bottles and breast pump equipment, leading to excessive washing) and concerns about sudden infant death and the newborn's breathing at night (leading to compulsive checking of the infant and compulsive Googling/forum checking often interfering with sleep or other function).

- Intrusive thoughts/images often include ego-dystonic thoughts of harming the baby, such as dropping them down the stairs/window, crushing them, cutting them, and the like. These thoughts can lead to avoidance and checking compulsions [22]. Most women are not familiar with these types of thoughts and thus often feel guilt and shame. Additionally, they fear sharing these thoughts with a practitioner could endanger their relationship with their child (i.e., a call to child protective services).

Intrusive thoughts/images are present for almost all women postpartum [22]. It is important to note that intrusive thoughts/images to harm an infant do not mean there is intent to harm the infant. Quite the opposite, many mothers then avoid their infant. Evaluation should include assessment of avoidance, how the infant is being cared for, and a careful ruling out of any delusions related to the infant that may indicate a psychotic phenomenon rather than pOCD.

Treatment
- See **Risk Discussions**
- Cognitive behavioral therapy (CBT) with exposure response prevention (ERP)
- Treatment similar to outside of pregnancy with close monitoring or safety

13.6.3 Bipolar Disorder

Bipolar disorder (BPAD) in pregnancy and postpartum is diagnosed with the same criteria as it is outside of pregnancy. There are, however, special considerations:

> Pre-conception: Women should be counseled on the risks of common treatment options such as valproic acid, lithium, and carbamazepine. These should be considered when prescribing for any woman of reproductive age regardless of their plan for pregnancy. For those planning for pregnancy, a discussion of postpartum psychosis (PPP) is also imperative, as BPAD is a risk factor of PPP.

Perinatal: Without treatment, an estimated 66% of women will have a relapse of illness in the postpartum. The vast majority will be a depressive episode.

Treatment
- Risk discussions
- BPAD1: Lithium, neuroleptics, sleep
- BPAD2: Lamotrigine, neuroleptics, sleep
- Attempts to avoid valproic acid and carbamazepine should be made, though there can be isolated cases where these are the only effective treatment for a patient and thorough conversation with documentation should be done.

13.6.4 Postpartum Psychosis

Postpartum psychosis is a true psychiatric emergency, occurring in approximately 1–2 per 1,000 live births. Classic PPP is not a primary thought disorder, but better conceptualized as occurring within the bipolar spectrum as an affective psychosis or manic delirium. Onset is usually within days of delivery, though can be seen in first months.

PPP has a waxing and waning characteristic, which can make it difficult to diagnose on a single cross-sectional emergency evaluation.

For those diagnosed with PPP, approximately 20–50% will have only an isolated PPP episode, while the remaining 50–80% of women will likely have mood episodes outside of the perinatal period and meet criteria for BPAD.

PPP requires careful interview of the patient but also an understanding of patient's baseline with collateral information around sleep/insomnia, irritability, mood lability, new beliefs, new behaviors, and psychiatric history. PPP is an emergency because of delusions of infanticide/suicide – the most common delusion is altruistic in nature, specifically that the patient must "save" the neonate via death.

The Mood Disorder Questionnaire (MDQ) is one of the most widely used screening tools to assess for emerging bipolar illness and may be a helpful screening tool when assessing for potential PPP [11]. We also recommend a full medical workup including lab monitoring (CMP, CBC, TSH), urinalysis with toxicology, brain imaging, as well as physical and neurological exams.

Treatment
- Hospitalization
- Lithium
- Benzodiazepines
- Other neuroleptics
- ECT

13.6.5 Psychotic Disorders
Psychotic disorders often require continued treatment during pregnancy, including long-acting injectables. Consult resources mentioned earlier to review specifics of medications. Efforts to avoid clozapine should be made.

13.6.6 Attention Deficit Hyperactivity Disorder
ADHD can remain the same or worsen in the peripartum period. Many women come into pregnancy already on stimulants for treatment. In women who abuse stimulants, preterm birth and low birthweight are some of the adverse outcomes reported [23].

Treatment
The results of two large studies have not shown an overall increase in risk of major malformations with prenatal exposure to prescription doses of amphetamines or methylphenidate [24, 25]. But there is a dose-dependent increase in gestational hypertension [23].
- Taper stimulant medications (if possible), use the lowest stimulant dose, or use medication on an as-needed basis.
- Consider work/school accommodations in perinatal period.
- Consider bupropion.
- In cases of severe ADHD leading to motor vehicle accidents, severe dysfunction in relationships or inability to maintain employment or narcolepsy, continuation of stimulants is warranted.

13.7 Treatment during Pregnancy: Special Considerations

13.7.1 Risk Discussions and Medication Considerations

Treatment in pregnancy is a discussion of relative risks rather than "safety." There are risks to untreated mental illness and there are risks to treatment. A discussion must include both. One of the biggest mistakes that we see is undertreated illness in pregnancy. This results in two exposures in pregnancy: illness and treatment. Additionally, we have minimal data on the risks of polypharmacy and cannot confidently say that the risk of each medication is the same as the risk of a combination of medications. Efforts to limit polypharmacy while maximizing treatment response are critical.

All medications pass through the placenta, and there are currently no medications approved by the Federal Drug Administration (FDA) for treatment during pregnancy. Additionally, most medications pass into breastmilk, though the majority are at levels considered low risk (relative infant dose <10% is considered likely safe for the infant).

The following is a broad discussion of some medication classes. For some in-depth knowledge, we recommend helpful resources such as Reprotox, LactMed, MotherToBaby, your state's referral line, and the PSI resource line.

13.7.2 Selective Serotonin Reuptake Inhibitors

SSRIs are typically first-line in treatment of perinatal depression and anxiety [26]. Newer SSRIs have less evidence in pregnancy and should be considered after older medications are trialed. Outcomes that are commonly included in risk conversations:

Congenital malformations: Current data has not demonstrated an increased risk [26].
Poor neonatal adaption syndrome (PNAS): Occurs in approximately 30% of children exposed to SSRIs in utero, within minutes to hours of delivery [26]. There is no consistent definition of this syndrome or blinded assessment of it. Most cases are mild (irritability, difficulty feeding, and changes in muscle tone), though rare cases can be more severe (difficulty breathing, hypoglycemia, cardiac arrhythmias). Symptoms are typically self-correcting are not associated with long-term complications or poor outcomes [26]. Tapering antidepressants in late pregnancy to prevent PNAS does not decrease the risk of its development and increases subsequent risk of developing PPD [27]. Breastfeeding is thought to be helpful in alleviating PNAS symptoms [28].

Long-Term Neurodevelopmental Outcomes

- A recent large cohort study did not show an association between SSRIs and long-term neurodevelopmental outcomes (ADHD, ASD, learning and speech disorders, among others) in children up to age 14 [29].
- This data is reassuring and should be included in shared decision-making with patients.

Breastfeeding

SSRIs are considered safe in breastfeeding. They fall below what the American Academy of Pediatrics considers a concerning relative infant dose of 10%. Sertraline has the lowest passage through breastmilk.

13.7.3 Serotonin and Norepinephrine Reuptake Inhibitors

The data on SNRIs with regard to **teratogenicity, PNAS, long-term development outcomes,** and **breastfeeding** safety is fairly similar to that of SSRIs though with fewer available studies than SSRIs. Unlike SSRIs, there is a risk of gestational hypertension associated with use of venlafaxine. Blood pressure should be closely monitored.

13.7.4 Bupropion, Mirtazapine, Tricyclic Antidepressants

TCAs have not been associated with teratogenicity. Bupropion and mirtazapine have limited human data but no known teratogenicity in animal studies or case reports. The decision to use these agents is determined by target symptom(s), tolerability and side effect profile, and risk of switching to another agent. As an example of available TCAs, desipramine and nortriptyline have fewer anticholinergic effects and are less likely to cause constipation and orthostatic hypotension (which can occur in normal pregnancy). There is minimal research on the use of MAOIs in pregnancy.

13.7.5 Lithium

Lithium clearance increases substantially during pregnancy due to renal blood flow and increased glomerular filtration rate [30], so levels must be checked frequently including close to pregnancy, during any episodes of dehydration/illness, immediately after delivery, and in the postpartum. A structured plan for dosing during delivery and the postpartum are imperative as the fluid changes at delivery and postpartum can risk toxicity. Coordination with obstetrics is recommended for optimal treatment during labor, delivery, and early postpartum. Wesseloo et al. published helpful strategies for lithium use in pregnancy in 2017 [31].

The risk of malformations, including cardiac ones, is present but much less than previously reported (cumulative OR < 2) and is likely dose dependent [1]. High-resolution ultrasounds and fetal echocardiogram should be performed at 16–20 weeks' gestation. Other risks include infant diabetes insipidus leading to polyhydramnios and a rare risk of decreased muscle tone and difficulty breathing in the infant.

Breastfeeding: There is risk of toxicity in an infant that is dehydrated or when a mother's dose is toxic (due to not lowering during delivery). Coordination of a pediatrician is vital. Lithium use is not an absolute contraindication to breastfeeding, and there are interdisciplinary ways to support successful breastfeeding.

13.7.6 Lamotrigine

Data on lamotrigine is also reassuring and it is becoming increasingly used in pregnancy [23]. Clearance is increased up to 300% in pregnancy, so dose increases can be guided by clinical judgment or, with preconception planning, by pre-pregnancy serum levels. Folate supplementation beyond that present in a prenatal vitamin is no longer necessary (1 mg/day).

13.7.7 Valproic Acid

Valproic acid should be avoided in reproductive-age women and should be discontinued in pregnancy whenever possible. Risks of major malformation are reported at 5–11% and are dose dependent. There is also an association with neurodevelopmental delays and cognitive defects. If this is the only effective agent and its use is absolutely necessary, augment with 4–5 mg/day of folate [1]. It is compatible with breastfeeding, though there is theoretical concern for hepatotoxicity.

13.7.8 Other Mood Stabilizers

Carbamazepine carries a risk of neural tube defects. Avoid, if possible, otherwise augment with 4–5 mg/day of folate. Gabapentin has limited data, though some animal studies show fetal growth impairment and developmental delay. Topiramate has limited evidence regarding its use and safety in pregnancy.

13.7.9 Neuroleptics/Antipsychotics

Data on atypical antipsychotics is limited but reassuring with regard to child development [26]. Extrapyramidal symptoms in newborns have been reported in some cases of third-trimester exposure. In breastfeeding, most antipsychotics increase prolactin and thus breastmilk. Aripiprazole does not impact prolactin and may, in fact, reduce lactation. Clozapine is not considered compatible with breastfeeding. Other antipsychotics are largely compatible with breastfeeding.

13.7.10 Benzodiazepines (BZDs)

Some of the benzodiazepines used in pregnancy include lorazepam, clozapine, and alprazolam typically in combination with SSRIs/SNRIs for the treatment of anxiety, insomnia, and phobias not responding completely with first-line treatment (SSRIs/ SNRIs). Ideally, BZDs are used sparingly and at low doses both for risks to mother in general and for risk of neonatal withdrawal and respiratory depression at birth. Use in the postpartum should be weighed against the risks of sedation while caring for a newborn.

13.8 Reproductive Psychiatry Outside of Pregnancy

13.8.1 Premenstrual Dysphoric Disorder / Premenstrual Exacerbation of Underlying Illness

Premenstrual dysphoric disorder (PMDD) is characterized by a combination of affective and physical or somatic symptoms that are only present during the luteal phase of the menstrual cycle and largely absent the remainder of the month [16]. This disorder impacts about 3–8% of women, and symptoms must be present for most menstrual cycles during a year-long period [32]. Affective symptoms commonly include dysphoric mood, changes in energy, sleep disruption, cognitive symptoms, and can include suicidal ideation. Physical or somatic symptoms may include gastrointestinal discomfort, fatigue, bloating, breast pain, and back pain, among others. To qualify for a PMDD diagnosis, patients must have both types of symptoms and they must cause clinically significant distress or impairment. Further, PMDD is a clinical diagnosis best identified through prospective tracking of daily symptoms over two to three cycles using the DSRP [33]. There are currently no laboratory tests needed to diagnose this disorder. Reproductive hormones levels do not provide insight into severity or illness. When making this diagnosis, consider a diagnosis of an underlying affective illness (such as major depressive disorder or bipolar disorder) with premenstrual exacerbation (PME) in the differential if there are symptoms present at other times of the month with worsening in the luteal phase.

Treatment

- Therapy.
- SSRI, either during the luteal phase or continuously.
- Hormonal birth control, though this treatment can also worsen symptoms.
- Augmenting agents, particularly to protect sleep in the luteal phase.
- Magnesium can be helpful for physical symptoms such as breast tenderness.
- In severe cases, hormonal suppression, such us with leuprolide, and possible oophorectomy have been considered but must be weighed against the risks associated with premature menopause.

13.8.2 Perimenopause

Women are at elevated risk for depressive symptoms during the perimenopausal transition, with some studies showing prevalence rates of up to 60% [1]. Most commonly, women experience sub-syndromal depressive symptoms that do not meet full criteria for a major depressive episode. Women with a history of prior affective illness (including PMAD, PMDD, and/or PME) are at risk of recurrent mood episodes during perimenopause. Common mood symptoms can include depressed mood, but also irritability and anxious distress. These symptoms often correspond with typical symptoms of menopause related to estradiol withdrawal, including hot flashes, vaginal dryness, and joint pain. Sleep disruption is a common source of functional impairment even in the absence of mood symptoms and most frequently manifests as sleep fragmentation. While psychological distress is commonly identified in relation to perimenopause, anxiety has not been as well studied. Cognitive symptoms are common and not as well studied but of major concern to many patients in this population.

There is not currently a widely used validated tool to screen for perimenopausal mood disorders specifically; however, several commonly available scales (PHQ-9, GAD-7, Greene) can be helpful to characterize the type and severity of symptoms present. However, a thorough psychiatric and reproductive history is still needed to establish the diagnosis.

Treatment

- SSRI/SNRIs, clonidine, and gabapentin have a role in treating mood, irritability, anxiety, and vasomotor symptoms.
- Addressing sleep, including orexin antagonists.
- CBT.
- Hormone placement therapy can be helpful for mood and cognitive symptoms in close collaboration with a gynecologist.
- Less studied, but combined OTCs can have some utility.
- Stimulants have pros and cons for cognitive fog.

13.9 Final Considerations

This is an expansive and nuanced specialty, and every topic/medication risk cannot be covered here. We recommend the following textbooks for deeper knowledge:

1. Hutner LA, Catapano LA, Nagle-Yang SM, Williams KE, Osborne LM, editors. *Textbook of Women's Reproductive Mental Health*. American Psychiatric Pub; 2021.
2. Cox E, ed. *Women's Mood Disorders: A Clinician's Guide to Perinatal Psychiatry*. Springer Nature; 2021.

References

1. L. A. Hutner, L. A. Catapano, S. M. Nagle-Yang, K. E. Williams, & L. M. Osborne, *Textbook of Women's Reproductive Mental Health* (American Psychiatric Pub, 2021).

2. J. L. Cox, J. M. Holden, & R. Sagovsky, Detection of Postnatal Depression: Development of the 10-item Edinburgh Postnatal Depression Scale. *The British Journal of Psychiatry*, **150** (1987) 782–786.

3. B. N. Gaynes, N. Gavin, S. Meltzer-Brody, K. N. Lohr, T. Swinson, G. Gartlehner, S. Brody, & W. C. Miller, Perinatal Depression: Prevalence, Screening Accuracy, and Screening Outcomes: Summary. *AHRQ Evidence Report Summaries* (Agency for Healthcare Research and Quality (US), 2005).

4. D. Gjerdingen, S. Crow, P. McGovern, M. Miner, & B. Center, Postpartum Depression Screening at Well-Child Visits: Validity of a 2-Question Screen and the PHQ-9. *The Annals of Family Medicine*, 7 (2009) 63–70.

5. B. P. Yawn, W. Pace, P. C. Wollan, S. Bertram, M. Kurland, D. Graham, & A. Dietrich, Concordance of Edinburgh Postnatal Depression Scale (EPDS) and Patient Health Questionnaire (PHQ-9) to Assess Increased Risk of Depression among Postpartum Women. *The Journal of the American Board of Family Medicine*, 22 (2009) 483–491.

6. S. Somerville, K. Dedman, R. Hagan, E. Oxnam, M. Wettinger, S. Byrne, S. Coo, D. Doherty, & A. C. Page, The Perinatal Anxiety Screening Scale: Development and Preliminary Validation. *Archives of Women's Mental Health*, **17** (2014) 443–454.

7. W. Simpson, M. Glazer, N. Michalski, M. Steiner, & B. N. Frey, Comparative Efficacy of the Generalized Anxiety Disorder 7-Item Scale and the Edinburgh Postnatal Depression Scale as Screening Tools for Generalized Anxiety Disorder in Pregnancy and the Postpartum Period. *The Canadian Journal of Psychiatry*, **59** (2014) 434–440.

8. E. B. Foa, J. D. Huppert, S. Leiberg, R. Langner, R. Kichic, G. Hajcak, & P. M. Salkovskis, The Obsessive-Compulsive Inventory: Development and Validation of a Short Version. *Psychological Assessment*, **14** (2002) 485–496.

9. E. A. Storch, S. A. Rasmussen, L. H. Price, M. J. Larson, T. K. Murphy, & W. K. Goodman, Development and Psychometric Evaluation of the Yale–Brown Obsessive-Compulsive Scale: Second Edition. *Psychological Assessment*, **22** (2010) 223–232.

10. L. H. Chaudron & N. Nirodi, The Obsessive-Compulsive Spectrum in the Perinatal Period: A Prospective Pilot Study. *Archives of Women's Mental Health*, **13** (2010) 403–410.

11. D. M. Millan, C. T. Clark, A. Sakowicz, W. A. Grobman, & E. S. Miller, Optimization of the Mood Disorder Questionnaire in Identification of Perinatal Bipolar Disorder. *American Journal of Obstetrics & Gynecology MFM*, 5 (2023) 100777.

12. C. J. Miller, J. Klugman, D. A. Berv, K. J. Rosenquist, & S. Nassir Ghaemi, Sensitivity and Specificity of the Mood Disorder Questionnaire for Detecting

Bipolar Disorder. *Journal of Affective Disorders*, **81** (2004) 167–171.

13. J. Endicott, J. Nee, & W. Harrison, Daily Record of Severity of Problems (DRSP): Reliability and Validity. *Archives of Women's Mental Health*, **9** (2006) 41–49.

14. J. G. Greene, A Factor Analytic Study of Climacteric Symptoms. *Journal of Psychosomatic Research*, **20** (1976) 425–430.

15. N. Leistikow, E. B. Baller, P. J. Bradshaw, J. N. Riddle, D. A. Ross, & L. M. Osborne, Prescribing Sleep: An Overlooked Treatment for Postpartum Depression. *Biological Psychiatry*, **92** (2022) e13–e15.

16. *Diagnostic and Statistical Manual of Mental Disorders: DSM-5^{TM}, 5th ed* (American Psychiatric Publishing, Inc., 2013).

17. E. Cox, ed., *Women's Mood Disorders: A Clinician's Guide to Perinatal Psychiatry* (Springer International Publishing, 2021).

18. E. Robertson, S. Grace, T. Wallington, & D. E. Stewart, Antenatal Risk Factors for Postpartum Depression: A Synthesis of Recent Literature. *General Hospital Psychiatry*, **26** (2004) 289–295.

19. S. Meltzer-Brody, H. Colquhoun, R. Riesenberg, C. N. Epperson, K. M. Deligiannidis, D. R. Rubinow, H. Li, A. J. Sankoh, C. Clemson, A. Schacterle, J. Jonas, & S. Kanes, Brexanolone Injection in Post-Partum Depression: Two Multicentre, Double-Blind, Randomised, Placebo-Controlled, Phase 3 Trials. *The Lancet*, **392** (2018) 1058–1070.

20. V. A. Canady, FDA Approves First Drug for Postpartum Depression Treatment. *Mental Health Weekly*, **29** (2019) 6–6.

21. K. S. Garcia, P. Flynn, K. J. Pierce, & M. Caudle, Repetitive Transcranial Magnetic Stimulation Treats Postpartum Depression. *Brain Stimulation*, **3** (2010) 36–41.

22. N. Hudepohl, J. V. MacLean, & L. M. Osborne, Perinatal Obsessive-Compulsive Disorder: Epidemiology, Phenomenology, Etiology, and Treatment. *Current Psychiatry Reports*, **24** (2022) 229–237.

23. E. R. Raffi, R. Nonacs, & L. S. Cohen, Safety of Psychotropic Medications During Pregnancy. *Clinics in Perinatology*, **46** (2019) 215–234.

24. L. Kolding, V. Ehrenstein, L. Pedersen, P. Sandager, O. B. Petersen, N. Uldbjerg, & L. H. Pedersen, Associations between ADHD Medication Use in Pregnancy and Severe Malformations Based on Prenatal and Postnatal Diagnoses: A Danish Registry-Based Study. *The Journal of Clinical Psychiatry*, **82** (2021) 437.

25. K. F. Huybrechts, G. Bröms, L. B. Christensen, K. Einarsdóttir, A. Engeland, K. Furu, M. Gissler, S. Hernandez-Diaz, P. Karlsson, Ø. Karlstad, H. Kieler, A.-M. Lahesmaa-Korpinen, H. Mogun, M. Nørgaard, J. Reutfors, H. T. Sørensen, H. Zoega, & B. T. Bateman, Association between Methylphenidate and Amphetamine Use in Pregnancy and Risk of Congenital Malformations: A Cohort Study from the International Pregnancy Safety Study Consortium. *JAMA Psychiatry*, **75** (2018) 167–175.

26. M. C. Kimmel, E. Cox, C. Schiller, E. Gettes, & S. Meltzer-Brody, Pharmacologic Treatment of Perinatal Depression. *Obstetrics and Gynecology Clinics*, **45** (2018) 419–440.

27. W. Warburton, C. Hertzman, & T. F. Oberlander, A Register Study of the Impact of Stopping Third Trimester Selective Serotonin Reuptake Inhibitor Exposure on Neonatal Health. *Acta Psychiatrica Scandinavica*, **121** (2010)

28. N. Kieviet, K. M. Dolman, & A. Honig, The Use of Psychotropic Medication During Pregnancy: How about the Newborn? *Neuropsychiatric Disease and Treatment*, **9** (2013) 1257–1266.

29. E. A. Suarez, B. T. Bateman, S. Hernández-Díaz, L. Straub, K. L. Wisner, K. J. Gray, P. B. Pennell, B. Lester, C. J. McDougle, Y. Zhu, H. Mogun, & K. F. Huybrechts, Association of Antidepressant Use during Pregnancy with Risk of Neurodevelopmental Disorders in Children. *JAMA Internal Medicine*, **182** (2022) 1149–1160.

30. K. M. Deligiannidis, N. Byatt, & M. P. Freeman, Pharmacotherapy for Mood Disorders in Pregnancy. *Journal of Clinical Psychopharmacology*, **34** (2014) 244–255.

31. R. Wesseloo, A. I. Wierdsma, I. L. van Kamp, T. Munk-Olsen, W. J. G. Hoogendijk, S. A. Kushner, & V. Bergink, Lithium Dosing Strategies during Pregnancy and the Postpartum Period. *The British Journal of Psychiatry*, **211** (2017) 31–36.

32. L. Dennerstein, P. Lehert, & K. Heinemann, Epidemiology of Premenstrual Symptoms and Disorders. *Menopause International*, **18** (2012) 48–51.

33. L. Hantsoo & C. N. Epperson, Premenstrual Dysphoric Disorder: Epidemiology and Treatment. *Current Psychiatry Reports*, **17** (2015) 87.

Psychomotor Agitation

Olusegun Adebisi Popoola and Nidal Moukaddam

14.1 Introduction

Psychomotor agitation refers to a state of increased motor activity, restlessness, and emotional tension that can impair a person's ability to function, hence requiring prompt assessment and intervention [1]. It is often characterized by restless movements, such as pacing, fidgeting, wringing of hands, or meaningless verbal activity, along with rapid speech and other signs of hyperactivity. Psychomotor agitation can be a symptom of several mental disorders, including bipolar disorder, major depressive disorder, anxiety disorders, and schizophrenia, as well as certain medical conditions such as hyperthyroidism, delirium, and substance intoxication or withdrawal [2].

While psychomotor agitation can be of abrupt onset, it can also develop gradually, resulting in a disruption in service delivery, patient care, and staff safety.

Psychomotor agitation is associated with several negative outcomes, including:

- Increased health care utilization: Agitated patients may require more frequent hospitalizations, longer hospital stays, and more intensive treatments.
- Higher mortality rates: Agitation can lead to physical harm, self-injury, and increased risk of medical complications, all of which can increase the risk of death.
- Decreased quality of life: Agitation can interfere with social functioning, relationships, and activities of daily living, leading to decreased quality of life for patients and their families.

Understanding the epidemiology of agitation can help clinicians identify at-risk patients, implement preventive measures, and provide appropriate treatment. Epidemiological studies have investigated the prevalence, risk factors, and outcomes associated with psychomotor agitation in different populations. Despite psychomotor agitation being encountered daily at different levels of care, the prevalence varies depending on the population studied, definition used, and the settings. The prevalence ranges between 10% and 80% [3–5]. In general, psychomotor agitation is more common in acute settings such as emergency departments, hospitals, and intensive care units, compared with other clinical settings.

14.2 Pathophysiology

The pathophysiology of psychomotor agitation is not fully understood. However, research has suggested that multiple neurotransmitter systems are involved [2]. Psychomotor agitation is a complex phenomenon with multiple contributing factors. While the exact pathophysiology is not fully understood, various neurotransmitter systems, including serotonin, dopamine, norepinephrine, and gamma-aminobutyric acid

(GABA), as well as the hypothalamic-pituitary-adrenal (HPA) axis, play important roles. The abnormalities in the neurotransmitter do not represent a distinctive clinical presentation or associated disorder. Additionally, psychological and environmental factors such as anxiety, stress, trauma, and substance use can also contribute to the development of psychomotor agitation [2].

Individuals with bipolar disorder who experienced psychomotor agitation had increased dopamine activity in the brain, as measured by positron emission tomography (PET) imaging [6]. Individuals with major depressive disorder who experienced psychomotor agitation had decreased GABA activity in the brain, as measured by magnetic resonance spectroscopy (MRS) [7]. These findings suggest that dysregulation of these neurotransmitter systems may play a role in the development of psychomotor agitation. Serotonin plays a key inhibitory role in aggressive behavior. For example, low levels of 5-hydroxyindolacetic acid (5-HIAA) in the cerebrospinal fluid are significantly correlated with impulsive aggressive behavior rather than with premeditated aggression [8]. This adds to the importance of identifying early signs of agitation in prevention and management of aggression in clinical settings.

Research has also suggested that abnormalities in the HPA axis may contribute to psychomotor agitation. A study by Swann and colleagues found that individuals with bipolar disorder who experienced psychomotor agitation had increased cortisol levels, which is a marker of HPA axis dysregulation [9].

The etiology of psychomotor agitation varies greatly depending on the age of the individual, preexisting psychiatric disorder, substance use history, and medical history, the majority of which can be co-occurring in nature. As a result, specific considerations must be made during the assessment and management of psychomotor agitation.

14.3 Etiology

Several identified risk factors for psychomotor agitation include:

- Age:
  - Older adults, particularly those with dementia or delirium, are at higher risk of agitation [10].
  - In children, psychomotor agitation could be due to behavioral disinhibition and impulsivity in the context of parent–child relational problem, DMDD, conduct disorder, ODD, adjustment disorder with disturbance of conduct, psychotic disorder, depressive disorder (which more often presents in children with irritability), or substance intoxication or withdrawal.
  - Medical illness: Patients with medical conditions such as Parkinson's disease, traumatic brain injury, epilepsy, delirium, or stroke are more likely to experience agitation.

- Psychiatric disorders: Patients with bipolar disorder, major depressive disorder, schizophrenia, and substance use disorders are at increased risk of agitation [11–13].
- Medications: Certain medications such as stimulants, gabapentin, antipsychotics, and corticosteroids can cause or exacerbate agitation [14].
- Environmental factors: Overstimulation, noise, and lack of privacy or personal space can contribute to agitation.

14.4 Treatment/Management

The management approach for psychomotor agitation requires the use of multiple modalities. The goal is to ensure the safety of the patient and other individuals present through the identification of risk factors for psychomotor agitation, the cause, and the implementation of the appropriate treatment in a timely and efficient manner. The prompt identification of psychomotor agitation is crucial to prevent or minimize negative outcomes. A prompt evaluation of the patient to ensure safety is paramount.

Several rating scales are available that can be used to evaluate the future risk of agitation, aggression, and associated violence in psychiatric inpatient settings. This includes the Broset Violence checklist [9, 15]. Another is the CGI, which is composed of a 5-point Likert scale and is a simple and quick tool that can be completed by a clinician and provide a rapid assessment of a patient [16].

Other tools for assessing for agitation is PANSS-EC, which assesses five items on a scale of 1 to 7, and the BARS, which rates the severity of agitated behavior using a seven-level single item [1]. The Modified Overt Aggression Scale, consisting of four items rated on a 4-point scale, can also be used to track the changes in the severity of aggression [17].

14.5 Therapeutic and Nontherapeutic Approach to the Management of Psychomotor Agitation

The effective expected outcome in the management of psychomotor agitation is not clearly defined. However, while patient participation is most desired, implemented intervention can result in sleep. This is not a desirable outcome because it will make evaluation impossible. Therapeutic outcomes such as oversedation can result in a need for constant monitoring and assistance with activities of daily living, such as toileting, resulting in an increased burden on the staff.

While it might be challenging to identify the etiology of psychomotor agitation, certain circumstances can hint at the cause in the absence of a prior diagnosis. Most situations in which PA presents have specific risk factors; for example, a patient who is presenting in the emergency room with substance intoxication or withdrawal might be easily identified. These individuals might also have a co-occurring medical or psychiatric diagnosis that could predispose them to PA; stabilizing the patient promptly regardless of the location of treatment – whether in the medical or psychiatric emergency ward – should the goal. Transferring patients between these units may be appropriate when possible. In the inpatient medical unit, PA can have varied etiology, and making a differential diagnosis can help stabilize the individual. Also, respecting the patient's autonomy by not using coercive measures is important.

The objective is to use the least restrictive means initially and only proceed to use the more restrictive means as a last resort in the context of imminent danger to self and to others.

Environment Approach: In the management of a patient with psychomotor agitation, modification to the environment should be attempted to achieve a therapeutic outcome [18]. The aim of this intervention is to ensure the safety of patients, anyone around them, and the staff. These interventions are not mutually exclusive but rather may need to be carried out simultaneously. This includes making sure that the patient is comfortable and does not feel threatened through safe communication and showing a caring attitude. Also, providing prompt responses to a patient can help reduce the risk of psychomotor agitation. Objects that can be easily used as a weapon, such as blood pressure machines, computers, and computer accessories, should be removed from and kept out of reach of the patient. Minimizing external stimuli such as noise and light, as in the case of phencyclidine intoxication, is another potentially helpful environmental modification.

Verbal de-escalation: Verbal de-escalation should be attempted because it provides an avenue to interact with the patient, which also provides diagnostic clues to the cause of psychomotor agitation. There should be a point person attempting verbal de-escalation, not multiple individuals at the same time. This intervention should be aimed at showing the patient the staff genuinely care about their well-being to establish a therapeutic alliance. Approaches for safe verbal de-escalation include maintaining a safe distance while respecting the patient's personal space, ensuring that the staff are at the egress using a nonthreatening postures, staff maintaining calmness, and ensuring that eye contact is adequate but not too extreme. This is also the time to set behavioral limits with the patient [1, 19, 20].

14.6 Psychopharmacological Intervention

The choice of medication that should be used in psychomotor agitation should be tailored to the population being treated, considering the least restrictive means, choosing between oral medication, intranasal inhalation (IN), and more invasive means such as intramuscular (IM) and intravenous intervention (IV).

14.7 Route of Administration of Medication

14.7.1 Less Invasive Route

The oral and intranasal route requires the full cooperation of the patient. This should be offered after verbal de-escalation, depending on the severity of PA. While this is less restrictive, it must be used with great caution in patients who have regained self-control because it brings the staff into physical proximity to the patient. This will require the patient to consent to medication administration. This poses a challenge to the implementation of treatment. It also applies to different patient populations differently [19]. In the pediatric population obtaining consent from the parent to administer oral medication in the case of agitation is important, and this should be taken into consideration.

14.7.2 More Invasive Routes

IM or IV intervention is often required in a severe form of psychomotor agitation and in those who did not respond to less restrictive means. The medication to be used in this situation must be easy to administer. IM administration may be preferred over IV route in most situations because of this. However, in the medical unit or the intensive care unit where an IV line is in place, the use of this route may be appropriate.

In most cases, a combination of medications is used, and the clinician should be aware of medications that can be combined in a syringe for administration and those that cannot be combined and will require two different syringes to be used, and the consequent need for two injections. Having to give two injections may pose a risk of harm to the staff that will administer the medication. In practice, haloperidol and lorazepam are commonly combined in the same syringe [21]. However, the combination of high-potency first-generation antipsychotics such as fluphenazine or haloperidol with lorazepam and diphenhydramine, which is commonly used in a syringe, can result in precipitation of the solution in the syringe or even in the muscles after administration, thereby affecting the efficacy of the combination; hence this trio has to be administered twice. Other combinations that are not commonly encouraged include the addition of low-potency first-generation antipsychotics such as chlorpromazine and lorazepam. Most second-generation antipsychotics must be given with two syringes when being used in combination with other medications. See Tables 14.1 and 14.2 for a more comprehensive list of interventions.

In the management of psychomotor agitation of the elderly in a medical unit or nursing facility, a considerable amount of medical and nursing supervision is needed. Additionally, there should be a high index of suspicion for delirium as a differential diagnosis.

Seclusion: When a patient presents with severe psychomotor agitation and does not respond to less restrictive means, it may be necessary to use seclusion. After receiving emergency IM medication, some patients may remain disruptive, posing a danger to themselves and others. As a result, there might be a need for prolonged manual holding by support staff, posing more harm to the patient and staff. Also, this approach will require more staffing. In this situation, placing a patient in seclusion is appropriate while waiting for the patient to become calm. The patient should be informed of the reason for seclusion and the condition for the discontinuation of seclusion. One can continue to engage a patient in seclusion as verbal de-escalation to promote the achievement of the desired outcome. Seclusion requires specially equipped rooms, and the patient has to be under constant observation while in seclusion [1]. After seclusion is discontinued, a debrief should be conducted with the treatment team and support staff.

Restraint: Restraint is used as a last resort in the management of psychomotor agitation as a safety measure. In some cases, a patient might be brought in already in restraint. When using restraint, a proper restraint bed and equipment should be used. Restraint has adverse psychological and physical outcomes [28]. Hence, the patient should be engaged by informing, to the extent allowed, of the need for restraint, and of the expected behavior required to discontinue restraint. The term *chemical restraints*, previously used, is no longer in use, and the practice is not considered humane or up to current standards.

Diagnostic workup: When possible, it is important to conduct a full physical examination as well as bloodwork and urine toxicology. This can help identify the likely differentials.

Once the differential is made, treating the underlying cause promptly is necessary to prevent the recurrence of psychomotor agitation.

14.7.2.1 Vignettes

Case 1: A young man in the emergency room was brought in by emergency medical services (EMS) and the police in handcuffs and leg shackles. He was noted to have a spit screen over his face. He was not in police custody. Upon presentation, EMS and police were unable to provide any personal information about the patient. The report stated that the patient was picked from the street yelling and throwing objects around.

Table 14.1 Pharmacological interventions

Medication Class	Medication	Dose Range/Route	Adverse Effect	Contraindication
Benzodiazepines	Lorazepam	– 1–8 mg/day – PO/SL/IM/IV	– Respiratory depression – Risk of fall and unsteady gait – Oversedation – Memory loss – Paradoxical disinhibition	– Use in neonates or infants unless in the ICU – Acute narrow-angle glaucoma – Severe respiratory depression – Alcohol dependence and abuse – Sleep apnea – Avoid in patient who is already on medication that are sedating.
	Midazolam	– 1–10 mg IM – 0.01–0.05 mg/kg q 10–15 mins until sedation – 5–15 mg IM [22]	–	
	Diazepam	– 10mg – 40mg IV	–	
First-Generation Atipsychotic	Haloperidol	– 2.5– 40 mg/day – Can be repeatead after 14 min	– Extrapyramidal side effects – Neuroleptic malignant syndrome – Torsade de pointes – QT prolongation – Sudden death	– Cardiovascular disease – Dementia-related psychosis – Parkinson's disease – History of seizures – History or allergic reaction
	Fluphenazine	– 2.5– 40 mg/day – Can be repeat after 14 min	– Extrapyramidal side effects – Neuroleptive malignant syndrome – Torsade de pointes – QT prolongation – Sudden death	– Hemodynamic instability
	Chlorpormazine	– 25–150 mg –	– Hypotension – Syncope – Extrapyramidal side effects – Alpha-adrenergic effects	Hemodynamic instability
	Lofexidine	– 9.1–18.2 mg	– Extrapyramidal side effects	– Bronchial asthma – Chronic obstructive pulmonary disease

	Drug	Dosing	Side effects	Contraindications
Second-Generation Antipsychotic	Aripiprazole	– 9.75–30 mg/day [23] – Can be repeated every 2 h	– Headache – Nausea – Dizziness – Somnolence – Akathisia or dystonia – Nonakathisia-related EPS (risk is low)	– Cardiovascular diseases – Documented alergic reaction – Avoid combining with benzodiazepine. – If administered together, monitor for orthostatic hypotension and oversedation.
	Olanzapine	– 2.5–20 mg IM – May use lower doses in the elderly – Can be repeated after 2 hr – Easy to reach maximum dose quickly	– Hypotension – Bradycardia – Excessive sedation – Cardiorespiratory depression	– Substance or alcohol intoxication – Avoid combination with benzodiazepine – Documented alergic reaction
	Ziprasidone	– 10–40 mg/day	– Tosades de pointes – QTc prolongation – Extrapyramidal symptoms – Syncope – Hypertension	– Abnormally elevated QTc interval – Cardiovascular disease – Documented alergic reaction
Ketamine	Ketamine	– 4 mg/kg IM or 1–2 mg/kg IV [24]. – Patient often requires repeated dosing for agitation	– Decreased oxygen saturation – Respiratory depression – Worsening of tachycardia and hypertension – Dissociation – Worsening psychosis (at subanesthetic doses). – Post administration, dysphoric emergence phenomena [25]	– Hypersensitivity. – Pt < 3 years old – Acute alcohol intoxication – Head trauma – HTN – Stroke

ICU, Intensive care unit; IM, intramuscular; IV, intravenous; PO, oral; SL, sublingual.

Table 14.2 Pharmacological interventions for specific considerations

Group	Commonly Used Medications/Combinations

Pediatric	IM
	– Chlorpromazine often starting at a low dose of 25 mg PO/IM to 50 mg PO/IM.
	– Diphenhydramine 25 mg PO or IM to 50 mg PO/IM.
	– Ativan 1 mg PO/IM.
	– Oral
	– Pediatric patients can be offered oral antipsychotic they are on as a treatment option in the case of psychomotor agitation, e.g.:
	  – Risperidone PO
	  – Aripiprazole PO
	
	– Thorazine IM or haloperidol IM at a low dose as a second option

Elderly	– For elderly patients, the risk of sudden death with antipsychotics must be considered clearly prior to use. – Low dose of antipsychotics should be used. – Avoid medication with cholinergic side effect. – Aripiprazole 2 mg PO can be used. – Risperidone 0.5 mg to 1 m q12h. – Seroquel 25–50 mg PO q8h prn. Consider the risk of QTc prolongation. – Olanzapine 2.5 mg PO q12h prn (5 mg max); can be given IM. – Haloperidol started as low as 1–2.5 mg PO q8h prn; can be given IM. – Use benzodiazepines with caution, starting with a low dose of 0.5–1 mg PO or IM [8].
Pregnancy	– Medication must be used with caution due to paucity of data [26]. – Haloperidol alone as first line. – Benzodiazepines alone have been used, but there is no supporting literature – Avoid using multiple medications if possible.
Healthy Adult	Oral/Intramuscular combination: – Haloperidol 5 mg + Lorazapem 2 mg [8]. Patients who received haloperidol + ativan combination alone have lower incidence of hypotension, shorter length of stay, and lower risk of oxygen desaturation [27]. – Adding diphenhydramine does not have added sedation/calming benefit. – Chlorpromazine + diphenhydramine. – Olanzapine + diphenhydramine. – Ziprasidone + ativan.

IM, Intramuscular; *PO*, oral; *prn*, as needed; *q8h*, every 8 hours; *q12h*, every 12 hours.

He was given a single dose of ketamine 200g IM about 20 minutes before arriving in the emergency room.

Treatment Consideration and Discussion

At presentation, the initial goal was to assess the patient and have the handcuffs removed. To achieve this, the patient was wheeled into a quiet room that had been cleared of all dangerous objects. He was engaged verbally to provide information about the reason he was brought in and the plan to remove his handcuffs and leg shackles. While the staff addressed the patient compassionately and professionally, the patient remained loud. The direction was to have the handcuffs removed. After a few minutes the patient started pacing. He refused to give any information about himself or to engage with the treatment team. Despite extensive verbal redirection, he remained uncooperative, attempting to leave the room and to attack the staff when prevented from doing so. As a result, the support staff was forced to restrain the patient manually. He was informed of the need for IM injections. Considering the lack of information about his medical and psychiatric history or allergies, the choice of medication to control the agitation was restricted to lorazepam 2 mg IM stat.

While the standard haloperidol + lorazepam or haloperidol + lorazepam + diphenhydramine was considered, the goal of medication was to maintain calmness and afford the staff to complete the evaluation of the patient. He was also offered oral medication and he refused. After the next modality would have been to place the patient in seclusion to ensure his safety as well as the safety of those in the emergency room while waiting for the medication to take effect. The patient then was noted to be feeling sleepy and seclusion was discontinued, and he was offered a bed.

Differential Diagnosis

Substance-induced disorders

Primary psychiatric diagnosis

Delirium/agitation due to another medical condition

Personality disorder (e.g., antisocial personality disorder)

Medication consideration: Benzodiazepines are the preferred medication when psychomotor agitation is due to either psychiatric causes or substance use. While adding haloperidol is a safe option in most healthy adults, and it can help in the case of psychosis, the lack of information about drug reactions or allergies raises the question about the added benefit.

Case 2: A 71-year-old man was being managed in the medical floor for atrial fibrillation. The patient has a prior psychiatric history of bipolar 1 disorder, cannabis use disorder, severe alcohol use disorder, severe tobacco use disorder, and a prior medical history of hypertension and arrhythmia with an AICD in place. He has no documented allergies. On day 13 of admission, he presents with agitation.

Treatment Consideration and Discussion

The consideration in managing this patient includes age, medical history, and psychiatric history.

Differential Diagnosis

Hyperactive delirium

Substance-related

Anger

Secondary to psychiatric diagnosis

Agitation due to medical condition – medication, medical diagnosis.

Rule out: Due to the length of stay, it is unlikely that the patient's presentation is alcohol related.

The initial approach will be to attempt environmental modification and verbal de-escalation. If both approaches fail and the patient is imminent danger to himself and/or others, a medication approach will be considered. The medication to be used and the dose must be carefully considered because of the risk factors. Medication with minimal cardiovascular risk must be considered. Options with be aripiprazole 2 mg oral, risperidone 0.5 mg oral, olanzapine 2.5 mg oral, or haloperidol 2 mg oral. Options of last resort will be olanzapine IM or haloperidol IM, avoiding benzodiazepines due to their significant adverse effect in advanced age.

References

1. Vieta E, Garriga M, Cardete L, Bernardo M, Lombraña M, Blanch J, et al. Protocol for the management of psychiatric patients with psychomotor agitation. *BMC Psychiatry*. 2017;17(1):1–11.

2. Lindenmayer J.-P. The pathophysiology of agitation. *J Clin Psychiatry*. 2000;61:5–10.

3. Pacciardi B, Mauri M, Cargioli C, Belli S, Cotugno B, Di Paolo L, et al. Issues in the management of acute agitation: how much current guidelines consider safety? *Front Psychiatry*. 2013;4:26.

4. Mansutti I, Venturini M, Palese A. Episodes of psychomotor agitation among medical patients: findings from a longitudinal multicentre study. *Aging Clin Experiment Res*. 2020;32:1101–1110.

5. Jaber S, Chanques G, Altairac C, Sebbane M, Vergne C, Perrigault P-F, et al. A prospective study of agitation in a medical-surgical ICU: incidence, risk factors, and outcomes. *Chest*. 2005;128 (4):2749–2757.

6. Anand A, Verhoeff P, Seneca N, Zoghbi SS, Seibyl JP, Charney DS, et al. Brain SPECT imaging of amphetamine-induced dopamine release in euthymic bipolar disorder patients. *Am J Psychiatry*. 2000;157(7):1108–1114.

7. Sanacora G, Gueorguieva R, Epperson CN, Wu Y-T, Appel M, Rothman DL, et al. Subtype-specific alterations of γ-aminobutyric acid and glutamatein patients with major depression. *Archiv Gen Psychiatry*. 2004;61(7):705–713.

8. Hughes DH. Emergency psychiatry: acute psychopharmacological management of the aggressive psychotic patient. *Psychiatr Serv*. 1999;50(9):1135–1137.

9. Steinert T. Prediction of inpatient violence. *Acta Psychiatrica Scandinavica*. 2002;106:133–141.

10. Agüera-Ortiz L, García-Ramos R, Grandas Pérez FJ, López-Álvarez J, Montes Rodríguez JM, Olazarán Rodríguez FJ, et al. Depression in Alzheimer's disease: a Delphi consensus on etiology, risk factors, and clinical management. *Front Psychiatry*. 2021;12:638–651.

11. Angst J, Gamma A, Benazzi F, Ajdacic V, Rössler W. Does psychomotor agitation in major depressive episodes indicate bipolarity? Evidence from the Zurich Study. *Europ Archiv Psychiatry Clin Neurosci*. 2009;259:55–63.

12. Day R. Psychomotor agitation: poorly defined and badly measured. *J Affective Disorders*. 1999;55(2–3):89–98.

13. Iwanami T, Maeshima H, Baba H, Satomura E, Namekawa Y, Shimano T, et al. Psychomotor agitation in major depressive disorder is a predictive factor of mood-switching. *J Affective Disorders*. 2015;170:185–189.

14. Childers MK, Holland D. Psychomotor agitation following gabapentin use in brain injury. *Brain Injury*. 1997;11 (7):537–540.

15. Woods P, Almvik R. The Brøset violence checklist (BVC). *Acta Psychiatrica Scandinavica*. 2002;106:103–105.

16. Huber CG, Lambert M, Naber D, Schacht A, Hundemer H-P, Wagner TT, et al. Validation of a Clinical Global Impression Scale for Aggression (CGI-A)

in a sample of 558 psychiatric patients. *Schizophrenia Res.* 2008;100 (1–3):342–348.

17. Kay SR, Wolkenfeld F, Murrill LM. Profiles of aggression among psychiatric patients: I. Nature and prevalence. *J Nerv Mental Dis.* 1988;176(9):539–546.

18. Zeller SL, Rhoades RW. Systematic reviews of assessment measures and pharmacologic treatments for agitation. *Clin Therapeutics.* 2010;32(3):403–425.

19. Marder SR. A review of agitation in mental illness: treatment guidelines and current therapies. *J Clin Psychiatry.* 2006;67(Suppl 10):13–21.

20. Richmond JS, Berlin JS, Fishkind AB, Holloman Jr GH, Zeller SL, Wilson MP, et al. Verbal de-escalation of the agitated patient: consensus statement of the American Association for Emergency Psychiatry Project BETA De-escalation Workgroup. *West J Emerg Med.* 2012;13 (1):17.

21. Citrome L. New treatments for agitation. *Psychiatric Quarterly.* 2004;75:197–213.

22. Kousgaard SJ, Licht RW, Nielsen RE. Effects of intramuscular midazolam and lorazepam on acute agitation in non-Elderly Subjects: a systematic review. *Pharmacopsychiatry.* 2017;50(4):129–135.

23. Josiassen RC, Shaughnessy RA. IM aripiprazole for acute agitation. *Curr Psychiatry.* 2007;6(7):103–107.

24. Riddell J, Tran A, Bengiamin R, Hendey GW, Armenian P. Ketamine as a first-line treatment for severely agitated emergency department patients. *Am J Emerg Med.* 2017;35(7):1000-1004.

25. Hopper AB, Vilke GM, Castillo EM, Campillo A, Davie T, Wilson MP. Ketamine use for acute agitation in the emergency department. *J Emerg Med.* 2015;48(6):712–719.

26. Allen MH, Currier GW, Carpenter D, Ross RW, Docherty JP. The expert consensus guideline series: treatment of behavioral emergencies 2005. *J Psychiatric Pract.* 2005;11:5–108.

27. Jeffers T, Darling B, Edwards C, Vadiei N. Efficacy of combination haloperidol, lorazepam, and diphenhydramine vs. combination haloperidol and lorazepam in the treatment of acute agitation: a multicenter retrospective cohort study. *J Emerg Med.* 2022;62 (4):516–523.

28. Hamers JP, Huizing AR. Why do we use physical restraints in the elderly? *Zeitschrift für Gerontologie und Geriatrie.* 2005;38(1):19–25.

The Suicidal Patient

Ryan E. Lawrence

15.1 Introduction

Suicide is an adverse event with devastating consequences for all persons involved: the victim, family and friends, the community, and any treating clinicians. Suicide has been a difficult problem for clinicians and researchers to study and improve, not only because of the high stakes involved but also because suicide has a low base rate, making it challenging to study with quantitative methods. Nevertheless, suicide and the suicidal patient are common enough that all clinicians are likely to encounter it regularly. The more clinicians can educate themselves about risk factors, engage patients in screening and assessment, and implement appropriate interventions, the more they will position themselves to interrupt the pathway from suicide ideation to suicidal behavior to death by suicide.

15.2 Epidemiology and Risk Factors

Suicide is a major problem around the globe. While precise data are difficult to collect, the World Health Organization has estimated that more than 700,000 people died from suicide in 2019, with 77% of these suicides occurring in low-and middle-income countries [1]. Moreover, the World Health Organization estimates that for every suicide death there are more than 20 suicide attempts.[2] The severe impact of suicide on families and communities around the world is beyond measure.

The risk of suicide is higher among some populations compared with others. Table 15.1 lists several commonly identified risk factors.

An especially strong link exists between mental health problems and suicide risk, as demonstrated in a recent case-control study among a general population sample in the United States (N = 2,674 persons who died by suicide and 267,400 patients who did not die from suicide) [3]. An estimated 51.3% of persons who died by suicide had a diagnosed mental health condition (an anxiety disorder, attention deficit–hyperactivity disorder, bipolar disorder, depressive disorder, or schizophrenia spectrum disorder; substance use and personality disorders were not analyzed) versus 12.7% of the control population (adjusted odds ratio [aOR] 6.84). Among the five disorders analyzed, patients with schizophrenia spectrum were the most likely to die by suicide (aOR 15.00), followed by bipolar disorder (aOR 13.17), depressive disorders (aOR 7.20), anxiety disorders (aOR 5.84), and attention deficit–hyperactivity disorder (aOR 2.37). When integrating the relative odds and the prevalence of these disorders, an estimated 27% of suicide deaths were attributable to depressive disorders, 22% to anxiety disorders, 8% to bipolar disorder, 2% to schizophrenia spectrum disorders, and 1% to attention deficit–hyperactivity disorder.

Table 15.1 Suicide related risk and protective factors

Risk Factors		Potential Protective Factors*
Mood disorders	Psychosocial stressors (e.g., relationship disruptions, financial problems)	Social connections
Anxiety disorders	Recent loss or humiliation	Strong relationships
Psychosis	Isolation	Religious and cultural beliefs
Substance use	High impulsivity	Reasons for living
Personality disorders	Agitation	Having goals for the future
Prior self-harm or suicide attempt	Access to lethal means (e.g., gun, pesticide)	Mental health care engagement
Recent psychiatric hospitalization	Attention deficit– hyperactivity disorder	Prior adaptive responses to similar circumstances
History of trauma	Chronic pain	
Family history of suicide	Traumatic brain injury	
Lesbian, gay, bisexual, transgender, intersex, other sexual minorities	Experiencing discrimination (e.g., migrants, refugees, indigenous people)	
Incarcerated persons		

* These factors may or may not be relevant or protective for specific individuals. A follow-up conversation about how each factor is helpful to the person is necessary before considering it a true protective factor.
Sources: Ryan & Oquendo 2020 [9]; World Health Organization 2022 [21]; Mann & Rizk 2020 [4].

Importantly, while suicidal behavior occurs in many psychiatric disorders, most persons with these disorders never attempt suicide. Many factors contribute to suicidal behavior, not simply the presence or severity of a psychiatric illness [4].

15.3 Clinical Presentation and Diagnosis

15.3.1 Screening and Assessment

While many risk factors have been identified, predicting suicide with any degree of precision (both who will die from suicide and in what time frame) is notoriously difficult. A study by Olfson et al. illustrates this [5]. The study followed Medicaid recipients for 1 year after an episode of deliberate self-harm (N = 61,297 adults, ages 18–64, with a clinical diagnosis of deliberate self-harm). Among this very high-risk cohort, 12,015 persons were treated for a subsequent episode of deliberate self-harm (nonfatal) and another 243 died from suicide during that year. While this corresponds to persons with deliberate self-harm having a 1-year suicide rate 37 times greater than the general population, it is still a very small number of suicide deaths spread across a large population and an extended time frame (much can happen in a person's life over 1 year). Trying to predict who will die by suicide is a daunting task (in this dataset, approximately 4 per 1,000 high-risk patients per year).

Many screening and risk assessment tools have been developed in an effort to aid researchers and clinicians in identifying persons at risk for suicide. Unfortunately, these tools have generally performed poorly in assessments of their predictive validity. In one systematic review of 15 instruments, none of the instruments assessed met the authors' predetermined utility benchmarks (80% sensitivity and 50% specificity) for suicide attempt or suicide [6]. Positive predictive value was low for both suicide attempt (7–40%) and suicide (1–13%). The authors commented that they found no scientific support for the use of suicide risk instruments for predicting suicidal acts.

On the other side, there is a risk that screening and assessment tools can be falsely reassuring. In one study of question 9 on the Patient Health Questionnaire ("Over the last 2 weeks, how often have you been bothered by thoughts that you would be better off dead or thoughts of hurting yourself?" N = 509,945 adult outpatients in various settings), 39% of suicide attempts and 36% of suicide deaths occurring within 30 days of completing the Patient Health Questionnaire happened among persons who responded "not at all" to this question [7].

Despite many controversies surrounding their use and interpretation, regulatory bodies have moved forward with mandating suicide screening and assessment tools in a variety of settings. For example, The Joint Commission requires that all patients who are being evaluated or treated for behavioral health conditions be screened for suicidal ideation using a validated screening tool [8].

As these tools are deployed, it is important for clinicians to maintain a balanced view of their benefits and limitations. Screening and assessment tools likely have value as educational aides for less experienced staff and as pedagogical tools [6]. For all clinical staff, regardless of experience level, there is value in having a consistent and structured way of eliciting information and weighing risk and protective factors [9]. At the same time, clinicians should keep in mind the gaps in the evidence base supporting their use [10], their reliance on patients' willingness to divulge sensitive information about suicidal thoughts or impulses [4], and their vulnerability to missing suicide thoughts during intervening periods between assessments (e.g., during the same 1-week period, 58% of persons who denied any past-week ideation on the Scale for Suicide Ideation reported ideation when assessed 6x per day via ecological momentary assessment [11]). Additionally, many of the studies validating screening and assessment tools were carried out in research settings, leaving open questions about how these tools perform when paired with more global clinical assessments [6].

15.3.2 Clinical Assessment

Best practice for evaluating suicide risk is to conduct a full clinical assessment [9]. This usually incorporates screening and assessment tools as well as a medical and psychiatric history, a family history, an assessment of current symptoms, a mental status exam, and collateral history (usually from a family member, friend, or another clinician). The goals are to elicit risk and protective factors (see Table 15.1), to distinguish between what is acute and what is chronic, to identify treatable or modifiable risk factors, and to make a

Table 15.2 Suggestions for framing the suicide risk assessment conversation

Goal	Possible Wording
Normalize the conversation	"Suicide thoughts are common enough that we make a point of asking everybody some safety questions."
Establish the stakes	"We have had people come through here who have gone on to hurt themselves. If there is an opportunity to reduce the chances of that happening, I want to take the opportunity."
Validate the patient's concerns	"I recognize this can be a hard topic to speak about. Please let me know if there are any topics that are especially difficult for you, and I will try to be sensitive."
Establish that the clinician and patient are on the same team	"I am going to do what I can to be helpful. I can make better recommendations if I know what you have been experiencing than if I do not know."

clinical judgment about the short- and long-term risk and the most appropriate clinical intervention.

Throughout the process clinicians must remain as sensitive as possible to what patients want, which may occasionally depart from what patient safety and good clinical practice require [9]. This can create a complicated dynamic between the patient and the clinician, especially when clinicians ask probing questions to elicit risk factors and patients fear their answers will lead to an involuntary trip to the emergency department or inpatient hospitalization [4]. Framing the conversation may help build an alliance and orient the patient to the goals of the conversation (Table 15.2). In light of the complicated relationship dynamic and competing incentives at play, clinicians should notice verbal and nonverbal cues, paying attention not only to what patients say but also to how they say it (e.g., patients may be engaged or disengaged; transparent and forthcoming or guarded and minimizing; insightful and self-reflective or superficial and dismissive; treatment seeking or discharge focused; helpful in facilitating the assessment or obstructive).

Identifying protective factors is an important part of the overall assessment. It is important to recognize that many putative protective factors are context dependent, and what is protective for one person may not be protective for another. For example, there is evidence that religious affiliation can protect against suicide attempts and possibly suicide [12], and also evidence that religion can be associated with increased risk of suicide ideation and suicide among some populations [13]. Engaging patients in a discussion of how a particular factor is protective for them will help the clinician appreciate the context, role, and relative importance of each protective factor.

When suicide thoughts are identified, they should be classified across several domains [9]:

- Activity level – ranging from a passive wish for nonexistence to active thoughts of killing oneself
- Intensity – ranging from weak and easily dismissed to strong and consuming
- Duration – ranging from fleeting to long-lasting

- Frequency – ranging from rare to chronic
- Planning stage – ranging from no method or plan to a detailed plan with a clear timeline and preparatory steps taken

  The clinical assessment should make special note of proximal warning signs [9]:
- Frank suicide ideation and planning
- Talking or writing about suicide (including text messages and social media posts)
- Increasing substance use
- Worsening psychiatric symptoms (depression, anxiety, psychosis)
- Hopelessness, feeling trapped
- Feeling there are no reasons for living
- Agitation, anger, rage
- Social withdrawal
- Feeling like a burden on others
- Insomnia

When present, these proximal warning signs should be explored and discussed further and may be grounds for escalating to a higher level of care.

15.4 Pathophysiology and Neurobiology of Suicidal Behavior

Multiple lines of research have shown that whether or not an individual progresses from a major life stressor to a suicide attempt or death by suicide depends in large part on underlying biological factors. The stress-diathesis model for suicidal behavior proposes that suicidal behavior is the result of a complex interaction between an acute stressor (sometimes called a proximal risk factor) and a diathesis (sometimes called distal factors suggestive of an underlying vulnerability) [4].

- Examples of acute stressors include relationship or financial problems (external stressors) or severe depressive symptoms (internal stressors).
- Examples of a high-risk diathesis include excessive subjective distress when depressed, attentional bias toward negative stimuli, altered decision-making with a tendency toward impulsivity and aggression, learning difficulties including cognitive rigidity and memory problems, and social distortions including a perceived lack of reciprocal caring relationships and increased rejection sensitivity.

With the stress-diathesis model in mind, a growing body of research is examining the various states and traits that lead some persons to progress toward suicidal behavior while others do not. To date, a large number of biological findings have been reported describing genetic vulnerabilities, disrupted neural circuitry, neurotransmitter dysfunction (especially serotonin), the hypothalamic–pituitary–adrenal axis, and neuroinflammation (Table 15.3).

Findings from neuroimaging are especially suggestive of an underlying neurobiological diathesis among some high-risk populations [4]. These include (1) enhanced negative affective and self-referential processing networks that may underlie excessive subjective distress, (2) structural and functional deficits that correlate with more subjective depression and potentially less top-down control, (3) differential response to pleasant versus negative facial expressions that may correspond to social distortions, (4) serotonergic release deficits, and (5) glutamate and opioid abnormalities that may affect memory, learning, and reward (Table 15.3).

Table 15.3 Neurobiological observations associated with increased suicide risk

Genetics:
- Twin studies have long suggested a heritable component to suicidal behavior.
- At least 40 genes have been associated with suicidal behavior, independent of psychiatric diagnosis.
- Candidate genes appear to be involved with inflammation, gamma-aminobutyric acid and glutamate neurotransmission, hypothalamic–pituitary–adrenal axis, neurogenesis, anerobic energy production, circadian clock regulation, and tyrosine catabolism.
- DNA methylation patterns among suicide decedents show alterations at genetic loci in the prefrontal cortex, cerebellum, and globally in the brain.

Neural circuits and findings from brain imaging studies:
- Neural circuitry dysfunction likely includes enhanced negative affective and self-referential processing networks, perhaps leading to excessive subjective distress. Implicated regions include the ventromedial prefrontal cortex, medial orbitofrontal cortex, rostral anterior cingulate cortex, insula, and ventral striatum.
- Structural and functional defects of several regions (dorsomedial prefrontal cortex, dorsolateral prefrontal cortex, ventrolateral prefrontal cortex, dorsal anterior cingulate cortex) may contribute to more severe subjective depression symptoms and less top-down control over ventromedial prefrontal cortex regions, affecting decision-making.
- Affected persons show differential activation of the orbitofrontal cortex in response to negative versus pleasant facial expressions, which may be related to excessive distress and social distortions.
- Persons with high-lethality suicidal behavior and death by suicide show serotonergic release deficits in the ventral prefrontal cortex and anterior cingulate cortex.
- Abnormalities of the glutamate and opioid systems may affect memory, learning, and reward mechanisms.
- Persons who died from suicide tend to have smaller gray matter volume in the dorsolateral prefrontal cortex and hippocampus, suggesting impaired decision-making, learning, and memory.
- High-lethality suicide attempters have larger prefrontal cortex and insula volumes. Violent attempters have greater caudate volume.
- Suicide attempters with a family history of suicidal behavior have smaller volumes in temporal regions, the dorsolateral prefrontal cortex, and the putamen.
- For persons with mood disorders, a prior suicide attempt is associated with impaired white matter integrity (lower fractional anisotropy on diffusion tensor imaging studies) suggesting impaired top-down executive control and increased impulsivity.
- Adolescent and adult suicide attempters show lower functional connectivity in the default mode network during resting-state functional MRI.
- Task-based functional MRI studies suggest suicide attempters have less activity in the dorsolateral prefrontal cortex, rostral anterior cingulate cortex, dorsal anterior cingulate cortex, thalamus, and insula when performing decision-making tasks.

Neurotransmitter disruptions:
- Depressed persons with low cerebrospinal fluid levels of 5-hydroxyindoleacetic acid (a serotonin metabolite) have increased suicide risk. Serotonin deficits likely involve reduced serotonin neuron firing and less release.
- Suicidal behavior is associated with increased raphe nucleus serotonin 1A receptor binding.

Table 15.3 (cont.)

- Depressed persons who died from suicide show less noradrenergic activity (fewer brain-projecting noradrenergic neurons in the rostral locus coeruleus and increased beta-adrenergic receptor binding in the prefrontal cortex). Depressed suicide attempters show less urinary and plasma levels of 3-methoxy-4-hydroxyphenylglycol, a metabolite of norepinephrine.
- Suicidal behavior is associated with altered expression of the glutamate receptor N-methyl-D-aspartate, alpha-amino-3-hydroxy-5-methyl-4-isoxazolepropionic acid, and kainite glutamate receptors.
- Suicidal individuals with post-traumatic stress disorder show increased metabotropic glutamate receptor type 5.
- The kappa opioid receptor system may be involved in the negative affect that often accompanies suicidal ideation. The mu opioid system is related to suicide risk, perhaps through regulation of reward circuits and social functions.

Hypothalamic–pituitary–adrenal axis and the stress response:
- Non-suppression on the dexamethasone suppression test predicts death by suicide.
- In the Trier Social Stress Test, suicide attempters show lower pre-task baseline cortisol and blunted total cortisol output.
- Suicide attempters with high levels of aggression and impulsivity have the strongest cortisol response, suggesting a subset of suicide attempters where this stress response is especially significant.

Apoptosis and neurotrophic pathways:
- Brain-derived neurotrophic factor and expression of its receptor tyrosine kinase B genes is reduced among persons who died from suicide.

Neuroinflammation:
- Multiple inflammatory markers are associated with increased suicide risk (e.g., C-reactive protein, neutrophil-to-lymphocyte ratio, proinflammatory interleukins, cytokines that regulate the immune response, tumor necrosis factor – alpha, tissue growth factor beta 1, vascular endothelial growth factor).
- Suicidal individuals show reduced anti-inflammatory markers (e.g., interleukin 2 and 4, interferon-gamma).
- Activated microglia and brain translocator protein (found in mitochondria of activated glial cells) are associated with increased suicide risk independent of whether a psychiatric disorder is present.

Lipids:
- Associations may exist between lipids (triglycerides, total cholesterol, high- and low-density lipoprotein cholesterol, polyunsaturated fatty acids, apolipoproteins) and suicide risk, possibly via their roles in neuroinflammation or the hypothalamic–pituitary–adrenal axis

Sources: Mann & Rizk 2020 [4]; Ryan & Oquendo 2020 [9].

Important goals for this line of research are to improve risk stratification, to identify novel treatment targets and to enable patients and clinicians to select more individualized and targeted therapies [4].

15.5 Treatment and Management
Many interventions have been tried in an effort to reduce suicide risk. Among those with the strongest evidence base are: (1) training non-psychiatrist physicians to diagnose and

treat depression; (2) improving outreach during high-risk periods (e.g., after discharge from hospitals or emergency departments); and (3) means restriction focusing on the most common methods in each country [4]. Within these broad categories, several specific interventions have been found to be especially helpful.

15.5.1 Restriction of Lethal Means

Modifying the environment to restrict access to common methods of suicide has some of the strongest empirical support of any intervention [14]. It is likely effective because it does not require speed or specificity (identifying and connecting with high-risk persons during a moment of crisis). Suicide attempts are usually method-specific, and suicidal individuals rarely switch methods in a moment of crisis, and if suicidal persons do change methods, they frequently use less lethal means. Limiting access to pesticides, carbon monoxide, jumping points, firearms, and other methods have been associated with reductions in suicide rates in countries around the world. Methods that are common, highly lethal, and account for a substantial proportion of suicide deaths are excellent candidates for means restriction initiatives.

15.5.2 Outreach after Discharge

Suicide risk is especially high in the weeks to months after patients are discharged from an inpatient hospital or an emergency room following treatment for a suicide attempt or intense suicide ideation. Follow-up contact and active outreach during this period are associated with reductions in suicide risk [4, 15]. These contacts may be as basic as sending a postcard, making a phone call, or sending a caring text message. Depending on how they are structured, they present an inexpensive and scalable method for correcting social cognitive distortions (for persons at risk of perceiving the social network as hostile or unhelpful), projecting helpful options to patients in crisis, identifying symptom recurrence, or improving engagement with treatment services.

15.5.3 Antidepressant Medication

Data describing the relationship between antidepressant medication and suicide risk are complex and difficult to interpret due to many factors including inconsistent definitions of suicide risk, the rarity of suicide, diverse study designs, different patient populations, and active exclusion of suicidal patients from many research trials. Consequently, analyses can be found suggesting that antidepressants increase, decrease, or have no direct effect on suicide risk. Even so, there is likely some reduction in suicide risk among depressed persons taking antidepressants [16].

15.5.4 Lithium

Lithium is the only somatic treatment with high-quality data documenting its anti-suicide effects in mood disorders [16]. Across all mood disorders, lithium has shown superiority to placebo for both suicide and all-cause mortality. The anti-suicide effect of lithium occurs rapidly (measurable within a month) and can occur independently from its effect on mood in patients with recurrent affective disorders. Long-term lithium treatment may be necessary, as stopping lithium is associated with a return to pre-treatment levels of suicide risk. Its benefits for suicide risk should be weighed against the need for close clinical monitoring due to the risk of toxicity, its potential to cause thyroid or kidney problems, and the possibility of interactions with other medications.

15.5.5 Clozapine

Clozapine is the only somatic treatment with high-quality data showing anti-suicide effects in schizophrenia [16]. Among persons with schizophrenia, treatment with clozapine is associated with significant decrease in overall mortality, and this effect occurs largely through its effect on suicidal behavior. Clozapine is superior to no treatment and to treatment with other antipsychotic medications. In one multinational, randomized, 2-year study comparing clozapine versus olanzapine, in which all patients were seen using the same visit frequency schedule (to account for the closer monitoring required of clozapine patients), persons randomized to clozapine had fewer suicide attempts, fewer hospitalizations and other rescue interventions, and fewer antidepressant prescriptions [16].

15.5.6 Ketamine

Low-dose ketamine (often 0.5 mg/kg delivered by intravenous infusion) differs from other somatic treatments in that it can produce rapid improvement in suicide risk among some patients with depression and suicide ideation [16]. Symptom reduction is often measurable by post-treatment day 1, with improvements lasting for approximately 1–2 weeks. Ketamine can improve both depressive symptoms and suicide risk, and these effects appear to be at least partially independent. An intranasal formulation of Esketamine (the S enantiomer of ketamine) is approved by the US Food and Drug Administration for use in the treatment of patients with depression and suicide ideation.

15.5.7 Psychotherapy

Cognitive behavioral therapy has been shown to decrease suicidal behavior in adolescents and adults with depression, in adults with borderline personality disorder, and in adolescents with substance use disorders [15]. It likely works by promoting more effective coping strategies (e.g., cognitive restructuring), improving negative problem orientation and emotion regulation, reducing impulsivity, and attenuating suicide ideation.

Dialectical behavioral therapy reduces suicide attempts, reduces hospitalizations for suicide ideation, and lessens medical consequences from self-harm behaviors [15]. It is a skills-based approach that teaches mindfulness, distress tolerance, interpersonal effectiveness, and emotional regulation. Core elements include a skills training group, individual therapy, phone coaching, and a consultation team that provides support for the treating therapists.

15.5.8 Safety Planning Intervention

The Safety Planning Intervention is a written, prioritized list of coping skills and supportive resources that patients can utilize during a suicidal crisis. Its basic elements include (1) recognizing warning signs of an impending suicidal crisis, (2) employing internal coping strategies, (3) using social contacts and social settings as a way of distracting from suicidal thoughts and impulses, (4) turning to family members or friends to help resolve the crisis, (5) contacting mental health professionals, and (6) restricting access to lethal means [17]. In a sample of patients discharged from emergency departments following a suicide-related visit, persons who received a combination of Safety Planning Intervention and follow-up phone calls (at least two contacts, occurring weekly until the patient began treatment or withdrew) were half as likely to engage in suicidal behaviors over the next 6 months compared with patients who received usual care (3.03% versus 5.29%) and were approximately twice as likely to engage in outpatient behavioral health care [18].

15.5.9 Zero Suicide Model

The Zero Suicide Model is a framework and toolkit promoted in the United States by the National Action Alliance for Suicide Prevention that integrates many of the evidence-based interventions described in the preceding sections. Its name represents an aspirational goal of preventing all suicides by patients engaged in health care systems. Its four clinical components are (1) suicide screening and risk assessment, (2) systematic suicide care protocols that include safety planning and lethal means reduction, (3) evidence-based treatments targeting suicidal thoughts and behaviors and other mental health issues, and (4) support during care transitions (including follow-up after discharge from acute care settings). It also includes three administrative components focused on leadership, training, and quality improvement. In a sample of 110 community-based outpatient clinics, greater fidelity to Zero Suicide organizational practices was associated with lower risk for suicide attempts and suicide deaths [19].

15.6 Support Following a Suicide Death

A clinician's risk of having a patient die by suicide increases the longer the clinician is in practice [20]. Toolkits and manuals have been developed that provide structure and guidance in the aftermath of a suicide death. These include the Texas postvention toolkit, evidence-based practices endorsed by the Suicide Prevention Resource Center, and the Loving Outreach to Survivors of Suicide Program. They promote practical interventions and best practices that are applicable to both lay and professional caregivers. They are intended to foster relationships among survivors, to build community resources, and to decrease the risk of contagion. Survey evidence suggests these toolkits are underutilized [20].

15.7 Conclusion

The process of identifying, assessing, and managing suicide risk is both an art and a science [9]. Clinicians who undertake this important responsibility are increasingly supported by a body of evidence-based best practices. Moreover, organizational practices are coalescing around a standard of care. By focusing on good processes and embracing ongoing quality improvement, there is reason for optimism that suicidal behavior can be reduced and countless lives can be saved.

References

1. World Health Organization. Suicide worldwide in 2019: global health estimates. 2021 https://www.who.int/publications/i/item/9789240026643 (accessed December 22, 2022).

2. World Health Organization. Suicide Prevention. 2022. www.who.int/health-topics/suicide#tab=tab_1 (accessed December 22, 2022).

3. H.-H. Yeh, J. Westphal, Y. Hu, et al. Diagnosed mental health conditions and

risk of suicide mortality. *Psychiatr Serv* 2019; **70(9)**: 750–757.

4. J. J. Mann, M. M. Rizk. A brain-centric model of suicidal behavior. *Am J Psychiatry* 2020; **177(10)**: 902–916.

5. M. Olfson, M. Wall, S. Wang, et al. Suicide following deliberate self-harm. *Am J Psychiatry* 2017; **174(8)**: 765–774.

6. B. Runeson, J. Odeberg, A. Pettersson, et al. Instruments for the assessment of suicide risk: a systematic review evaluating the certainty of the evidence. *PLoS ONE* 2017; **12(7)**: e0180292.

7. G. E. Simon, K. J. Coleman, R. C. Rossom, et al. Risk of suicide attempt and suicide death following completion of the Patient Health Questionnaire depression module in community practice. *J Clin Psychiatry* 2016; **77(2)**: 221–227.

8. The Joint Commission. National Patient Safety Goals Effective January 2023 for the Hospital Program. 2022 www .jointcommission.org (accessed December 27, 2022).

9. E. P. Ryan, M. A. Oquendo. Suicide risk assessment and prevention: challenges and opportunities. *Focus* 2020; **18**: 88–99.

10. E. O'Connor, M. Henninger, L. A. Perdue, et al. Screening for depression, anxiety, and suicide risk in adults: a systematic evidence review for the U.S. Preventive Services Task Force. Evidence Synthesis Number 223. AHRQ Publication No 22-05295-ER-1, August 2022 www.uspreventiveservicestaskforce .org (accessed December 27, 2022).

11. I. Gratch, T.-H. Choo, H. Galfalvy, et al. Detecting suicidal thoughts: the power of ecological momentary assessment. *Depress Anxiety* 2021; **38(1)**: 8–16.

12. R. E. Lawrence, M. A. Oquendo, B. Stanley. Religion and suicide risk: a systematic review. *Arch Suicide Res* 2016; **20(1)**: 1–21.

13. R. E. Lawrence, D. Brent, J. J. Mann, et al. Religion as a risk factor for suicide attempt and suicide ideation among depressed patients. *J Nerv Ment Dis* 2016; **204(11)**: 845–850.

14. P. S. F. Yip, E. Caine, S. Yousuf, et al. Means restriction for suicide prevention. *The Lancet* 2012; **379(9834)**: 2393–2399.

15. J. J. Mann, C. A. Michel, R. P. Auerbach. Improving suicide prevention through evidence-based strategies: a systematic review. *Am J Psychiatry* 2021; **178(7)**: 611–624.

16. E. M. Hawkins, W. Coryell, S. Leung, et al. Effects of somatic treatments on suicidal ideation and completed suicides. *Brain Behav* 2021; **11(11)**: e2381.

17. B. Stanley, G. K. Brown. Safety planning intervention: a brief intervention to mitigate suicide risk. *Cogn Behav Pract* 2012; **19(2)**: 256–264.

18. B. Stanley, G. K. Brown, L. A. Brenner. Comparison of the safety planning intervention with follow-up vs usual care of suicidal patients treated in the emergency department. *JAMA Psychiatry* 2018; **75(9)**: 894–900.

19. D. M. Layman, J. Kammer, E. Leckman-Westin, et al. The relationship between suicidal behaviors and Zero Suicide organizational best practices in outpatient mental health clinics. *Psychiatr Serv* 2021; **72(10)**: 1118–1125.

20. M. D. Erlich, S. A. Rolin, L. B. Dixon, et al. Why we need to enhance suicide postvention: evaluating a survey of psychiatrists' behaviors after the suicide of a patient. *J Nerv Ment Dis* 2017; **205(7)**: 507–511.

21. World Health Organization. Suicide. 2022. www.who.int/news-room/fact-sheets/detail/suicide (accessed December 22, 2022).

Depressive Disorders

Carolina Olmos and Joao Quevedo

16.1 Introduction

According to the World Health Organization (WHO), depression is a leading cause of disability worldwide and greatly contributes to the global burden of disease. In a WHO report released in 2019, the global prevalence of depression in adults estimated at 5%. Moreover, in an international survey with communities from 14 different countries, the lifetime prevalence of unipolar depressive disorder was of 12% [1]. It has been estimated that during the initial year of the COVID-19 pandemic, the global prevalence of anxiety and depression increased by an impressive 25% according to the WHO report released in March 2022. In the face of this massive increase in prevalence and lack of sufficient resources to effectively treat all patients suffering from depressive disorders, it is of utmost importance that depressive disorders are well understood, screened for, recognized and treated by physicians in the community.

Worldwide, women have a twofold higher prevalence of major depressive disorders (MDD) than men. Potential reasons for this difference are thought to involve differing psychosocial stressors for women and men, hormonal differences, childbirth effects, and behavioral models of learned helplessness. Another well-known risk factor for depression is lacking close interpersonal relationships and being separated, divorced, or widowed [2]. In regards to socioeconomic status, data differs. Some authors find there is no correlation between socioeconomic status and MDD [2], while others have found that the 12-month prevalence of MDD is higher in lower-income households [3].

Across all the depressive disorders, the common presented feature is that of sad, empty, or irritable moods to a degree that would significantly affect the patient's ability to function. This group of disorders include disruptive mood dysregulation disorder, major depressive disorder, persistent depressive disorder, premenstrual dysphoric disorder, substance-/medication-induced depressive disorder, depressive disorder due to another medical condition, other specified depressive disorder, and unspecified depressive disorder. The main differences between them are timing, duration, and/or presumed etiology [4]. Disruptive mood dysregulation disorder (DMDD) and premenstrual dysphoric disorder (PMDD) are addressed in other chapters of this book.

16.2 Clinical Presentation/Diagnosis

16.2.1 Major Depressive Disorder

A major depressive episode can be defined as a period of at least 2 weeks' duration, with the patient presenting at least one of the following symptoms: having depressed mood or

Table 16.1 Characterization of the severity of major depressive disorder episodes

Mild	Few, if any, symptoms in excess of those required to make the diagnosis are present, the intensity of the symptoms is distressing but manageable, and result in minor impairment in social or occupational functioning.
Moderate	Number and intensity of symptoms and/or functional impairment are between those specified for "mild" and "severe."
Severe	Number of symptoms is substantially in excess of that required to make the diagnosis, intensity of the symptoms is seriously distressing and unmanageable, and there is a marked interference with social and occupational functioning.

Reproduced from DSM-5-TR [4].

loss of interest or pleasure for most of the day, nearly every day. Additionally, the patient must have at least four other symptoms from the following list: appetite and unintentional weight changes, sleep changes (either insomnia or hypersomnia), activity level changes (psychomotor agitation or retardation), lack of energy, intense feelings of inappropriate guilt or worthlessness, difficulties concentrating and making decisions, and recurrent thoughts of death or suicide. These symptoms must also cause a change from previous levels of functioning in social, occupational, or other important areas of the patient's life [2, 4].

For diagnostic purposes, clinicians should be certain that those symptoms are not better explained by any other medical condition or represent the effects of any substance use. It should also be noted that symptoms appearing in the context of a significant loss, such as in bereavement, may resemble a depressive episode. Clinicians should evaluate if symptoms, including their intensity and duration, are compatible with the personal and cultural aspects involved in the expression of grief in a particular patient. Last, for a diagnosis of MDD, the patient should not have a history of manic or hypomanic episodes.

In order to better describe and characterize the depressive episode, the provider should investigate and document if the episode was a single episode or recurrent. An episode is considered recurrent when there is a period of at least 2 consecutive months between episodes without significant symptoms. It is also necessary to gather information about the severity, presence or absence of psychotic symptoms, and the patient's current remission level. Severity is assessed based on the number of symptoms and the degree of functional disability they cause, as described in Table 16.1.

Major depressive episodes, as per DSM-5-TR, can also be classified according to different specifiers (Table 16.2). Last, when describing a patient with a recent major depressive episode that no longer meets the acute criteria, the terms "full remission" (no symptoms are currently present) or "partial remission" (some symptoms are still present but not enough to meet the full criteria for a current depressive episode) can be utilized.

16.2.2 Persistent Depressive Disorder

The main feature of persistent depressive disorder (PDD) is having depressed mood occurring for most of the day, for more days than not, for at least 2 years or at least 1 year in children or adolescents (for the latter, mood can be irritable instead of depressed).

Table 16.2 DSM-5-TR specifiers for major depressive disorder

With anxious distress	Presence of two or more symptoms from the following list, during most days of the current MDD episode or persistent depressive disorder: • Feeling keyed up or tense • Feeling unusually restless • Decreased concentration due to worry • Fear something awful might happen • Feeling that the individual might be of losing self-control Specify current severity: Mild: two symptoms Moderate: Three symptoms Moderate-severe: Four to five symptoms Severe: Four to five symptoms and motor agitation
With mixed features	Presence of three or more of the following hypomanic or manic symptoms during most days of the current MDD episode (or most recent episode): • Expansive, elevated mood • Increased self-esteem or grandiosity • Presence of pressure of speech or being more talkative • Subjective experience of racing thoughts or flight of ideas • Increased energy or goal-directed activities • Excessive involvement in or increased activities that have high potential for painful consequences • Decreased need for sleep Those symptoms must be observable by others and be a change from the usual self. If the individual meets full criteria for a manic or hypomanic episode, the diagnosis should be changed to bipolar I or bipolar II. The symptoms are not attributable to effects of a substance use. Since mixed features have been shown to be a risk factor for development of bipolar disorder, it is clinically useful to note this specifier and adequately monitor treatment planning and response to treatment.
With melancholic features	Presence of at least four of the following symptoms during the most severe period of the current MDD episode, which must include either loss of pleasure or lack of reactivity: • Loss of pleasure in most activities or all activities • Unreactive to usually pleasurable stimuli (does not feel better even when positive things happen) • A distinct quality of depressed mood that is characterized by despair, profound despondency, and/or moroseness or by so-called empty mood • Depressive symptoms usually worse in the morning • Early-morning awakening (at least 2 hours before usual) • Psychomotor retardation or agitation • Significant weight loss or anorexia • Excessive/ inappropriate guilt
With atypical features	Presence of at least three of the following symptoms most days of the current MDD episode or current persistent depressive disorder, with at least one of them being reactivity to pleasurable stimuli:

Table 16.2 (cont.)

	• Mood reactivity to pleasurable stimuli • Significant increased appetite or weight gain • Hypersomnia • Heavy or leaden feeling in arm and legs (Leaden paralysis) • Long-standing pattern of interpersonal rejection sensitivity that results in social or occupational issues and are not limited to the depressive episodes Criteria cannot be met for "with melancholic features" or "with catatonia" during the episode
With psychotic features	Presence of delusions and/or hallucinations at any time during the MDD episode. If present, specify if psychotic features are mood-congruent or mood-incongruent: • With mood-congruent psychotic features: Content of the hallucinations or delusions is consistent with typical depressive themes such as excessive guilt, disease, death, nihilism, inadequacy or deserved punishment. • With mood-incongruent psychotic features: Content of the hallucinations or delusions do not involve the typical depressive themes.
With catatonia	Presence of catatonic features during most of the current or more recent MDD episode, which consists of prominent psychomotor disturbances (either increased or decreased activity).
With peripartum onset	Peripartum onset is applied to current or more recent MDD episode if the onset of mood symptoms occurs either during pregnancy or within four weeks of childbirth.
With seasonal pattern	This specifier refers to a regular temporal relationship between the onset of MDD episodes with a particular time of the year, for at least the past 2 years, two MDD episodes must have occurred to demonstrate the temporal seasonal relationships and no nonseasonal episodes must occur at the same period. Remission is also achieved at specific time of the year, and the seasonal MDD episodes must have outnumbered the nonseasonal MDD episodes.

Reproduced from DSM-5-TR [4].

While these individuals are experiencing a depressive episode, at least two of the following symptoms must be present:

– Decreased appetite or overeating
– Insomnia or hypersomnia
– Low self-esteem
– Low energy or fatigue
– Feelings of hopelessness
– Poor concentration or difficulty in decision-making

During this 2-year period (or 1 year for children and adolescents), any periods without symptoms should not last longer than 2 months. Major depressive episodes could precede PDD or occur during the illness. In individuals that meet the criteria for MDD for 2 years, a diagnosis of PDD should be also given. Patients should not be diagnosed with PDD if they ever meet the criteria for a manic or hypomanic episode [4].

16.2.3 Substance-/Medication-Induced Depressive Disorder

This diagnosis requires a prominent and persistent disturbance in mood predominating in the clinical presentation characterized by depressed mood or significant decreased interest or pleasure in all or almost all activities due to direct effects of a substance. The depressive symptoms must develop during or soon after the substance/medication intoxication or withdrawal as evidenced by clinical history, laboratory findings, and physical examination, and the substance/medication must be capable of producing such depressive symptoms. Symptoms should not occur exclusively during delirium and should not be better explained by a non-medication-/substance-induced depressive disorder. The disturbance should also cause clinically significant distress and/or impairment in functionality.

The most likely categories to cause substance-/medication-induced depressive disorders are the so-called depressants including alcohol, benzodiazepines and sedatives, hypnotic or anxiolytic drugs (that cause symptoms during intoxication), and stimulants such as amphetamine-type and cocaine (causing symptoms during its withdrawal) [4].

16.3 Course and Prognosis

16.3.1 Major Depressive Disorder

Despite having significant symptoms before an episode is identified, the first depressive episode is diagnosed before 50 years old in about 50% of patients [2]. However, MDD can appear at any age, with a significant increase in likelihood of onset with puberty. Its course might reflect social and structural adversities that can be linked to poverty, racism, or marginalization [4].

MDD is highly recurrent. Following recovery from a single episode, the estimated rate of recurrence over 2 years is greater than 40%, and after two episodes, risk of recurrence within 5 years is approximately 75% [5].

In most cases, untreated depressive episodes last from 6 to 13 months, and the majority of treated episodes last around 3 months. Stopping antidepressants before those 3 months almost always results in return of the symptoms. For about 40% of individuals, recovery starts within 3 months and for 80% within 1 year. The more recent the onset of depressive symptoms, the more likely a patient is to recover sooner. With the progression of the disorder, patients tend to have more frequent, longer-lasting episodes. Over a period of 20 years, the mean number of episodes is between five and six.

MDD tends to be chronic, and patients tend to relapse. Generally, as a patient experience more episodes, the time between them decreases and their severity increases, but the risk of recurrence is lower the longer the duration of the remission period. Higher risk of recurrence is noted in patients whose most recent episode was severe, who were younger, and had already presented multiple past episodes. In individuals with chronic symptoms, there is an increased chance of underlying comorbidities with anxiety, personality or substance use disorders and also a decreased chance that treatment will achieve full remission. That said, it is very important to ask the patients when was the last time they've experienced a period of 2 months or longer without any symptoms.

Lower recovery rates are associated with duration of an episode, psychotic features, prominent anxiety, personality disorders, and severity of symptoms. Persistence of symptoms during remission is also a significant predictor of recurrence [2, 4].

Approximately 5–10 % of patients initially diagnosed with unipolar MDD will develop a manic episode in the next 6–10 years after their first episode of depression. The mean age for this switch is 32 years old, and tends to occur after two to four depressive episodes [2] .

16.3.2 Persistent Depressive Disorder

Persistent depressive disorder (PDD) includes certain previously utilized diagnostic categories, such as dysthymia or dysthymic disorder, characterized by prolonged depressive symptoms that do not meet the full criteria for a major depressive episode. This condition often has an insidious onset and, by definition, a chronic course. If the onset is early (before age 21 years), it is associated with a greater chance of comorbidity with substance use disorders and personality disorders. The depressive symptoms in these patients are much less likely to fully resolve at any given period in the context of this diagnosis than in a patient with a non-chronic MDD episode. Symptoms can at times progress to the level of a full major depressive episode but are likely to return to a lower level later [4].

Predictive factors for poorer long-term outcome include greater severity of symptoms, higher levels of negative affectivity (neuroticism), poorer global functioning, and comorbidity with anxiety disorder or conduct disorder. PDD is also associated with elevated risk of suicidal outcomes and high levels of disability [4].

16.3.3 Substance-Induced Depressive Disorder

The depressive disorder associated with substance use must have its onset either while the individual is using the substance or during withdrawal. Most commonly the symptoms appear within the initial few weeks to 1 month of heavy use. After discontinuation, depending on the half-life of the substance and withdrawal syndrome, symptoms usually cease within days to weeks. If symptoms persist for longer than 4 weeks beyond the expected withdrawal course of a certain substance, other possible causes should be investigated [4].

16.4 Pathophysiology of Depressive Disorders

16.4.1 Neurochemistry

The dysfunction of the monoamine neurotransmitter systems (i.e., serotonin, norepinephrine, dopamine) has been associated with depression. Of those systems, serotonin is the recipient of the greatest attention, since there is strong evidence that its dysfunction plays a major role in the pathophysiology of depression. More recently, there has been growing evidence that the glutamatergic system also plays a significant role in depression [6].

To date, more limited data have been found supporting the importance of norepinephrine and dopamine dysfunction in depression pathophysiology, but these data suggest that they do play a significant role [7]. It can also be noted that medications selectively blocking norepinephrine reuptake, such as Bupropion or Mirtazapine, are effective in treating depression, and medications that target the dopamine system, such as monoamine oxidase inhibitors (MAOIs), have also shown to be very effective.

The excitatory neurotransmitter glutamate has also been implicated in memory, cognition, and mood disorders [8], and individuals with depression have been shown to present changes in glutamate levels in cerebrospinal fluid, plasma concentration, and brain tissue. Adding to those findings, patients with major depressive disorders were also noted to have decreased glutamate and glutamine in the hippocampus, amygdala, anterior cingulate cortex, left dorsolateral prefrontal cortex, dorsomedial prefrontal cortex, and ventromedial prefrontal cortex [9]. An increasing number of studies have explored medication targeting a specific glutamate receptor type, N-methyl-D-aspartate (NMDA) receptor, and emerging evidence is suggesting that medications antagonizing the NMDA receptor have antidepressant effects.

Acetylcholine (Ach) is found diffusely in neurons through the cerebral cortex, and we know that cholinergic neurons interact with the three monoamine systems. Agonist and antagonist cholinergic drugs have clinical effects on mania and depression. Agonists are able to produce anergia, lethargy, and psychomotor retardation and can also reduce manic symptoms and exacerbate depressive symptoms. However, these effects are not sufficient for clinical application, and the side effects are too problematic. In animal models, some strains of mice with different sensitivity to cholinergic agonists were found also to have different susceptibility to learned helplessness. Cholinergic agonists also can potentially induce hypothalamic–pituitary–adrenal (HPA) activity changes and sleep changes that can mimic depressive symptoms [2].

The γ-Aminobutyric acid (GABA) is inhibitory to ascending monoamine pathways, especially in the mesolimbic and mesocortical systems. Lower levels of GABA have been documented in cerebrospinal fluid (CSF), plasma, and the brain in depression. In animal studies, chronic stress was found to potentially lower or deplete GABA levels. Antidepressants, by contrast, can upregulate GABA receptors, and some GABAergic medications were observed to have some weak antidepressant results [2].

The neuroendocrine system is also involved in the pathophysiology of mood disorders, with the HPA axis noted to be dysfunctional in some depressed patients [10]. Increased HPA activity is one of the clearest links between depression and chronic stress as well as a hallmark of stress responses in mammals [2]. Patients who are severely depressed with a history of unsuccessful medication trials may also have a hyperactive HPA axis, as evidenced by changes in cortisol levels and feedback response impairments with the prednisolone suppression test. Recently reported alterations in cortisol regulation that were associated with history of abuse or early-life trauma may suggest HPA axis dysregulation could be a marker of vulnerability for affective disorders later in life, and also suggests this dysregulation could be the cause for specific types of depression (not the reverse) [9, 11]. It is also noteworthy that the corticotropin-releasing factor is an important monoaminergic activity modulator [9]. There is data indicating that about 5–10% of individuals who had undergone evaluation for depression had a previously undetected thyroid dysfunction: either an elevated thyroid-stimulating hormone (TSH) level or an increased response of TSH to thyroid-releasing hormone (TRH). Those alterations, if not treated, can compromise the response to treatment [2].

16.4.2 Sleep Alterations

Sleep neurophysiology alterations are also noticeable in depressed patients. The sleep changes associated with depression are a premature loss of deep (slow-wave) sleep and increased nocturnal arousal. The increased nocturnal arousal can be evidenced by the following changes:

- Increase in nocturnal awakenings
- Reduction in total time of sleep
- Increased rapid eye movement (REM) sleep
- Increased core body temperatures

Due to the decreased slow-wave sleep and increased REM sleep time, there is a significant decrease in the first period of non-REM sleep, referred to as reduced REM latency. Such changes can persist even after recovering from a depressive episode.

16.4.3 Inflammation

All mood disorders have been increasingly recognized to have a strong correlation with a pro-inflammatory state, an understanding that is providing the basis for new therapeutic targets [12].

Ever-increasing data support the role of inflammatory processes in depression, for instance the elevated levels of inflammatory markers with increased incidence of mood symptoms, notably acute C-reactive protein (CRP), prostaglandin E2 (PGE2), TNF-α, IL-1β, IL-2, and IL-6 both in peripheral blood and CSF. This relationship between inflammation and mood symptoms appears to be bidirectional, since psychological stress may also be associated with an acute inflammatory response [13]. Some inflammatory markers and immune mediators have been linked to depressive symptoms, and investigations continue with more studies evaluating the use of anti-inflammatory medications such as celecoxib, acetylsalicylic acid, antitumor necrosis factor α agents, minocycline, and omega-3 polyunsaturated fatty acids for mood disorders [9].

16.4.4 Neuroanatomical Findings

Recent advances in structural and functional neuroimaging have permitted increasing detail-oriented findings of brain anatomy and improved our understanding of how certain portions of the brain are involved in the pathophysiology of depression [9].

Decreased volumes of the prefrontal cortex, hippocampus, amygdala, and various basal ganglia structures are the most common structural abnormalities associated with depression, despite inconsistent data [14].

16.4.5 Genetic Factors

The heritability of depression was found to be 33–50% [15]; however, given the complexity of the inheritance patterns and variability of presentations, it should be noted that mood disorders likely involve significant genetic environmental interactions and multiple genes [9].

First-degree relations of individuals with MDD have a two- to fourfold higher risk of developing MDD than the general population. There is also a higher relative risk for early-onset and recurrent forms of MDD. Heritability is approximately 40%, and the neuroticism personality trait seems to account for substantial portion of it. Women are also at increased risk of developing depressive symptoms during specific reproductive stages including premenstrual, postpartum, and perimenopausal [4].

16.4.6 Psychosocial Factors

Social determinants of mental health, including low income, limited formal education, racism, and/or other forms of discrimination, are associated with higher risk of developing MDD. Adverse childhood experiences are another significant risk factor, especially if there are multiple and diverse types of adversities. Women may be at disproportionately higher risk for childhood adversity including sexual abuse, potentially contributing to the higher rates of depression observed in this group. Women are also more affected by main risk factors, including interpersonal trauma. Stressful events in life are well documented as precipitants for MDD episodes [4]. The stressor most often related to the onset of an episode of depression is the loss of a spouse; another very significant risk factor is unemployment [2].

16.5 Treatment/Management

Most studies use the terms *response* and *remission* when describing a treatment outcome, based on the degree of improvement from baseline on administered depression rating scales [16, 17] as follows:

- Response – Improvement $\geq$ 50% but less than the threshold for remission
- Remission – Resolution of the depression symptoms identified by a depression rating scale $\leq$ to the specific cutoff defining normal range

The main goal of treating depression is remission of symptoms and restoration of the functioning baseline for the patients [18, 19]. In one of the most significant studies in the field, a prospective study (Sequenced Treatment Alternatives to Relieve Depression STAR*D) outpatients with MDD were followed up to 12 months after improvement due to treatment with pharmacotherapy and/or psychotherapy [20].

According to randomized trials, the combination treatment of pharmacotherapy with psychotherapy is more effective than either treatment alone; therefore, it is used as the first treatment option [21, 22]. However, a reasonable alternative for initiating treatment is psychotherapy alone or pharmacotherapy alone, since each has demonstrated efficacy as monotherapy as well and with comparable results [23, 24]. In summary, choosing between pharmacotherapy plus psychotherapy combined, pharmacotherapy alone, and psychotherapy alone in treating an MDD episode is consistent with both the American Psychiatric Association practice guidelines and the United Kingdom National Institute for Health and Care Excellence (NICE), despite NICE having the initial recommendation of psychotherapy for patients presenting with initial mild depression.

Selective serotonin reuptake inhibitors (SSRIs) are the initial treatment option for patients with MDD that will include antidepressants, due to their efficacy and tolerability, making them the most widely prescribed class of antidepressants [25–27]. Other reasonable alternatives include serotonin and norepinephrine reuptake inhibitors (SNRIs), atypical antidepressants, and serotonin modulators, since many reviews concluded that the efficacy of different antidepressants is comparable within and across classes with no replicated meaningful differences [28–30]. Therefore, when selecting a medication, the clinician should base the decision on other factors, such as safety, side effects profile, comorbid illnesses, specific depressive symptoms, medications the patient is already using (potential drug–drug interactions), ease of use, patient's preference and expectations, previous response to antidepressants, costs, and even family history of response to antidepressants [31]. Antidepressants frequently used to treat MDD are listed in the Appendix (Table A.1). Please note that not all of them carry FDA approval for the treatiun of depression in the United States, although off-label use is common. Furthermore, the list does not include certain classes of medications such as tricyclic antidepressants and monoamine oxidase inhibitors, which are difficult to manage and usually reserved for more severe, resistant cases.

The medication trial should proceed for 6–12 weeks before determining whether the antidepressant has provided a significant response; however, patients with little improvement after 4–6 weeks can be advanced to the next step [20, 32–34]. In that case, several options are available, including switching to another antidepressant (usually from a different class), adding another antidepressant, or adding a different pharmacological agent (e.g., atypical antipsychotics) as augmentation.

There are many psychotherapies that can be used for the treatment of MDD, including cognitive behavioral therapy, interpersonal psychotherapy, behavioral activation, psychodynamic psychotherapy, problem-solving therapy, and family and couples' therapy, to name a few. Among the major lines of evidence-based psychotherapies, there is no evidence of any modality being superior to another, therefore the choice should be based on availability and patient's preference [35–38].

In addition, patients with persistent depressive disorder historically have been treated with long-term insight-focused psychotherapy. More recent data, however, support the value and efficacy of cognitive behavioral therapy in conjunction with pharmacotherapy for the treatment of these patients [2, 39].

Last, in some cases, a major depressive episode may be classified as **difficult-to-treat depression** or, more commonly, **treatment-resistant depression**. There is no consensus about the definition of treatment-resistant depression, but it is commonly characterized as the depression that fails to respond to at least two different antidepressants. Different combination and augmentation strategies can be used for the treatment of treatment-resistant depression, as well as other treatment options including esketamine or ketamine administration, transcranial magnetic stimulation, electroconvulsive therapy, and vagal nerve stimulation. As a last resource, deep brain stimulation has been used experimentally in the treatment of resistant depression, with variable degrees of success.

References

1. R. M. Pluta, Development of lifetime comorbidity in the World Health Organization world mental health surveys. **305** (2011), 870.

2. R. Boland, M. Verdiun, P. Ruiz, *Kaplan and Sadock's Synopsis of Psychiatry,* Twelfth edition. (Philadelphia: Wolters Kluwer Health, 2021).

3. D. S. Hasin, A. L. Sarvet, J. L. Meyers, T. D. Saha, W. J. Ruan, M. Stohl, B. F. Grant, Epidemiology of adult DSM-5 major depressive disorder and its specifiers in the United States. **75** (2018), 336–346. https://doi.org/10.1001/jamapsychiatry.2017.4602.

4. *Diagnostic and statistical manual of mental disorders: DSM-5-TR,* 5th edition, text revision. (Washington, DC: American Psychiatric Association Publishing, 2022).

5. D. A. Solomon, M. B. Keller, A. C. Leon, T. I. Mueller, P. W. Lavori, M. T. Shea,

W. Coryell, M. Warshaw, C. Turvey, J. D. Maser, J. Endicott, Multiple recurrences of major depressive disorder. **157** (2000), 229–233. https://doi.org/10.1176/appi.ajp .157.2.229.

6.   C. Caddy, G. Giaroli, T. P. White, S. S. Shergill, D. K. Tracy, Ketamine as the prototype glutamatergic antidepressant: pharmacodynamic actions, and a systematic review and meta-analysis of efficacy. **4** (2014), 75–99. https://doi.org/ 10.1177/2045125313507739.

7.   D. A. Morilak, A. Frazer, Antidepressants and brain monoaminergic systems: a dimensional approach to understanding their behavioural effects in depression and anxiety disorders. **7** (2004), 193–218. https://doi.org/10.1017/ S1461145704004080.

8.   G. Sanacora, G. Treccani, M. Popoli, Towards a glutamate hypothesis of depression: an emerging frontier of neuropsychopharmacology for mood disorders. **62** (2012), 63–77. https://doi .org/10.1016/j.neuropharm.2011.07.036.

9.   D. B. Arciniegas, S. C. Yudofsky, R. E. Hales, *Textbook of Neuropsychiatry and Clinical Neurosciences*, Sixth edition (Washington, DC: American Psychiatric Association Publishing, 2018).

10. C. M. Pariante, S. L. Lightman, The HPA axis in major depression: classical theories and new developments. **31** (2008), 464–468. https://doi.org/10.1016/j.tins .2008.06.006.

11. C. Heim, E. B. Binder, Current research trends in early life stress and depression: review of human studies on sensitive periods, gene–environment interactions, and epigenetics. **233** (2012), 102–111. https://doi.org/10.1016/j.expneurol.2011 .10.032.

12. R. K. McNamara, F. E. Lotrich, Elevated immune-inflammatory signaling in mood disorders: a new therapeutic target? **12** (2012), 1143–1161. https://doi.org/10 .1586/ern.12.98.

13. J. D. Rosenblat, D. S. Cha, R. B. Mansur, R. S. McIntyre, Inflamed moods: a review of the interactions between inflammation and mood disorders. **53** (2014), 23–34. https:// doi.org/10.1016/j.pnpbp.2014.01.013.

14. T. Wise, A. J. Cleare, A. Herane, A. H. Young, D. Arnone, Diagnostic and therapeutic utility of neuroimaging in depression: an overview. **10** (2014), 1509–1522. https://doi.org/10.2147/NDT .S50156.

15. D. F. Levinson, The genetics of depression: a review. **60** (2006), 84–92. https://doi.org/10.1016/j.biopsych.2005 .08.024.

16. S. A. Montgomery, M. Åsberg, A new depression scale designed to be sensitive to change. **134** (1979), 382-389. https:// doi.org/10.1192/bjp.134.4.382.

17. M. Hamilton, A rating scale for depression. **23** (1960), 56–62. https://doi .org/10.1136/jnnp.23.1.56.

18. A. Cleare, C. M. Pariante, A. H. Young, I. M. Anderson, D. Christmas, P. J. Cowen, C. Dickens, I. N. Ferrier, J. Geddes, S. Gilbody, P. M. Haddad, C. Katona, G. Lewis, A. Malizia, R. H. McAllister-Williams, P. Ramchandani, J. Scott, D. Taylor, R. Uher, Evidence-based guidelines for treating depressive disorders with antidepressants: a revision of the 2008 British Association for Psychopharmacology guidelines. **29** (2015), 459–525. https://doi.org/10.1177/ 0269881115581093.

19. M. Bauer, A. Pfennig, E. Severus, P. C. Whybrow, J. Angst, H. J. Möller, World Federation of Societies of Biological Psychiatry (WFSBP) guidelines for biological treatment of unipolar depressive disorders, part 1: update 2013 on the acute and continuation treatment of unipolar depressive disorders. **14** (2013), 334–385. https://doi .org/10.3109/15622975.2013.804195.

20. A. J. Rush, M. H. Trivedi, S. R. Wisniewski, A. A. Nierenberg, J. W. Stewart, D. Warden, G. Niederehe, M. E. Thase, P. W. Lavori, B. D. Lebowitz, P. J. McGrath, J. F. Rosenbaum, H. A. Sackeim, D. J. Kupfer, J. Luther, M. Fava, Acute and longer-term outcomes in depressed outpatients requiring one or

several treatment steps: a STARD report. **163** (2006), 1905–1917. https://doi.org/10.1176/ajp.2006.163.11.1905.

21. P. Cuijpers, J. Dekker, S. D. Hollon, G. Andersson, Adding psychotherapy to pharmacotherapy in the treatment of depressive disorders in adults: a meta-analysis. **70** (2009), 1219–1229. https://doi.org/10.4088/JCP.09r05021.

22. P. Cuijpers, A. van Straten, L. Warmerdam, G. Andersson, Psychotherapy versus the combination of psychotherapy and pharmacotherapy in the treatment of depression: a meta-analysis. **26** (2009), 279–288. https://doi.org/10.1002/da.20519.

23. D. J. Kupfer, E. Frank, M. L. Phillips, Major depressive disorder: new clinical, neurobiological, and treatment perspectives. **379** (2012), 1045–1055. https://doi.org/10.1016/s0140–6736(11)60602-8.

24. P. Cuijpers, C. F. Reynolds, 3rd, T. Donker, J. Li, G. Andersson, A. Beekman, Personalized treatment of adult depression: medication, psychotherapy, or both? A systematic review. **29** (2012), 855–864. https://doi.org/10.1002/da.21985.

25. S. C. Marcus, M. Olfson, National trends in the treatment for depression from 1998 to 2007. **67** (2010), 1265–1273. https://doi.org/10.1001/archgenpsychiatry.2010.151.

26. R. Mojtabai, M. Olfson, National patterns in antidepressant treatment by psychiatrists and general medical providers: results from the national comorbidity survey replication. **69** (2008), 1064–1074. https://doi.org/10.4088/jcp.v69n0704.

27. J. Spijker, W. A. Nolen, An algorithm for the pharmacological treatment of depression. **121** (2010), 180–189. https://doi.org/10.1111/j.1600-0447.2009.01492.x.

28. G. E. Simon, R. H. Perlis, Personalized medicine for depression: can we match patients with treatments? **167** (2010), 1445–1455. https://doi.org/10.1176/appi.ajp.2010.09111680.

29. G. Gartlehner, R. A. Hansen, L. C. Morgan, K. Thaler, L. Lux, M. Van Noord, U. Mager, P. Thieda, B. N. Gaynes, T. Wilkins, M. Strobelberger, S. Lloyd, U. Reichenpfader, K. N. Lohr, Comparative benefits and harms of second-generation antidepressants for treating major depressive disorder: an updated meta-analysis. **155** (2011), 772–785. https://doi.org/10.7326/0003-4819-155-11-201112060-00009.

30. G. Gartlehner, *Second-Generation Antidepressants in the Pharmacologic Treatment of Adult Depression: An Update of the 2007 Comparative Effectiveness Review.* (Rockville, MD: Agency for Healthcare Research and Quality, 2011).

31. G. Gartlehner, K. Thaler, S. Hill, R. A. Hansen, How should primary care doctors select which antidepressants to administer? **14** (2012), 360–369. https://doi.org/10.1007/s11920–012-0283-x.

32. G. I. Papakostas, Managing partial response or nonresponse: switching, augmentation, and combination strategies for major depressive disorder. **70 Suppl 6** (2009), 16–25. https://doi.org/10.4088/JCP.8133su1c.03.

33. M. Fava, Diagnosis and definition of treatment-resistant depression. **53** (2003), 649–659. https://doi.org/10.1016/s0006–3223(03)00231-2.

34. R. S. McIntyre, When should you move beyond first-line therapy for depression? **71 Suppl 1** (2010), 16–20. https://doi.org/10.4088/JCP.9104su1c.03.

35. P. Cuijpers, E. Karyotaki, E. Weitz, G. Andersson, S. D. Hollon, A. van Straten, The effects of psychotherapies for major depression in adults on remission, recovery and improvement: a meta-analysis. **159** (2014), 118–126. https://doi.org/10.1016/j.jad.2014.02.026.

36. K. Shinohara, M. Honyashiki, H. Imai, V. Hunot, D. M. Caldwell, P. Davies, T. H. Moore, T. A. Furukawa, R. Churchill, Behavioural therapies versus other psychological therapies for depression. **2013** (2013), Cd008696. https://doi.org/10.1002/14651858.CD008696.pub2.

37. P. Cuijpers, A. van Straten, G. Andersson, P. van Oppen, Psychotherapy for depression in adults: a meta-analysis of comparative outcome studies. **76** (2008), 909–922. https://doi.org/10.1037/a0013075.

38. S. M. Stahl, M. M. Grady, *Stahl's Essential Psychopharmacology: Prescriber's Guide,* Seventh edition (Cambridge: Cambridge University Press, 2020).

39. P. Cuijpers, A. van Straten, J. Schuurmans, P. van Oppen, S. D. Hollon, G. Andersson, Psychotherapy for chronic major depression and dysthymia: a meta-analysis. **30** (2010), 51–62. https://doi.org/10.1016/j.cpr.2009.09.003.

Bipolar Disorders

Marsal Sanches and Jair C. Soares

17.1 Introduction

Bipolar disorder (BD) is one of the most important and potentially incapacitating mental disorders. It is typically characterized by the alternation of depressive symptoms with periods of elevated mood, called manic or hypomanic episodes [1]. Since the original descriptions by authors such as Falret, Kraepelin, and Leonard, the concept of BD has been progressively expanded and currently includes not only classic forms of the illness but also more subtle presentations when it comes to manic symptomatology [2]. Given its variable clinical presentation and the absence of established biomarkers to help with its diagnosis, the identification of BD is often challenging, with a high number of patients with BD being mistakenly diagnosed with major depressive disorder [3, 4]. Available evidence points to a several years gap between the onset of symptoms and the correct diagnosis of BD, leading to delays in the implementation of appropriate therapeutic strategies and higher levels of morbidity and functional impairment [5].

While epidemiological studies indicate a lifetime prevalence of BD ranging between 1% and 4%, those numbers vary widely, with different prevalence rates having been reported according to what presentations are considered [6, 7]. BD seems to equally affect men and women (albeit with differences regarding different subtypes) [8], and its onset usually happens in adolescence and early adulthood. Nevertheless, pediatric bipolar disorder is an area of growing interest, and the identification of prodromal symptoms and of predictors of future development of bipolar disorder among individuals with high genetic risk for the illness has been the focus of several recent studies [9, 10].

The last several decades have witnessed considerable advances in the understanding of the pathophysiology of BD. However, despite those advances, the management of BD remains challenging, with a high number of patients failing to properly respond to available treatments.

17.2 Clinical Presentation/Diagnosis

The clinical presentation of BD can vary considerably. In its most typical forms, patients with BD will alternate episodes of depression with periods of elevated mood, called manic or hypomanic episodes. During a depressive episode, patients may experience different symptoms such as sadness, anhedonia, low energy, appetite changes, sleep disturbances (with insomnia or excessive sleep), depressive thoughts, psychomotor slowness or agitation, poor concentration, and death thoughts / suicidal ideation. The number of symptoms and the duration necessary for the diagnosis of a depressive episode varies according to the classification system adopted. DSM-5, for example, requires a minimum of five symptoms for a period of at least 2 weeks [11]. While the clinical presentation of a depressive episode in BD can be indistinguishable from the ones observed in individuals suffering from major depressive disorder ("unipolar depression"), a growing amount of evidence points to certain features that are particularly common during a depressive episode in individuals with BD (see Section 17.2.3).

On the other hand, during a manic episode, patients often experience symptoms opposed to depression: mood is usually euphoric (although it can be irritable) with increase in goal-directed activity and, often, agitation. Energy levels are increased, and the patient usually reports decreased need for sleep when compared to their usual self, as well as marked distractibility. They may experience a rapid influx of thoughts, commonly translated into excessive talking with frequent topic switching ("flight of ideas"). Their thought process reflects their mood state, with ideas of excessive self-confidence, inflated sense of self, and multiple plans for the future. In severe forms of the illness, that can assume the form of delusions of grandiosity, when the patient mistakenly believes in having superpowers, being wealthy, having multiple talents, or living through mystical experiences. Hallucinations can also be present. Moreover, patients in manic states commonly show a variety of out-of-character behaviors, with prodigality (excessive spending/buying), hypersexual behavior, and risk-taking actions (such as driving at excessive speed or getting involved in fights), among others. According to DSM-5, for the formal diagnosis of a manic episode (Table 17.1), a specific period of elevated or irritable mood, associated with increase in activity and energy, is necessary [11]. Such episodes need to last at least 7 days and three additional symptoms are necessary, but if the mood is only irritable and not euphoric, four additional symptoms are necessary for the diagnosis [11]. For diagnostic purposes, manic episodes are necessarily associated with marked impairment in functioning, psychotic symptoms, and/or need for hospitalization. While the criteria for a hypomanic episode are similar to the ones for a manic episode, there are some key differences: hypomanic episodes do not produce significant functional impairment but still present a clear deviation from the patient's usual self, which is noticeable by others. A hypomanic episode lasts at least 4 days and, by definition, does not have psychotic symptoms such as delusions and hallucinations, does not require hospitalization, and is not associated with marked impairment in social or occupational functioning [11]. Despite these objective criteria, the distinction between mania and hypomania in clinical practice can be difficult, especially in cases of nonpsychotic mania.

In addition to its elevated level of psychological suffering and functional impairment, BD is strongly associated with suicidal behavior. Research findings indicate that one-third to one-half of patients with BD attempt suicide, with lifetime rates of complete suicide ranging from 15% to 20% [1]. Those numbers place BD among the most concerning psychiatric conditions with regards to suicide risk.

Last, a large amount of evidence points to marked associations between BD and medical conditions such as cardiovascular disease, diabetes, hypertension, and autoimmune diseases [12, 13]. Epidemiological data on patients with BD point to a lower life expectancy when compared to the general population, not only due to suicide but also due to "natural" causes of death [14]. The nature of the association between BD and medical illnesses is not yet totally clear and is likely multifactorial, including common pathophysiological mechanisms, such as inflammation (see Section 17.3) and side effects of medications, among other factors.

Table 17.1 DSM-5 criteria for a manic episode

A. A distinct period of abnormally and persistently elevated, expansive, or irritable mood and abnormally and persistently goal-directed behavior or energy, lasting at least 1 week and present most of the day, nearly every day (or any duration if hospitalization is necessary).

B. During the period of mood disturbance and increased energy or activity, three (or more) of the following symptoms have persisted (four if the mood is only irritable), are present to a significant degree, and represent a noticeable change from usual behavior:

1. Inflated self-esteem or grandiosity

2. Decreased need for sleep (e.g., feels rested after only 3 hours of sleep)

3. More talkative than usual or pressure to keep talking

4. Flight of ideas or subjective experience that thoughts are racing

5. Distractibility (i.e., attention too easily drawn to unimportant or irrelevant external stimuli), as reported or observed

6. Increase in goal-directed activity (either socially, at work or school, or sexually) or psychomotor agitation

7. Excessive involvement in activities that have a high potential for painful consequences (e.g., engaging in unrestrained buying sprees, sexual indiscretions, or foolish business investments)

C. The mood disturbance is sufficiently severe to cause marked impairment in social or occupational functioning or to necessitate hospitalization to prevent harm to self or others, or there are psychotic features.

D. The episode is not attributable to the direct physiological effects of a substance (e.g., a drug of abuse, a medication, or other treatment) or another medical condition.

Note: A full manic episode that emerges during antidepressant treatment (e.g., medication, electroconvulsive therapy) but persists at fully syndromal level beyond the physiological effect of that treatment is sufficient evidence for a manic episode and therefore a bipolar I diagnosis.

Note: Criteria A–D constitute a manic episode. At least one lifetime manic episode is required for the diagnosis of bipolar I disorder

Reproduced from DSM 5-TR [11]

17.2.1 Bipolar Disorder Subtypes and Clinical Course

DSM-5 recognizes two main specific subtypes of bipolar illness: BD type I, where the patient experiences at least one episode of mania during their lifetime; and BD type II, characterized by the presence of at least one episode of major depression and one episode of hypomania but no full manic episodes [11]. While technically a patient with BD type I could receive that diagnosis without ever experiencing a depressive episode, major depressive episodes are likely to be present at some point over the course of the illness.

The number of mood episodes experienced in BD varies, but virtually all patients with BD type I will have more than one manic episode, while those with BD type II usually experience a higher number of episodes of depression and an equally high number of hypomanic episodes. Nonetheless, patients with so-called rapid cycling have a significantly higher number of episodes and mood shifts. There are different definitions of rapid cycling, with the most frequently utilized one requiring at least four separate mood episodes over the course of 1 year [11, 15].

Moreover, while mood episodes usually last from weeks to months, there are cases of patients who experienced manic symptoms for as long as 2 years. In addition, despite the fact that, at least in theory, patients experience full remission between episodes, residual mood symptoms, especially depressive ones, are very common and seem to contribute to impairments in functional status associated with BD. Similarly, the functional impact of cognitive deficits in BD has been explored with great interest, as these deficits seem to be present not only in acute mood episodes but also during periods of euthymic mood [16].

17.2.2 Bipolar Spectrum

The term *bipolar spectrum* was popularized in the late 1990s and early 2000s and is based on the assumption that individuals with a high genetic load for BD, despite sometimes not fulfilling full criteria for BD type I or II, often experience subsyndromal symptoms of mania, leading to differences in terms of clinical presentation, prognosis, and treatment response [2, 17]. According to this concept, there is a *continuum* across different forms of BD with certain forms of BD being placed closer to unipolar major depressive disorder and others situated closer to BD type I, which would correspond to the prototypal form of BD. Some conceptualizations of the BD spectrum include the bipolar subtype of schizoaffective disorder as the other end of the bipolar continuum, in the so-called psychotic frontier. Moreover, the bipolar spectrum concept assumes that certain temperament patterns can actually be considered attenuated presentations of bipolar disorder. For example, cyclothymia, previously called cyclothymic temperament, is characterized by the chronic alternation of subthreshold depressive and hypomanic symptoms, is recognized by DSM-5 as an independent bipolar condition, and requires the presence of symptoms for at least 2 years [11]. Hagop Akiskal, one of the main proponents of the bipolar spectrum concept, suggested the existence of at least 10 different subtypes of BD in addition to the well-established BD types I and II [2]. Examples are individuals with BD type III, whose natural course includes only symptoms of depression but can experience hypomanic symptoms when exposed to antidepressants; and BD type IV, where patients with a so-called hyperthymic temperament experience overlapping depression. The concept of bipolar spectrum has generated considerable controversy. On the one hand, those who advocate for its existence argue that the categorical approach for BD (and for mental disorders in general) is artificial and does not account for all presentations of the illness, contributing to the misdiagnosis of BD and preventing individuals who do not meet full criteria for the typical presentations to receive proper treatment. In contrast, critics of the bipolar spectrum idea point out that this concept may weaken the core concept of BD, contributing to diagnostic confusions, especially with regards to the differential with unipolar major depressive disorder and certain personality disorders. While the concept of bipolar spectrum and several of its components are not officially recognized by DSM-5 as a formal diagnosis, many of them can be included in DSM categories such as "other specified bipolar and related disorders," "substance-/medication-induced bipolar and related disorders," or "unspecified bipolar and related disorders."

17.2.3 Bipolar Depression

Bipolar depression is a generic designation to episodes or symptoms of depression experienced by individuals with bipolar disorder [5, 18]. The correct identification of

Table 17.2 Features suggestive of bipolar disorder among patients with depression*

Early onset

Family history of bipolar disorder

Postpartum onset

Psychotic depression

History of suicidal attempts

Depression with mixed symptoms

Multiple depressive episodes

Atypical features

* None of these features is pathognomonic of bipolar disorder, and the strength of their association with a possible diagnosis of BD varies across different studies

bipolar depression has important therapeutic implications, as its management and treatment response are considerably different from the ones observed in non-bipolar depression. While the clinical presentation of bipolar depression, as stated above, can be very similar to those with unipolar depression, a growing amount of evidence indicates that certain features (Table 17.2), when present during a depressive episode, are highly suggestive of bipolar disorder [19–21]. Even though the presence of these features can increase the suspiciousness regarding a possible diagnosis of BD, especially among individuals with no previously identified history of manic or hypomanic symptoms, they are not pathognomonic of BD and should not be utilized, by themselves, to justify a diagnosis of BD.

17.2.4 Mixed Features

Despite its apparent contrast with the concept of BD as an illness that alternates mood states, the idea that symptoms of depression and mania can present simultaneously in patients with BD is not new, having been already proposed by Kraepelin in the early 20th century. Mixed features are of high clinical importance, as they can be associated with a higher risk of comorbid substance use, mood dysphoria, and higher rates of suicide [22–24]. One of the major changes from DSM-IV to DSM-5 with regards to the classification of BD was the removal of the "mixed episodes," which would automatically justify a diagnosis of BD type I, and its replacement with the "mixed features specifier" [11]. According to this concept, mixed features in BD can occur during any mood episode (depressive, manic, or hypomanic), and can also be present during depressive episodes in individuals with non-bipolar major depression.

17.3 Pathophysiology

The pathophysiology of BD is complex and has not yet been completely elucidated. From a biological standpoint, research findings in BD point to disruptions at different biological levels, including genetic, neurochemical, neuroanatomical, neurophysiological, and systemic processes. While several attempts have been made to integrate these different findings, no satisfactory single model for the pathophysiology of BD is currently available. Nonetheless, in the absence of a full understanding of the pathophysiology of BD, the generic "stress-diathesis model," according to which psychiatric conditions result from a combination of genetically predisposed factors and exposure to environmental triggers, continues to be utilized to summarize the different factors involved in the development of BD. While the following subsections provide some introductory information on these factors, a full discussion of the pathophysiological mechanisms involved in BD in light of available evidence is beyond the scope of this chapter.

17.3.1 Genetic Factors

It is well known that BD runs in families, although the exact nature of the genetic factors involved in BD is still under investigation. The concordance rates for BD in twin studies range from 40% to 70%, and the risk of BD in first-degree relatives of patients with BD is between 5% and 10%, with particularly high rates among offspring of parents with BD [25].

Furthermore, genome-wide association studies (GWAS), which compare individuals with and without the phenotype of interest (in this case, BD) with regards to the presence of specific genotypes, have identified several genetic markers associated with BD. Some of these genetic markers provide a direct link with pathophysiological processes putatively involved in BD [26, 27]. Nevertheless, the effect sizes associated with these findings are usually modest, suggesting that BD actually results from polygenic inheritance mechanisms, which have not yet been completed elucidated.

17.3.2 Environmental Factors and Systemic Processes in Bipolar Disorder

The role of environmental factors in BD is well established. During the 1990s, hypotheses such as the *kindling* model attempted to explain the frequent association of mood episodes with stressful life events. According to this model, stressful events could disrupt mood regulation mechanisms and trigger mood episodes (particularly depressive episodes) in individuals with genetic predisposition to BD; moreover, the repeated exposure to life stressors could gradually decrease the threshold necessary for the development of a mood episode, eventually leading to spontaneous mood episodes over the course of the illness [1].

More recently, researchers have focused on the hyperactivation of the hypothalamus–pituitary axis (HPA) in response to stressors in patients with mood disorders, including BD [28]. This model emphasizes the role of deficient glucocorticoid receptor regulation during exposure to stressors, leading to chronically elevated levels of cortisol and abnormal allostatic load, which could have repercussions not only at a neurobiological level (resulting, for example, in hippocampal atrophy) but also systemic ones, including hyperoxidating effects and chronic activation of inflammatory response, as described in the next paragraph.

Similarly, a large volume of evidence points to enhanced inflammatory processes among patients with BD, with elevated levels of markers of inflammatory activity (e.g., C-reactive protein) and inflammation mediators such as tumor necrosis factor (TNF-alpha) and interleukin 6 (IL-6) [29]. The causes of such enhanced inflammation in BD are not yet completely understood but likely include factors related to stress exposure and increased HPA activity (see earlier discussion), dietary features, genetic factors, and abnormalities in gut microbiota [29, 30]. The interface between BD and inflammation represents an interesting and promising area for treatment research.

17.3.3 Brain Circuit Abnormalities in Bipolar Disorder

Even though an extensive body of evidence supports the existence of neuroimaging abnormalities in BD, these findings are not usually identifiable in neuroimaging tests routinely performed in clinical practice, such as MRIs and CT scans [31]. Nevertheless, research with special measurement techniques applied to structural MRI scans, in addition to functional neuroimaging techniques such as functional MRI and positron emission tomography (PET) scan, points to abnormalities in the brain circuits involved in the regulation of emotions and cognitive processes in patients with BD.

These findings suggest that abnormalities in two brain circuits seem to be of particular importance in BD: disruption in the first circuit, which consists of the amygdala, anterior cingulate cortex, basal ganglia, and insula, are likely involved in the abnormal emotional processing observed in BD. On the other hand, abnormalities in the second circuit, comprised by the prefrontal cortex, the hippocampus, and the striatum, seem to play a role in the abnormal cognitive processes observed in this condition [31].

It is important to emphasize that, despite the importance of brain imaging research in BD and its contributions to understanding the pathophysiology of this condition, the clinical utility of neuroimaging in BD is at this point still modest and limited to helping in the differential diagnosis between BD and neurological conditions that could present with similar symptoms, such as brain tumors and certain neurodegenerative disorders.

17.4 Treatment/Management

The optimal treatment of BD is interdisciplinary and consists of medications and other biological approaches aiming at improving mood symptomatology and preventing relapse, as well as psychosocial interventions focusing on the different aspects of BD, including psychoeducation, family-oriented interventions, and a variety of psychotherapeutic approaches. In addition, several neurostimulation techniques have been utilized for the treatment of BD, especial in the management of resistant cases [32, 33]. Electroconvulsive therapy (ECT) remains one of the most effecting treatments for the management of depression and can also be of benefit in the treatment of resistant mania. Despite not being approved for the treatment of depression in BD, transcranial magnetic stimulation (TMS) is sometimes utilized off-label for that indication, with variable degrees of success. Of notice, TMS can induce manic switches in patients with BD. Vagus nerve stimulation is currently FDA approved for the treatment of depression in BD, but its effect can be small, and long latencies in treatment effects are commonly observed.

17.4.1 Pharmacological Treatment of Bipolar Disorder

Different medications (Table 17.3) are currently utilized for the treatment of BD with distinct profiles in terms of mechanism of action, tolerability, and efficacy across the different phases of the illness. While some of them are approved by the FDA for the

Table 17.3 Pharmacological agents commonly utilized in the treatment of bipolar disorder

| | | | Efficacy* | | |
Agent		Usual Total Daily Dose	Mania	Depression	Mixed Features	Maintenance
Mood Stabilizers	Lithium Carbonate	600–1,200 mg	+	+	–	+
	Divalproex	500–2,000 mg	+	–	+	+
	Carbamazepine	600–1,200 mg	+	+/–	+	+
	Lamotrigine	100–200 mg	–	+	+/–	+
	Oxcarbazepine	600–1,800 mg	+/–	–	+	+/–
Atypical antipsychotics	Olanzapine	5–20 mg	+	–	+	+
	Quetiapine	100–600 mg	+	+	+	+
	Risperidone	1–4 mg	+	+	+	+
	Ziprasidone	80–160 mg	+	–	+	+
	Lurasidone	40–80 mg	+	+	+	+
	Asenapine	10–20 mg	+	–	+	+
	Aripiprazole	10–30 mg	+	–	+	+
	Cariprazine	1.5–6 mg	+	+	+	+
Typical antipsychotics	Haloperidol	5–20 mg	+	–	–	–
	Chlorpromazine	100–300 mg	+	–	–	–

* Based on available evidence and clinical experience; includes both FDA-approved use and off-label use.

treatment of BD, several are utilized off-label, based on research findings and, some-times, anecdotal reports. More details about the different pharmacological agents that can be used in the treatment of BD are found in the Appendix.

Acute mania: The treatment of acute episodes of mania is usually based on the use of mood stabilizers and/or antipsychotics and on the discontinuation of medications that could be contributing to the manic state, such as antidepressants. Lithium and valproic acid seem to have similar anti-manic effects but may be less potent and have a longer latency of response when compared to antipsychotics [1]. In the past, typical antipsychotics as monotherapy or combined with mood stabilizers used to be reserved for more severe cases or for cases of mania with psychotic symptoms, due to concerns about extrapyramidal side effects (EPS), but that changed after the advent of atypical antipsychotics, which are now widely used in the treatment of patients with acute mania. Atypical antipsychotics, which include olanzapine, risperidone, quetiapine, and aripiprazole, among others, offer a lower risk of EPS, but there are concerns about their risk of metabolic syndrome, especially in the long term [34]. QTc prolongation is another concern when it comes to the use of certain antipsychotics [35]. With regards to the tolerability of mood stabilizers, lithium requires close monitoring due to the risk of acute toxicity, in addition to weight gain, hypothyroidism, kidney failure, and diabetes insipidus [34]. Valproic acid, the most currently prescribed medication for the treatment of BD, carries a risk of liver toxicity including, in rare cases, acute liver failure [36]. Other potential side effects include pancreatitis and thrombocytopenia [37]. Carbamazepine, another anticonvulsant with anti-manic properties, carries a risk of leukopenia and hyponatremia, in addition to liver toxicity and elevated rates of drug interactions [38]. While the same agents utilized for the treatment of mania may also be effective in the treatment of hypomania, most clinicians will act more conservatively when it comes to pharmacological choices for the management of hypomania, avoiding polypharmacy and choosing medications with a milder side effect profile whenever possible. Last, despite the fact that DSM-5 no longer considers the existence of mixed episodes, many of the agents approved for the treatment of acute mania are also approved for the treatment of mixed states and can be of particular benefit for the treatment of manic episodes with mixed symptomatology. Of notice, similarly to rapid cycling, the presence of mixed symptomatology is considered a predictor of poor response to monotherapy with lithium, although this assumption has been more recently brought into question, based on literature data [39].

Bipolar depression: The effective treatment of bipolar disorder during the depressive phase may be challenging, as there is a shortage of agents specifically approved for the management of this condition. While lithium and lamotrigine may offer some antide-pressive effect in patients with BD, their efficacy is variable. Certain atypical antipsychotics, such as quetiapine, lurasidone, and cariprazine, are specifically approved by the FDA for the treatment of depression in BD, although other atypicals may also be of benefit, based on available evidence [40]. Even though a combination of olanzapine and fluoxetine is currently approved for the treatment of bipolar depression, the use of antidepressants in bipolar disorder remains controversial, not only due to the risks related to the induction of manic switches, rapid cycling, and worsening of mixed symptomatology but also because of the limited evidence supporting their efficacy [41]. As a general rule, antidepressants should be avoided in patients with bipolar disorder and should not be used without being associated with a mood stabilizer or an atypical antipsychotic, especially in the case of BD type I [41–43]. In the rare instances where they are utilized, antidepressants should be kept for the shortest period of time possible, aiming at minimizing potentially negative effects associated with their use.

Maintenance treatment: Once improvement in the acute mood episodes is achieved, the treatment enters the so-called maintenance phase. At the present moment, in light of available evidence, patients with BD are recommended to remain on long-term pharmacological treatment [44]. While many clinicians tend to continue with the same agents utilized to achieve remission, the cycling nature of BD might complicate the decision-making process involved in the choice of the best maintenance agent for a patient with BD. Despite decreases in its utilization due to the availability of new agents, lithium remains the gold standard for long-term treatment for BD, not only due to its mood stabilizing properties but also because of its neuroprotective and anti-suicidal effects [45]. However, lithium, as previously explained, carries high risks of toxicity, and its chronic use may be associated with impairments in kidney and thyroid function. Valproic acid can be used as a maintenance treatment in BD but seems to be restricted to the prevention of mania. In contrast, lamotrigine is approved for maintenance treatment in BD, but its efficacy in preventing manic or hypomanic episodes is limited. Atypical antipsychotics can be used as maintenance treatment in BD, although several of them are not approved for that indication, and their efficacy in the prevention of different phases of the illness can be uneven. Last, despite the fact that some patients with BD type II might tolerate and benefit from antidepressants, most guidelines do not recommend maintenance with antidepressants in BD.

17.5 Conclusions

BD is a complex and potentially serious mental illness. Its diagnosis and management can be challenging, but ongoing research has led to considerable advances in our understanding of its pathophysiology. It is expected that, over the course of the next few years, some of these advances will result in improvements in the correct and early identification of BD, as well as more personalized treatments for this condition.

References

1. Grande I, Berk M, Birmaher B, Vieta E. Bipolar disorder. *Lancet.* 2016;387 (10027):1561–1572.

2. Akiskal HS, Pinto O. The evolving bipolar spectrum. *Psychiatr Clin North Am.* 1999;22(3):517–534.

3. Ghouse AA, Sanches M, Zunta-Soares G, Swann AC, Soares JC. Overdiagnosis of bipolar disorder: a critical analysis of the literature. *Sci World J.* 2013;2013:1–5.

4. Sanches M. Bipolar disorder: how to avoid overdiagnosis. *Curr Psychiatry.* 2018;17(6):29.

5. Baldessarini RJ, Vázquez GH, Tondo L. Bipolar depression: a major unsolved challenge. *Int J Bipolar Disord.* 2020;8 (1):1.

6. Merikangas KR, Akiskal HS, Angst J, Greenberg PE, Hirschfeld RMA, Petukhova M, et al. Lifetime and 12-month prevalence of bipolar spectrum disorder in the National Comorbidity Survey replication. *Arch Gen Psychiatry.* 2007;64(5):543–552.

7. Rowland TA, Marwaha S. Epidemiology and risk factors for bipolar disorder. *Ther Adv Psychopharmacol.* 2018;8 (9):251–269.

8. Diflorio A, Jones I. Is sex important? Gender differences in bipolar disorder. *Int Rev Psychiatry Abingdon Engl.* 2010;22 (5):437–452.

9. Sanches M, Soares JC. Prevention of bipolar disorder: are we almost there? *Curr Behav Neurosci Rep.* 2020;7 (2):62–67.

10. Post RM, Chang K, Frye MA. Paradigm shift: ultrahigh risk for childhood bipolar disorder to facilitate studies on prevention. *J Clin Psychiatry.* 2013;74 (2):167–169.

11. American Psychiatric Association, ed. *Diagnostic and statistical manual of mental disorders: DSM-5.* 5th ed. American Psychiatric Association; 2013.

12. Crump C, Sundquist K, Winkleby MA, Sundquist J. Comorbidities and mortality in bipolar disorder: a Swedish national cohort study. *JAMA Psychiatry.* 2013;70 (9):931–939.

13. Chen M, Jiang Q, Zhang L. The prevalence of bipolar disorder in autoimmune disease: a systematic review and meta-analysis. *Ann Palliat Med.* 2021;10(1):350–361.

14. Chan JKN, Tong CHY, Wong CSM, Chen EYH, Chang WC. Life expectancy and years of potential life lost in bipolar disorder: systematic review and meta-analysis. *Br J Psychiatry J Ment Sci.* 2022;221(3):567–576.

15. Schneck CD, Miklowitz DJ, Calabrese JR, Allen MH, Thomas MR, Wisniewski SR, et al. Phenomenology of rapid-cycling bipolar disorder: data from the first 500 participants in the Systematic Treatment Enhancement Program. *Am J Psychiatry.* 2004;161(10):1902–1908.

16. Osuji IJ, Cullum CM. Cognition in bipolar disorder. *Psychiatr Clin North Am.* 2005;28(2):427–441.

17. Ghaemi SN. Bipolar spectrum: a review of the concept and a vision for the future. *Psychiatry Investig.* 2013;10(3):218.

18. McIntyre RS, Calabrese JR. Bipolar depression: the clinical characteristics and unmet needs of a complex disorder. *Curr Med Res Opin.* 2019;35(11):1993–2005.

19. Hirschfeld RM. Differential diagnosis of bipolar disorder and major depressive disorder. *J Affect Disord.* 2014;169: S12–S16.

20. Kessing LV, Willer I, Andersen PK, Bukh JD. Rate and predictors of conversion from unipolar to bipolar disorder: a systematic review and meta-analysis. *Bipolar Disord.* 2017;19(5):324–335.

21. Stahl SM, Morrissette DA, Faedda G, Fava M, Goldberg JF, Keck PE, et al. Guidelines for the recognition and management of mixed depression. *CNS Spectr.* 2017;22(2):203–219.

22. Hu J, Mansur R, McIntyre RS. Mixed specifier for bipolar mania and depression: highlights of *DSM-5* changes and implications for diagnosis and treatment in primary care. *Prim Care Companion CNS Disord.* Apr 17, 2014 [cited Aug 5, 2018]. Available from: http://article.psychiatrist.com/? ContentType=START&ID=10008615

23. Jain R, Maletic V, McIntyre RS. Diagnosing and treating patients with mixed features: academic highlights. *J Clin Psychiatry.* 2017;78(8):1091–1102.

24. Tavormina G. From the temperaments to the bipolar mixed states: essential steps for the clinicians on understanding the mixity. *Psychiatr Danub.* 2021;33(Suppl 9):6–10.

25. Sanches M, Soares JC. Prevention of bipolar disorder: are we almost there? *Curr Behav Neurosci Rep.* 2020;7 (2):62–67.

26. Craddock N, Sklar P. Genetics of bipolar disorder. *Lancet.* 2013;381 (9878):1654–1662.

27. Goes FS. Genetics of bipolar disorder. *Psychiatr Clin North Am.* 2016;39 (1):139–155.

28. Daban C, Vieta E, Mackin P, Young AH. Hypothalamic-pituitary-adrenal axis and bipolar disorder. *Psychiatr Clin North Am.* 2005;28(2):469–480.

29. Barbosa IG, Machado-Vieira R, Soares JC, Teixeira AL. The immunology of bipolar disorder. *Neuroimmunomodulation.* 2014;21 (2–3):117–122.

30. Martins LB, Braga Tibães JR, Sanches M, Jacka F, Berk M, Teixeira AL. Nutrition-based interventions for mood disorders.

Expert Rev Neurother. 2021;21 (3):303–315.

31. Sanches M, Soares JC. Brain imaging abnormalities in bipolar disorder. In Soares JC, Young A, eds. *Bipolar Disorders.* 3rd ed. Cambridge University Press; 2016:102–110.

32. Loo C, Katalinic N, Mitchell PB, Greenberg B. Physical treatments for bipolar disorder: a review of electroconvulsive therapy, stereotactic surgery and other brain stimulation techniques. *J Affect Disord.* 2011;132(1–2):1–13.

33. Kim YK. *Treatment Resistance in Psychiatry: Risk Factors, Biology, and Management.* Springer Berlin Heidelberg; 2018.

34. Hales RE, Yudofsky SC, Roberts LW, American Psychiatric Publishing, eds. *The American Psychiatric Publishing Textbook of Psychiatry.* 6th ed. American Psychiatric Publishing; 2014.

35. Beach SR, Celano CM, Noseworthy PA, Januzzi JL, Huffman JC. QTc prolongation, torsades de pointes, and psychotropic medications. *Psychosomatics.* 2013;54(1):1–13.

36. Sadock BJ, Sadock VA, Ruiz P, Kaplan HI, eds. *Kaplan & Sadock's Comprehensive Textbook of Psychiatry.* 9th ed. Wolters Kluwer Health/Lippincott Williams & Wilkins; 2009.

37. Schatzberg AF, DeBattista C. *Schatzberg's Manual of Clinical Psychopharmacology.* 9th ed. American Psychiatric Association Publishing; 2019.

38. Stahl SM, Grady MM. *Stahl's Essential Psychopharmacology: Prescriber's Guide.* 6th ed. Cambridge University Press; 2017.

39. Fountoulakis KN, Tohen M, Zarate CA. Lithium treatment of bipolar disorder in adults: a systematic review of randomized trials and meta-analyses. *Eur Neuropsychopharmacol J Eur Coll Neuropsychopharmacol.* 2022;54:100–115.

40. Diaz AP, Fernandes BS, Quevedo J, Sanches M, Soares JC. Treatment-resistant bipolar depression: concepts and challenges for novel interventions. *Rev Bras Psiquiatr Sao Paulo Braz 1999.* 2022;44(2):178–186.

41. Antosik-Wójcińska A, Stefanowski B, Święcicki Ł. Efficacy and safety of antidepressant's use in the treatment of depressive episodes in bipolar disorder: review of research. *Psychiatr Pol.* 2015;49 (6):1223–1239.

42. Scaini G, Quevedo J. The conundrum of antidepressant use in bipolar disorder. *Mol Psychiatry.* 2023;28(3):972–973.

43. Goldberg JF, Nierenberg AA, Iosifescu DV. Wrestling With Antidepressant Use in Bipolar Disorder: The Ongoing Debate. J Clin Psychiatry. 2021 Jan 19;82(1):19ac13181.

44. Yatham LN, Kennedy SH, Parikh SV, Schaffer A, Bond DJ, Frey BN, et al. Canadian Network for Mood and Anxiety Treatments (CANMAT) and International Society for Bipolar Disorders (ISBD) 2018 guidelines for the management of patients with bipolar disorder. *Bipolar Disord.* 2018;20 (2):97–170.

45. Cipriani A, Hawton K, Stockton S, Geddes JR. Lithium in the prevention of suicide in mood disorders: updated systematic review and meta-analysis. *BMJ.* 2013;346(4):f3646.

Psychotic Disorders

Olaoluwa Okusaga and Gabriela Austgen

18.1 Introduction

Psychotic disorders are syndromes characterized by the presence of psychosis. The term *psychosis* denotes an abnormal mental status characterized by various forms of bizarre, disorganized behavior, disorganized or illogical thinking, misperceptions, and distortion of reality. Specific terms used to describe psychotic mental states include *delusions* and *hallucinations* [1]. Delusions are defined as fixed, false beliefs held by an individual despite clear and convincing evidence against the held beliefs. For example, a person experiencing psychosis might have a delusional belief (and stays convinced) that he/she is the current president of the United States, despite being shown a live televised speech by the (real) president. Hallucinations are defined as abnormal sensory perceptions occurring in the absence of actual stimulus, and they may occur in any sensory modality (auditory, visual, tactile, gustatory, or olfactory). For example, a person with a psychotic disorder might be hearing "voices" of people whispering or talking even though he/she is alone and no one is actually talking.

Psychosis, as a phenomenon, is not a specific diagnosis, and not pathognomonic of any specific health condition, nor does it indicate a specific etiology. To clarify, psychosis can be conceptualized as a psychiatric phenomenon analogous to fever in general medicine. Just as the presence of fever in an individual can be due to several health conditions, the presence of psychosis should prompt a search for the underlying etiology. Indeed, psychosis can result from numerous medical, neurological, and psychiatric illnesses. Historically, psychosis is considered "primary" when there is no identifiable inducing agent or medical condition. On the contrary, psychosis is considered "secondary" when the psychotic symptoms are induced by an identified medical/ neurological condition, prescribed medications, drugs of abuse, exposure to toxins, or other causes. Notably, in primary psychotic disorders, the most common type of hallucinations is auditory. However, visual, tactile, gustatory, or olfactory hallucinations in the absence of auditory hallucinations are more likely to be related to secondary psychotic disorders [1]. This chapter will focus on primary psychosis or primary psychotic disorders including brief psychotic disorder, schizophreniform disorder, schizophrenia, schizoaffective disorder, and delusional disorder. More space will be dedicated to schizophrenia, as it is the prototypical psychotic disorder.

18.2 Brief Psychotic Disorder

18.2.1 Diagnosis

According to the Diagnostic and Statistical Manual of Mental Disorders, Fifth Edition (DSM-5) [2], brief psychotic disorder is diagnosed when at least one psychotic symptom (hallucination, delusion, disorganized speech or behavior) occurs for at least 1 day and no more than 1 month. Patients are expected to return to premorbid functional status.

18.2.2 Epidemiology

The prevalence of brief psychotic disorder is estimated to range between 3% and 9% of all first-admission psychoses, making it rare among the other psychotic disorders [3]. The mean age of onset is mid-30s, and it is more prevalent among women.

18.2.3 Genetics

The genetic basis for brief psychotic disorder is not well understood.

18.2.4 Neurobiology

Abnormal frontal lobe volume as well as functional connectivity abnormalities between attentional and visual processing networks have been associated with brief psychotic disorder [4].

18.2.5 Clinical Manifestations

Symptoms may emerge abruptly, with disorganized thought process, bizarre behavior, psychomotor agitation, and elevated emotionality. Patients with brief psychotic disorder tend to have higher premorbid functioning than those with schizophrenia.

18.2.6 Treatment

Antipsychotic medications are first-line treatment. Psychoeducation is recommended for patients and their family.

18.3 Schizophreniform Disorder

18.3.1 Diagnosis

Schizophreniform disorder is diagnosed when an individual develops a psychotic syndrome consisting of criterion A signs and symptoms of schizophrenia (see Section 18.4) but for a shorter duration of time (less than 6 months).

18.3.2 Epidemiology and Genetics

The estimated lifetime prevalence of schizophreniform disorder was 0.07% in one sample [5]. Persons with schizophreniform disorder may be more likely to have relatives with schizophrenia but not affective disorders [6] – a finding suggestive of common genetic risk with schizophrenia.

18.3.3 Clinical Manifestations and Treatment

The clinical manifestations of schizophreniform disorder are similar to those in schizophrenia, with the exception of the duration of symptoms. As in schizophrenia, antipsychotic medications (the mainstay of treatment) should be combined with psychosocial interventions.

18.4 Schizophrenia

18.4.1 Historical Background

Before it was known as schizophrenia, Emil Kraepelin, a German psychiatrist, in the late 19th century, described a syndrome he termed *dementia praecox*, or precocious dementia, after noting a pattern of functional decline that occurred at variable speeds across cases [7]. Subsequently, Eugen Bleuler, a Swiss psychiatrist, in the early 1900s, coined the term *schizophrenia*, reframing the illness as a split of psyche (i.e., thought, emotion, and behavior) [7]. Thereafter, Kurt Schneider, a German psychiatrist, in the 1950s, introduced a set of first- and second-rank symptoms that he believed were pathognomonic for schizophrenia [8]. The use of first- and second-rank symptoms has subsequently been criticized after they were found to be present in only a subset of persons meeting criteria for schizophrenia, and because of the high frequency with which they are seen in other disorders [8].

18.4.2 Diagnosis

According to DSM-5, schizophrenia is diagnosed when at least two of the following symptoms are present for most of a 1-month period: delusions, hallucinations, disorganized speech, grossly disorganized or catatonic behavior, and negative symptoms (i.e., diminished emotional expression or avolition). At least one of the symptoms must be one of the first three listed. Furthermore, for a significant portion of time since symptom onset, functioning in a major area (such as work, relationships, or self-care) is markedly impaired. Also, signs of the mental disturbance must be present for at least 6 months; the 6-month period must include at least a 1-month period during which psychotic symptoms are obvious (the active phase) and may include periods when psychotic symptoms are attenuated (prodromal or residual phases). However, schizophrenia can still be diagnosed if the active phase is less than 1 month (e.g., in a situation where the psychotic symptoms were successfully treated).

18.4.3 Epidemiology

Median lifetime prevalence of schizophrenia is between 0.4% and 0.64 % and up to 1% [9]. Age of onset typically falls between late adolescence and the mid-20s. On average, women become symptomatic several years later than men do, and the age of onset for women has a second "peak" in the 40s.

18.4.4 Environmental Risk Factors and Genetics

The schizophrenia phenotype is now widely believed to result from an interaction between a person's genetic makeup and environmental exposures/stressors (risk factors) in utero, childhood, and early adolescence. Such risk factors include prenatal exposure to infectious agents (e.g., viruses, toxoplasma), maternal nutritional deficiencies during pregnancy, birth trauma, birth during late winter or early spring, childhood adversity, urban dwelling, immigration, advanced paternal age, and chronic/heavy use of cannabis. However, some of the aforementioned risk factors (e.g., childhood adversity) have a tenuous association with schizophrenia [10]. In contrast, a family history of schizophrenia is an established risk factor for schizophrenia. Indeed, the risk of schizophrenia in a person with a mother, father, or sibling suffering from schizophrenia is seven to nine times higher than in persons without a family history of schizophrenia [11]. Furthermore, schizophrenia is highly heritable, with a heritability (a statistical measure of how much of the variation in a given trait can be attributed to genetic differences between individuals in the population) estimate of approximately 80% [12].

Additionally, several alterations (referred to as *genomic variants*) in a single base pair of DNA (e.g., adenine, thymine, cytosine, or guanine) have been associated with schizophrenia. If the variants are present in at least 1% of the population, they are called *single-nucleotide polymorphisms* (SNPs), but *single-nucleotide variants* (SNVs) if present in less than 1% of the population. Currently, 329 SNPs in 270 independent loci have been associated with schizophrenia [13]. Importantly, each SNP independently is unlikely to result in the schizophrenia phenotype but may confer significant risk when multiple schizophrenia-associated SNPs are inherited together. In fact, the concept of polygenic risk score (PRS) has recently been introduced to estimate the risk of schizophrenia in a person based on the schizophrenia-associated SNPs inherited by the person [14]. Specifically, PRS is calculated as a weighted sum of SNPs found in the latest schizophrenia genome-wide association study (GWAS). Although there are limitations, higher PRS indicates a higher genetic susceptibility to schizophrenia.

In contrast to SNPs, inheritance of a copy number variant (CNV), which disrupts a large amount of genetic material, independently increases the risk of manifesting the schizophrenia phenotype (i.e., more clinically penetrant than SNPs). At least 15 CNVs associated with schizophrenia have been identified; of these, deletions at 22q11.2 and 3q29 are known to have the highest risk for schizophrenia (>50-fold risk). Moreover, some of the genetic risk factors associated with schizophrenia are known to be associated with dopamine and glutamate neurotransmission (specifically with respect to the N-methyl-D-aspartate, or NMDA, receptor), as well as immune system functioning, especially the major histocompatibility complex and the complement system, respectively [15] (see further discussion in the next section).

18.4.5 Neurobiology

The most well-known explanatory hypothesis for schizophrenia is the dopamine hypothesis, which posits that hallucinations and delusions are caused by excessive dopamine activity in the brain's mesolimbic pathway (Figure 18.1). The mesolimbic pathway consists of neurons projecting from the ventral tegmental area (dopamine-rich nucleus in the mid brain) to the ventral striatum (nucleus accumbens). The dopamine hypothesis is supported by the mechanism of action of antipsychotic medications (reduction of mesolimbic dopamine activity via blockade of dopamine-2 receptors) and by the fact that drugs that increase dopaminergic activity (e.g., CNS stimulants such as amphetamines) may induce psychotic symptoms. The dopamine hypothesis of schizophrenia also extends to the mesocortical pathway that projects from the ventral tegmental area to the frontal cortex; however, there is reduced dopaminergic transmission in this pathway. Reduced dopamine neurotransmission in the mesocortical pathway has been linked to cognitive impairment, now considered a core feature of schizophrenia.

However, the dopamine hypothesis is not sufficient to explain the full scope of neuropsychiatric dysfunction seen in individuals with schizophrenia, and NMDA receptor (NMDAR) dysfunction and aberrant glutamatergic transmission have emerged as

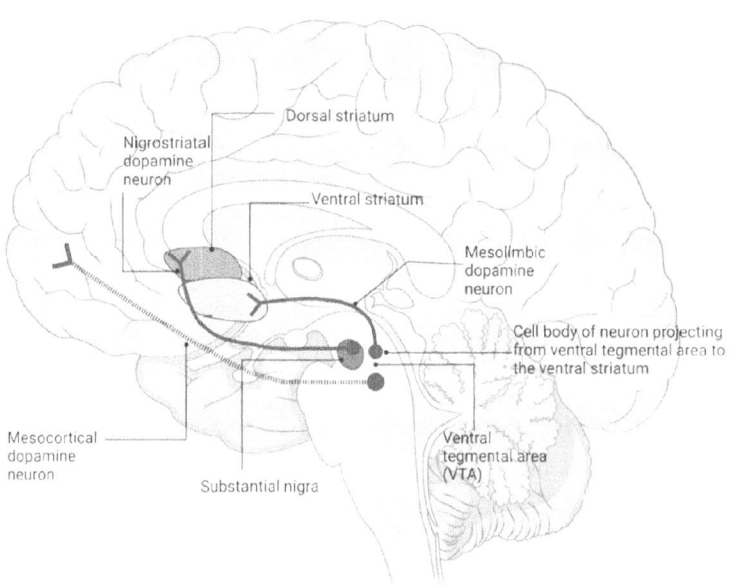

Figure created with BioRender.com

Figure 18.1 Dopamine hypothesis of schizophrenia. The projection from the ventral tegmental area (VTA) to the ventral striatum (mesolimbic pathway) is in bold, depicting increased dopamine neurotransmission in this pathway. However, in the axonal projection from the VTA to the frontal cortex (mesocortical pathway), the broken lines indicate reduced dopamine neurotransmission. Blockade of dopamine neurotransmission in the nigrostriatal pathway by antipsychotic medications can lead to movement side effects (acute dystonia, parkinsonism).
Created with BioRender.com.

complementary to the dopamine hypothesis. Specifically, the NMDA hypothesis of schizophrenia posits that NMDA receptors on parvalbumin-positive cortical inhibitory gamma-aminobutyric acid (GABA) interneurons are hypofunctional and are therefore unable to inhibit pyramidal (glutamatergic) neurons which project to the mesolimbic dopamine neurons (i.e., cortical-brainstem projection) in the VTA. As glutamate is excitatory, the uninhibited release of glutamate by the cortical-brainstem glutamate neurons that make connections with the mesolimbic dopamine neurons in the VTA results in excessive release of dopamine in the mesolimbic pathway (Figure 18.2), thereby worsening positive symptoms of psychosis (delusions and hallucinations).

NMDA receptor hypofunction of cortical GABA interneurons has also been linked to cognitive impairment via a pathway that involves another set of GABA inhibitory interneurons in the brainstem (Figure 18.3).

Additionally, muscarinic cholinergic receptor (M1 and M4) and trace amine-associated receptor 1 (TAAR-1) dysfunction have been implicated in the pathophysiology of schizophrenia. Medications that target these receptors are currently being tested for the treatment of symptoms of schizophrenia [16].

Importantly, the neuropathological processes that cause abnormal structure and functioning of brain networks in individuals with schizophrenia are thought to begin

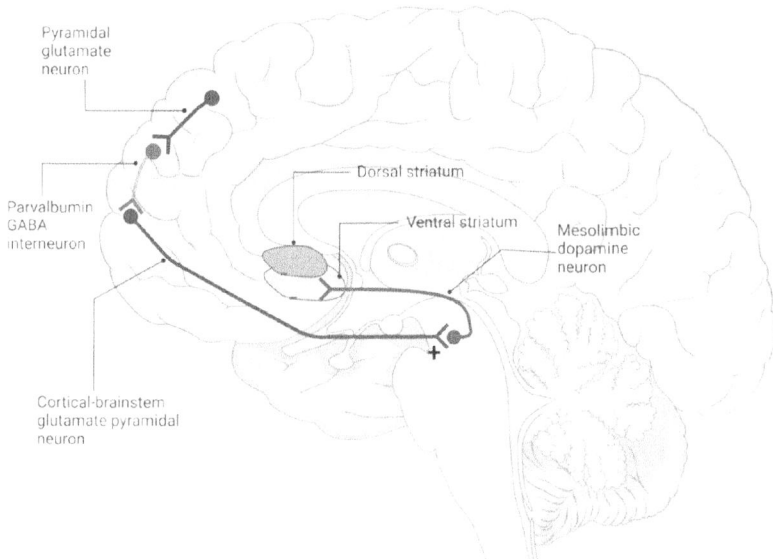

Figure created with BioRender.com

Figure 18.2 NMDA hypothesis of schizophrenia (direct pathway). The GABA interneuron with abnormal NMDA receptors is depicted in gray and with broken lines. As a result of failure of the GABA interneuron to inhibit the glutamate neuron projecting from the cortex to the brain stem (making connection with the cell body of the mesolimbic dopamine neuron), there is excessive dopaminergic neurotransmission in the mesolimbic pathway, which subsequently results in positive symptoms of schizophrenia.
Created with BioRender.com.

years before the onset of psychotic symptoms and cognitive abnormalities – perhaps as early as the prenatal period. For this reason, schizophrenia is considered to be a neurodevelopmental disorder. Furthermore, early life exposure to infectious agents and other proinflammatory factors impacting the brain's immune system are thought to promote increased proinflammatory activity and dysfunction of microglia (the brain's immune cells). Consequently, during childhood and adolescence, the dysfunctional microglia excessively remove or prune synapses (synaptic pruning is a major mechanism of brain maturation). Moreover, excessive synaptic pruning has been linked to loss of gray matter volume and abnormal white matter integrity (particularly in frontal and temporal lobes) and to complement component 4 abnormalities in schizophrenia [17].

18.4.6 Clinical Manifestations

Schizophrenia is heterogeneous in its clinical manifestations, course, and outcomes. Oftentimes, there is a prodromal period of several months to years prior to the emergence of prominent psychotic symptoms. During the prodromal period, patients might exhibit social withdrawal, cognitive disturbance (difficulty concentrating or paying attention), and diminishing interest in personal hygiene. During the active phase of

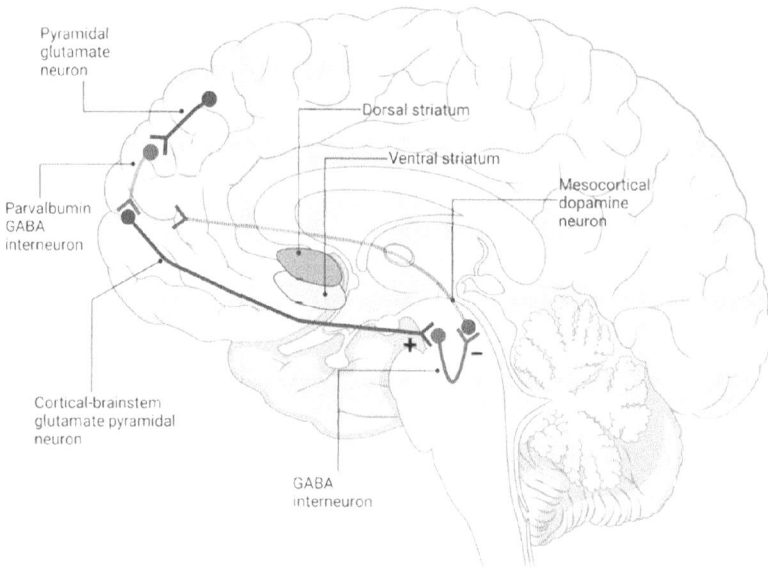

Figure 18.3 NMDA hypothesis of schizophrenia (indirect pathway). A second set of GABA interneurons are located in between the cortical-brainstem glutamate neuron and the mesocortical dopamine neurons. Unlike the ones in the cortex, the brainstem GABA interneurons have normal NMDA receptors and effectively provide inhibitory signals to the mesocortical dopamine neurons. Excessive inhibition of the mesocortical neuron (depicted by the broken lines) is believed to underlie the cognitive symptoms of schizophrenia. Created with BioRender.com.

illness when psychotic symptoms become prominent, patients can report delusional ideas and experience hallucinations. Patients also exhibit disorganized speech (tangential, incoherent speech) and behavior. Delusions, hallucinations, and disorganized speech and behavior are all referred to as *positive symptoms*. However, some patients exhibit *negative symptoms* such as abnormally reduced speech with little or no elaboration (referred to as poverty of speech) and lack of normal emotional reaction and variation in facial expression in response to emotion-evoking stimuli (referred to as blunted affect). Some patients may also exhibit agitated or hostile behavior secondary to delusions or hallucinations. Suicidal ideation and suicide attempt can also accompany positive psychotic symptoms.

18.4.7 Treatment

Antipsychotic medications are the mainstay of psychopharmacological management of schizophrenia. Antipsychotics are effective for both acute and long-term management, prevent relapse, reduce hospitalizations, and improve functioning in persons with schizophrenia. Antipsychotic medications are divided into first-generation (or "typical") and second-generation (or "atypical") classes (please see Chapter 7 on psychopharmacology). Most patients are now started and maintained on the second-generation antipsychotic medications due to their lower liability for movement side effects (acute dystonia, akathisia, parkinsonism, and tardive dyskinesia) relative to the first-generation antipsychotic medications. However, most second-generation medications have a higher risk of metabolic syndrome (obesity, dyslipidemia, diabetes, hypertension) relative to first-generation medications. Clozapine is a particularly notable drug in that it is considered to be the most effective pharmacological treatment for schizophrenia, and the only one approved for treatment-resistant schizophrenia. A patient is labeled as being treatment-resistant if psychotic symptoms are not controlled by at least two different antipsychotic medications sequentially prescribed at optimal doses for an adequate period of time (at least 6 weeks). Electroconvulsive therapy (ECT), either alone or in combination with clozapine, has also been shown to be effective in treatment-resistant cases. Of note, none of the currently available antipsychotic medications has been shown to be clinically effective for treating negative or cognitive symptoms of schizophrenia. Adjunctive medications that are sometimes prescribed alongside antipsychotic medications include mood stabilizers (for mood lability or aggression), antidepressants (to target depressive symptoms), and short-term sedative-hypnotics (to target anxiety and insomnia).

Psychological and social (psychosocial) interventions such as family interventions, psychoeducation, cognitive behavioral therapy, vocational rehabilitation and supported employment, social skills training, appropriate housing (e.g., supervised group/personal care homes), and cognitive remediation are also important for achieving the best outcomes in patients with schizophrenia. Furthermore, since patients (especially in the chronic phase of illness) often present with metabolic abnormalities including overweight/obesity, dyslipidemia, insulin resistance/diabetes, hypertension, and chronic inflammation [18], liaison with a primary care physician is advisable.

18.5 Schizoaffective Disorder

18.5.1 Diagnosis

Schizoaffective disorder is diagnosed when an individual meets criterion A for schizophrenia and concurrently experiences a major mood episode (depression or mania). The psychotic symptoms must occur for at least 2 consecutive weeks in the absence of a major mood episode. Importantly, mood symptoms may still be present for most of the illness. However, the distinction between schizoaffective disorder and schizophrenia has been questioned, as both disorders were found to be identical to one another on key cognitive, social cognitive, and neural measures [19]. Subtypes of schizoaffective disorder include bipolar type (in which there are manic episodes, with or without depressive episodes) and depressive type (in which there are only depressive episodes).

18.5.2 Epidemiology

The lifetime prevalence of schizoaffective disorder is estimated to range between 0.3% and 0.5%, and it appears to be more commonly diagnosed in women. Younger individuals are more likely to be diagnosed with the bipolar subtype, and the depressive subtype is more commonly diagnosed in older individuals.

18.5.3 Neurobiology

Results of structural and functional neuroimaging studies indicate that persons with schizoaffective disorder and schizophrenia have similar changes in gray matter volume, and these changes are greater than those in patients with bipolar disorder.

18.5.4 Genetics

The genetics of schizoaffective disorder has been less investigated relative to those of schizophrenia, but the disease seems to share genetic correlation with both schizophrenia and bipolar disorder [20].

18.5.5 Clinical Manifestations

Patients present with psychotic symptoms similar to those seen in patients with schizophrenia but with affective (mood) episodes. However, in general, both cognitive and social impairments are less severe in schizoaffective disorder, compared to schizophrenia – but more severe than in mood disorders.

18.5.6 Treatment

Antipsychotic medications are first line, but they are often prescribed in combination with mood stabilizers or antidepressants. Paliperidone is the only FDA-approved medication for schizoaffective disorder and has the benefit of being available in a long-acting injectable formulation. Electroconvulsive therapy can also be an effective treatment for schizoaffective disorder, especially in treatment-resistant cases. As in schizophrenia, psychosocial interventions are also included in the treatment plan of patients with schizoaffective disorder.

18.6 Delusional Disorder

Delusional disorder is diagnosed when a person has one or more delusions for at least 1 month, and when criterion A for schizophrenia has never been met. Grossly bizarre behavior, as in schizophrenia, must not be present. DSM-5 subtypes of delusional disorder (according to the type of delusion) include persecutory, jealous, erotomanic, grandiose, somatic, mixed, or unspecified.

18.6.1 Epidemiology

The prevalence of delusional disorder is estimated to be 0.2%. Mean age of onset is between the late 30s and 40s, but some patients may have initial onset in midlife or old age.

18.6.2 Genetics

The genetics of delusional disorder is not well understood, but a family history of schizophrenia has been found to increase the risk of delusional disorder [21].

18.6.3 Neurobiology

Abnormalities in dopamine and serotonin neurotransmission as well as abnormalities in the medial frontal/anterior cingulate cortex and insula (key nodes in the salience network) have been linked to delusional disorder [22].

18.6.4 Clinical Manifestations

Psychotic features may not be apparent initially, especially if the delusions are not being discussed. Delusions negatively impact work and interpersonal relations (e.g., false accusations that coworkers are intentionally trying to make life difficult for him/her). Delusional disorder can be accompanied by mood symptoms (e.g., depression) and aggressive/violent behavior.

18.6.5 Treatment

Delusional disorder is difficult to treat due to lack of insight, which makes patients resistant to any treatment recommendation. Nevertheless, some evidence supports the use of both first and second-generation antipsychotics [23]. Psychological interventions such as cognitive-behavioral strategies may also help improve a patient's insight in addition to symptom reduction.

References

1. Arciniegas DB. Psychosis. Contin. Lifelong Learn. *Neurol.* 2015;**21**:715–736.

2. American Psychiatric Association. DSM-5 Diagnostic Classification. In *Diagnostic and Statistical Manual of Mental Disorders.* APA Publishing; 2013.

3. Susser E, Fennig S, Jandorf L, Amador X, Bromet E. Epidemiology, diagnosis, and course of brief psychoses. *Am J Psychiatry.* 1995;**152**:1743–1748.

4. Li H, Kéri S. Regional brain volumes in brief psychotic disorder. *J Neural Transm.* 2020;**127**:371–378.

5. Perälä J, Suvisaari J, Saarni SI, Kuoppasalmi K, Isometsä E, Pirkola S, et al. Lifetime prevalence of psychotic and bipolar I disorders in a general population. *Arch Gen Psychiatry.* 2007;**64**:19–28.

6. Kendler KS, Walsh D. Schizophreniform disorder, delusional disorder and psychotic disorder not otherwise specified: clinical features, outcome and familial psychopathology. *Acta Psychiatr Scand.* 1995;**91**:370–378.

7. Ebert A, Bär KJ. Emil Kraepelin: a pioneer of scientific understanding of psychiatry and psychopharmacology. *Indian J. Psychiatry.* 2010;**52**:191–192.

8. Lake CR. Kurt Schneider (1887–1967): First- and Second- Rank Symptoms, Not Pathognomonic of Schizophrenia, Explained by Psychotic Mood Disorders. In: Lake CR (editor). Schizophrenia Is a Misdiagnosis: Implications for the DSM-5 and the ICD-11. Springer, New York, 2012. Pages 137–150

9. Saha S, Chant D, Welham J, McGrath J. A systematic review of the prevalence of schizophrenia. *PLoS Med.* 2005;**2**:e141.

10. Jauhar S, Johnstone M, McKenna PJ. Schizophrenia. *Lancet.* 2022;**399**:473–486.

11. Mortensen PB, Pedersen CB, Westergaard T, Wohlfahrt J, Ewald H, Mors O, et al. Effects of family history and place and season of birth on the risk of schizophrenia. *N Engl J Med.* 1999;**340**:603–608.

12. Hilker R, Helenius D, Fagerlund B, Skytthe A, Christensen K, Werge TM, et al. Heritability of schizophrenia and schizophrenia spectrum based on the nationwide Danish twin register. *Biol Psychiatry.* 2018;**83**:492–498.

13. Consortium TSWG of the PG, Ripke S, Walters JT, O'Donovan MC. Mapping genomic loci prioritises genes and implicates synaptic biology in schizophrenia. *medRxiv* 2020;2020.09.12:20192922.

14. Weinberger DR. Polygenic risk scores in clinical schizophrenia research. *Am J Psychiatry.* 2019;**176**:3–4.

15. Howes OD, McCutcheon R, Owen MJ, Murray RM. The role of genes, stress, and dopamine in the development of

schizophrenia. *Biol Psychiatry*. 2017;**81**:9–20.

16. Krogmann A, Peters L, Von Hardenberg L, Bödeker K, Nöhles VB, Correll CU. Keeping up with the therapeutic advances in schizophrenia: a review of novel and emerging pharmacological entities. *CNS Spectr*. 2019;**24**:41–68.

17. Sekar A, Bialas AR, De Rivera H, Davis A, Hammond TR, Kamitaki N, et al. Schizophrenia risk from complex variation of complement component 4. *Nature*. 2016;**530**:177–183.

18. Boozalis T, Devaraj S, Okusaga OO. Correlations between body mass index, plasma high-sensitivity C-reactive protein and lipids in patients with schizophrenia. *Psychiatr Q*. 2019;**90**:101–110.

19. Hartman LI, Heinrichs RW, Mashhadi F. The continuing story of schizophrenia and schizoaffective disorder: one condition or two? *Schizophr Res Cogn*. 2019;**16**:36.

20. Cardno AG, Owen MJ. Genetic relationships between schizophrenia, bipolar disorder, and schizoaffective disorder. *Schizophr Bull*. 2014;**40**:504–515.

21. Chou IJ, Kuo CF, Huang YS, Grainge MJ, Valdes AM, See LC, et al. Familial aggregation and heritability of schizophrenia and co-aggregation of psychiatric illnesses in affected families. *Schizophr Bull*. 2017;**43**:1070.

22. Vicens V, Radua J, Salvador R, Anguera-Camós M, Canales-Rodríguez EJ, Sarró S, et al. Structural and functional brain changes in delusional disorder. *Br J Psychiatry*. 2016;**208**:153–159.

23. Muñoz-Negro JE, Cervilla JA. A systematic review on the pharmacological treatment of delusional disorder. *J Clin Psychopharmacol*. 2016;**36**:684–690.

Anxiety Disorders

Grace Kim, Vaishali Tirumalaraju, and Sudhakar Selvaraj

19.1 Introduction

Anxiety disorders, including social anxiety disorder, panic disorder (or attacks), generalized anxiety disorder, specific phobias (including agoraphobia), selective mutism, and separation anxiety disorder, constitute the largest group of mental disorders. These disorders impose a large burden on society due to their chronic nature, comorbidity with other conditions, and prevalence. According to the global burden of disease study, around 275 million people are affected by anxiety disorders. Furthermore, there are around 42 million newly diagnosed with anxiety disorders per year worldwide [1]. As a whole, patients who have anxiety disorders have significantly higher median medical care charges than patients without anxiety disorders, indicating a high individual economic burden of disease [2, 3]. Anxiety disorders are also a risk factor for suicidal behavior. Comorbidity with a mood disorder correlates with an even higher risk factor for suicidal behavior [4].

Despite their high prevalence, anxiety disorders have not always been well documented throughout history. Ancient Greek and Latin writings were first to describe anxiety as its own set of medical disorder, separating it from other mood disorders and detailing the disease as a negative influence and how to overcome it with cognitive techniques. There is a gap in history in which anxiety disorders are, for the most part, absent in writing. In the 19th and 20th centuries, anxiety disorders were diagnosed as "pantophobia," "neurasthenia," or "anxiety neurosis." Pantophobia refers to a generalized fear of everything and is included in the broad category of neurasthenia – nervous exhaustion. *Anxiety neurosis* is a term coined by Sigmund Freud, and he initially described it as an accumulation of sexual excitation that couldn't be released by sex. The term was later utilized by others but devoid of its sexual component [5]. The DSM-1, in 1952, had a category called "psychoneurotic disorders" and placed "anxiety reaction" in this category, describing it as anxious expectation often associated with somatic symptoms. The DSM-II revised these symptoms as "neuroses" in which the main symptom was anxiety. Starting with the DSM-III, anxiety disorders were classified into distinct disorders, including generalized anxiety disorder and panic disorder. From then on, further editions of the DSM have grouped anxiety disorders into different stratifications (anxiety, obsessive-compulsive disorder, and trauma/stress-related disorders) [6].

The defining characteristics of anxiety disorders include extreme or excessive fear and anxiety that persists and/or avoidance of perceived threats. These disorders are diagnosed in accordance with either the Diagnostic and Statistical Manual of Mental Disorders, Fifth Edition (DSM-5) or the International Classification of Disease, Tenth Edition (ICD-10). Some traits that differentiate anxiety disorders from more typical or transient fear or anxiety are the length of anxiety (usually lasting 6 months or more) and if the anxiety that the patient feels is disproportionate to the realistic level of danger they are in. Additionally, in disorders such as selective mutism or separation anxiety disorder, which are more common in childhood, it is important to distinguish if the level of anxiety that the patient displays is consistent with the patient's level of development [7].

The onset of anxiety disorders is often during childhood, adolescence, or early adulthood. Subsets of anxiety disorders have different average ages of onset, with separation anxiety disorder and phobias having early ages of onset (ages 7–14 median) and other anxiety disorders (generalized anxiety disorder, panic disorder) having later ages of onset (ages 24–50 median) [8]. Anxiety disorders also have a high prevalence, with an estimated prevalence of about 28.3% globally in 2012 [9]. Prevalence and burden highlight the importance of researching ideal intervention methods for anxiety disorders ranging from early intervention to cognitive behavioral therapy to pharmacological treatment. This chapter discusses the clinical presentation, epidemiology, pathophysiology, and management of anxiety disorders with additional emphasis on current and ongoing research on these disorders.

19.2 Clinical Presentation

The DSM-5 details 11 different types of anxiety disorders, each with distinct clinical presentations. Though all of them present with extreme anxiety, they differ in what causes the said anxiety as detailed in Table 19.1.

Additionally, many anxiety disorders are often comorbid with other anxiety disorders and mental disorders. Therefore, it is important to consider the clinical diagnosis of anxiety disorders even when treating other mental disorders. Cross-disorder comorbidity is often associated with more severe symptoms, longer duration, and greater rates of treatment than single anxiety disorders [17].

19.3 Diagnosis/Screening

Clinically diagnosing anxiety disorders as a whole can be difficult because of the reliance on history and lack of biomarkers to verify a diagnosis. It is helpful to use screening tools such as the Generalized Anxiety Disorder 7-item (GAD-7) and the Penn State Worry Questionnaire for Measuring Response (PSWQMR). These questionnaires help provide a more standardized response that can be used to diagnose the patient with anxiety disorders. These methods have been shown to be sensitive and specific to detecting anxiety disorders [18].

19.4 Epidemiology

Anxiety disorders are the most common group of disorders in mental health, with 1 out of 14 people meeting diagnostic criteria at any point in time [9]. However, there is variability in the prevalence of anxiety disorders among various countries and cultures. Non-Western cultures are associated with having a lower risk for anxiety disorders [9]. It remains to be seen whether these differences are legitimate or partly due to a lack of diagnosis, education, or cultural taboos [19]. There are also culture-specific anxiety disorders such as taijin hyo-fusho, a social anxiety disorder regional to East Asian cultures that stems from a fear of embarrassing others rather than themselves [20].

The onset of anxiety disorders is overall early in life, often manifesting in childhood or young adulthood. Specifically, separation anxiety disorder and specific phobia are

Table 19.1 Types of anxiety disorders according to DSM-5

Disorder	Age of Onset	Duration of Symptoms Necessary for Diagnosis	Clinical Symptoms	Prevalence
Separation anxiety disorder	Ages 7–14	More than 4 weeks in children 6 months or more in adults	Excessive fear and anxiety related to separation from home or people that the patient is attached to that is unreasonable to the person's developmental stage Can manifest as excessive worry about harm or death happening to an attachment figure, fear about leaving home, or extreme distress on being separated from attachment figures	Lifetime prevalence around the world 4.8% [10]
Selective mutism	Before 5 years of age	At least 1 month	Children fail to respond and speak to others in specific social interactions, even though they choose to speak at home or in other more comfortable situations	Relatively rare, 0.71% in a school-based study [11]
Specific phobia	Early childhood; median age 7–11 years	6 months or longer	Exaggerated fear and anxiety of a specific object or situation that occurs every time the person is presented with that object/situation that interferes with person's functioning	Lifetime prevalence around the world 3–15% [12]
Social anxiety disorder	Median age of onset 13 years	6 months or longer	Marked fear and anxiety in relation to social situations Difficulty maintaining social and professional relationships	Lifetime prevalence in the US 12.1% [13]
Panic disorder	Median age of onset 20–24 years	At least one of the attacks is followed by 1 month or more of persistent worry about additional panic attacks and consequences or significant maladaptive change in behavior related to the panic attack	Recurrent panic attacks that have four or more of the following symptoms: palpitations or racing heart, paresthesia, sweating, fear of losing control, chest pain, lightheadedness, shaking, shortness of breath, nausea, depersonalization, child, feelings of choking, fear of dying that can occur with or without known trigger	Lifetime prevalence in the US 4.7% [14]

Table 19.1 (*cont.*)

Disorder	Age of Onset	Duration of Symptoms Necessary for Diagnosis	Clinical Symptoms	Prevalence
Agoraphobia	Onset average 17 years of age; majority have initial onset before 35	6 months or longer	Irrational fear or anxiety of facing two or more of the following: using public transportation, being in open spaces, being outside of the home alone, being in a line or crowd	Lifetime prevalence in the US 1.3% [15]
Generalized anxiety disorder	Very broad age of onset; median age of onset 30 years	6 months or longer	Excessive worry and anxiety about various aspects of daily life including school, work, or personal relationships Three or more of the following (one in kids): difficulty concentrating, restlessness, irritability, muscle tension, fatigue, sleep disturbances	Lifetime prevalence in the US 5.7% [16]
Substance/medication-induced anxiety disorder			Symptoms of anxiety disorder that can't be explained by other disorders except by use of substance/medication Common substances include alcohol, stimulants, cannabis, hallucinogens Common medications include anesthetics, antipsychotics	Unclear
Anxiety disorders due to another medical condition			Anxiety disorders that are caused by a separate condition (not another mental disorder) Most commonly panic attacks and anxiety manifestations Commonly include metabolic disturbances, neurological illnesses, endocrine diseases	Unclear
Other specified anxiety disorder			Symptoms characteristic of an anxiety disorder that causes significant impairment in life, but doesn't meet criteria of other anxiety disorders and clinicians specify the reason why the patient doesn't meet the criteria	Unclear

Table 19.1 (*cont.*)

Disorder	Age of Onset	Duration of Symptoms Necessary for Diagnosis	Clinical Symptoms	Prevalence
Unspecified anxiety disorders			Similar as above but without the clinician specification	Unclear

Source: Anxiety Disorders. *Diagnostic and Statistical Manual of Mental Disorders* (American Psychiatric Association Publishing, 2022). https://doi.org/10.1176/appi.books.9780890425787.x05_Anxiety_Disorders.

shown to onset in childhood and early adolescence. In contrast, generalized anxiety disorder and panic disorder have later onsets in young adulthood [21]. Along with having early onset, anxiety disorders are highly chronic with high 12-month to lifetime prevalence ratios [19].

Anxiety disorders are more prevalent in women than in men, with women having higher rates of lifetime diagnosis for anxiety disorders. There are no gender differences in the age of onset or duration of the disorder [22]. Some socioeconomic components that increase the risk for anxiety disorders include unmarried status, low education, and low income [18].

Other risk factors for anxiety disorders include a parental history of mood or anxiety disorder and childhood adversities. In particular, history of childhood sexual abuse is associated with an increased risk for anxiety disorders including panic disorder, social anxiety disorder, and agoraphobia [23]. Parenting styles that are overbearing or rejective have also been seen to increase a child's risk of developing an anxiety disorder [23].

It is very important to remember that comorbidity is high in anxiety disorders. In the United States, the National Comorbidity Study has found that three-quarters of people with a chronic anxiety disorder also have another mental illness. Several people who have one anxiety disorder often fulfill the diagnostic criteria for another anxiety disorder. Some strong associations to take note of are that between generalized anxiety disorder and panic disorder as well as between panic disorder and agoraphobia. There is also high comorbidity between anxiety disorders and mood disorders and substance use disorders. In general, the onset of anxiety disorders either comes before or at the same time as the onset of mood disorders and before alcohol/substance use disorders [24].

19.5 Pathophysiology

19.5.1 Genetics

Anxiety disorders are known to have moderate to strong heritability, with twin studies suggesting that heritability ranges from 30% to 50%. Additionally, the risk of developing an anxiety disorder in someone who has a first-degree relative with an anxiety disorder is four to six times higher than in general population. The genetic risks also cross diagnoses lines, with family members having one anxiety disorder casting a greater probability for relatives to suffer from a range of anxiety disorders. However, the genetic risk of anxiety disorders is not simply caused by a single gene, and instead they are likely to come from a multitude of different genetic factors [25].

Many genetic studies for anxiety disorders have focused on candidate genes that relate to the hypothalamic–pituitary–adrenal (HPA) axis and the monoaminergic neurotransmitter system. Multiple lines of research focused on candidate gene variants of COMT (catechol-O-methyltransferase) and SLC6A4 (serotonin transporter allele) as biomarkers of anxiety disorders [25]. However, research studies suggest anxiety disorders are likely polygenic with anxiety-related phenotypes.

More comprehensive genome-wide association studies (GWAS) allow for the testing of genetic variants as they relate to anxiety disorders throughout the whole genome [25]. A recent GWAS study suggested used one of the world's largest biobanks – the Million Veterans Program – to find potential signals for a continuous trait of anxiety. Some significant signals that were found include on chromosome 3 near SATB1 (global regulator for gene expression) and chromosome 6 near ESR1 (estrogen receptor). Another locus – MAD1L1 on chromosome 7 – was found to be a significant signal for anxiety and has already been identified as a signal for bipolar disorder and schizophrenia. This creates avenues to explore genetic sources of comorbidity of mental disorders [26]. However, the process of conducting GWAS studies in relation to anxiety disorders has barriers. Two main challenges to be overcome are the small sample size and phenotypic heterogeneity. To counter the phenotypic heterogeneity barrier, it has been proposed that studying clusters of anxiety disorders with shared genetic risk factors rather than studying individual anxiety disorders may be beneficial [25]. It is also important to consider epigenetics, referring to the modification of genes through mechanisms such as methylation. Originally, many epigenetics studies were focused on candidate gene studies with how the brain changed due to stress response. However, with the advent of whole-genome epigenetic technology (EWAS – epigenome-wide association study), epigenetic research in anxiety disorders remains a hopeful area of research [25].

19.5.2 Environment

A person's environment can strongly influence their mental health and ability to manage stress. For example, specific environmental factors include high-stress situations and exposure to trauma, especially in early years of life. However, measuring these environmental factors objectively can be difficult, as most of them are measured through questionnaires. Retrospective bias and general invalidity of responses hinder the scaling of the impact of environmental measures. Research has shown that early childhood adversity, abuse, and trauma lead to higher risk for a wide variety of mental health disorders including anxiety disorders [27]. Epigenetics of gene and environment is an exciting area of research that can explain how genetic factors change the direction toward disorder risk or resilience. For example, high social support has been shown to mitigate the social anxiety disorder risk conferred by the gene 5-HTTLPR (serotonin-transporter-linked promoter region) [28]. These kinds of effects can be extended to epigenetics. An instance of this is that significantly increased methylation levels in the promoter region of the glucocorticoid gene (NR3C1) have been reported in medication-free GAD patients [28]. Discoveries in epigenetics of gene and environment in relation to anxiety disorders can potentially benefit patients in regard to personalized treatment based on each patient's epigenetic profile [28].

19.5.3 Neuroscience

Understanding the neurobiological mechanisms involved in the development of anxiety and stress-related disorders is of vital importance in effectively treating these conditions. Early animal studies postulated that the amygdala and its efferent projections to regions such as the stria terminalis, the hypothalamus, the hippocampus, the ventral striatum, the orbitofrontal cortex, and the periaqueductal gray was the main circuitry involved in fear conditioning [29]. However, it appeared there are possibly more complex mechanisms at play in the development and maintenance of a sustained threat response. This was evidenced by the preservation of defensive anxious responses in animals with amygdala lesions [30]. Newer animal studies provide evidence that the activation of corticotrophin receptors in the bed nucleus of the stria terminalis (BNST) and its GABA (gamma-aminobutyric acid) medicated projections to the cortical, limbic, and hindbrain structures are more instrumental in the maintenance of a sustained anxiety response that is characteristic of anxiety disorders [31, 32]. Furthermore, it appears different regions of the BNST are responsible for either the upregulation or downregulation of anxiety, the details of which are still unknown [33, 34].

Converging evidence from preclinical models suggests that the current hypothesis for development and maintenance of anxiety is that the perceived environmental threat processed through the ventral hippocampus and the interoceptive signals processed by the insula relay the signal to the medial prefrontal cortex (particularly the prelimbic cortex), which is the center for attention and affective information processing [35–37]. The prelimbic cortex in turn activates the amygdala and the BNST, which then produces the defensive anxious response [37]. In humans, the prefrontal cortex (PFC), particularly the dorsolateral PFC (dlPFC), appears to regulate the anxiety network and sustains the anxious response [38, 39]. Additionally, the dorsomedial PFC (dmPFC) and dorsal anterior cingulate cortex (dACC), which are responsible for goal-directed behaviors, emotional regulation, and interoceptive processing, are also implicated in this network [40–42]. Functional neuroimaging studies in humans link decreased connectivity between the amygdala and PFC with the development of generalized anxiety disorder (GAD) [43, 44]. Newer studies have shown an increase in ventrolateral PFC activity (vlPFC) following treatment intervention in individuals with GAD, implicating that it is possibly an important region that aids in compensatory self-regulation of anxiety [45].

Recent structural neuroimaging studies have shown reduced white matter organization in the fronto-limbic regions such as the uncinate fasciculus and anterior cingulate cortex [46]. Reduced white matter volumes in the midbrain, DLPFC, precentral gyrus, and anterior limb of the internal capsule have also been noted in other studies [46]. While these findings add to the growing body of evidence for the hypothesized neural circuitry involved, there is no clear consensus on structural neuroimaging changes in anxiety disorders [47].

Neuroimaging studies have also demonstrated decreased glucose metabolism in the basal ganglia and increased glucose metabolism in the cortex and other limbic areas in GAD patients versus controls [48]. There is limited and inconclusive evidence, however, regarding the involved neurotransmitters and biomarkers such as serotonin, norepinephrine, C-reactive protein, and other proinflammatory cytokines [49–52]. It has been hypothesized that selective serotonin reuptake inhibitors (SSRIs) likely alleviate anxiety by increasing the synaptic serotonin availability and thereby attenuating the engagement of this PFC-amygdala circuit [53, 54]; however, the exact pathophysiology is still elusive. On the other hand, neuroendocrine changes such as elevated cortisol secondary to sustained threat [43] have been more demonstrable in both animal and human studies, although hardly conclusive. Dysfunction of the HPA axis led to the development of corticotrophin release factor (CRF-1) antagonists to treat mood and anxiety disorders, and while these bore fruit in animal models, evidence from human models and clinical trials is inconclusive [55, 56]. This further leads to a hypothesis that although the initial response to anxiety involves increase in cortisol secondary to the activation of the HPA axis, there is likely an overall decrease in cortisol levels in chronic anxiety [57].

19.5.4 Management

Although anxiety disorders are among the most common of mental disorders, they are often underdiagnosed and consequently undermanaged. However, there are effective ways to manage anxiety disorders that improve the quality of life and symptoms. Both psychological and pharmacological treatments can be beneficial to the patient, and treatment varies per patient. The patient and the provider should participate in a shared decision-making process with side effects, cost, and time taken into account.

19.5.5 Pharmacology

Pharmacological therapies for anxiety disorder patients (Tables 19.2 and 19.3) are often viewed as joint first-line therapies with psychotherapy. Some factors that would prioritize pharmacological interventions include comorbidity with depression, unresponsiveness to psychotherapy, and chronic or severe illness.

Antidepressants are considered the first-line pharmacological therapy for patients with anxiety disorders. The most widely used antidepressants are SSRIs and serotonin noradrenergic reuptake inhibitors (SNRIs). SSRIs and SNRIs have shown efficacy in treating all anxiety disorders except for specific phobia [20]. Some side effects that may deter patients from taking these medications include diarrhea, gastrointestinal discomfort, sexual dysfunction, and insomnia [58]. Other antidepressants such as tricyclic antidepressants (TCA) and monoamine oxidase inhibitors (MAOs) have been used to treat anxiety disorders in the past but have largely been discontinued due to adverse side effects [20].

Benzodiazepines are commonly used in clinics for rapid symptomatic relief in anxiety disorders. However, benzodiazepine use is complicated by their short duration of action, side effect profile, and risk factors associated with dependency and co-intake with alcohol. Some of the side effects associated with benzodiazepines include drowsiness, dizziness, and the risk of falls in the elderly, thereby warranting their cautious use in vulnerable populations. Antiepileptic drugs that regulate GABA levels, such as gabapentin and pregabalin, can be used as an alternative to benzodiazepines in treating anxiety disorders when there is concern about side effects or dependency [20]. Buspirone is a 5-HT1A receptor partial agonist that has been shown to be effective in the treatment of GAD and anxiety symptoms in depression. Furthermore, Buspirone is generally well tolerated [59]. Beta-adrenergic blockers such as propranolol or atenolol are sometimes efficacious for patients with social anxiety disorder but haven't been seen to be effective treatments for other anxiety disorders [20].

Table 19.2 Medications FDA approved for the treatment of anxiety disorders

Drug	Recommended Dose for Adults (mg/day)	Treatment Response	Indications	Common Side Effects
SSRIs				
Fluoxetine	20–60	4–6 weeks	Panic disorder	Diarrhea, GI discomfort, sexual dysfunction, insomnia
Sertraline	50–200	4–6 weeks	Panic disorder, SAD	
Escitalopram	10–20	4–6 weeks	GAD	
Paroxetine	20–60	4–6 weeks	Panic disorder, SAD, GAD	
SNRIs				
Duloxetine	30–60	4–6 weeks	GAD	Diarrhea, GI discomfort, sexual dysfunction, insomnia
Venlafaxine	75–300	4–6 weeks	GAD	
Benzodiazepines				
Clonazepam	1–2	1–2 hours	Panic disorder	Risk of dependency, confusion, drowsiness, dizziness, falls in the elderly
Alprazolam	1–4	1–2 hours	Anxiety, panic disorder	
Lorazepam	2–6	1–6 hours	Anxiety	
Chlordiazepoxide	20–100	0.5–4 hours	Anxiety	
Oxazepam	30–60	1–4 hours	Anxiety	
5-HT1A Partial Agonists				
Buspirone	15–60	2–4 weeks	Anxiety	Dizziness, drowsiness, and nausea
H1 Antagonists				
Hydroxyzine	25–100	4–6 hours	Anxiety	Dry mouth, drowsiness
Antipsychotics				
Trifluoperazine	2–6	2–3 weeks	Anxiety	Extrapyramidal side effects, sedation, weight gain, anticholinergic effects

FDA, Food and Drug Administration; GAD, generalized anxiety disorder; GI, gastrointestinal; SAD, social anxiety disorder.

19.5.6 Psychotherapy

Psychotherapy is often the first-line therapy for most patients with anxiety disorders (Table 19.4). Among psychotherapies, the most efficacious and commonly used is cognitive-behavioral therapy (CBT). People with anxiety disorders typically tend to over-estimate the risk of the situation on hand while concurrently underestimating their own

Table 19.3 Medications frequently used off-label for the treatment of anxiety disorders

Drug	Recommended Dose for Adults (mg/day)	Treatment Response	Indications	Common Side Effects
SSRI				
Citalopram	20–40	4–6 weeks	GAD, Panic disorder, SAD	Diarrhea, GI discomfort, sexual dysfunction, insomnia
Fluoxetine	20–60	4–6 weeks	GAD, SAD	
Sertraline	50–200	4–6 weeks	GAD	
Escitalopram	10–20	4–6 weeks	Panic disorder, SAD	
Paroxetine ER	25–75	4–6 weeks	GAD	
SNRIs				
Duloxetine	30–60	4–6 weeks	Panic disorder, SAD	Diarrhea, GI discomfort, sexual dysfunction, insomnia
Venlafaxine	75–300	4–6 weeks	Panic disorder, SAD	
Desvenlafaxine	50–100	4–6 weeks	GAD, Panic disorder, SAD	
Tricyclic Antidepressants				
Clomipramine	100–250	2–4 weeks	GAD, Panic disorder, SAD	Drowsiness, headache, blurred vision, constipation, dry mouth
Nortriptyline	50–150	2–4 weeks	GAD, Panic disorder, SAD	
Imipramine	100–300	2–4 weeks	GAD, Panic disorder, SAD	
Desipramine	100–200	2–4 weeks	GAD, Panic disorder, SAD	
Atypical Antidepressants				
Mirtazapine	15–45	4–6 weeks	Anxiety, Panic disorder, GAD, SAD	Somnolence, weight gain, dry mouth, constipation

Table 19.3 *(cont.)*

Drug	Recommended Dose for Adults (mg/day)	Treatment Response	Indications	Common Side Effects
GABAergic Medications				
Gabapentin	600–2400	4–8 weeks	GAD, SAD, Panic disorder	Ataxia, dizziness drowsiness, fatigue, somnolence
Pregabalin	150–600	1 day – 4 weeks	GAD, SAD	
Benzodiazepines				
Clonazepam	1–2	1–2 hours	Anxiety, GAD	Risk of dependency, confusion, drowsiness,
Alprazolam	1–4	1–2 hours	SAD, Panic disorder	dizziness, falls in the elderly
Lorazepam	2–6	1–6 hours	GAD, SAD, Panic disorder	
Chlordiazepoxide	20–100	0.5–4 hours	GAD, SAD, Panic disorder	
Oxazepam	30–60	1–4 hours	GAD, SAD, Panic disorder	
Beta Blockers				
Propranolol	60–120	30 min–4 hours	Anxiety, Panic disorder, SAD	Bradycardia, dizziness, fatigue, hypotension
5-HT1A Partial Agonists				
Buspirone	15–60	2–4 weeks	GAD	Dizziness, drowsiness, nausea
H1 Antagonists				
Hydroxyzine	25–100	4–6 hours	GAD, SAD, Panic disorder	Dry mouth, drowsiness
Antipsychotics				
Olanzapine	5–15	1–2 weeks	Anxiety, GAD	Orthostatic hypotension, weight gain, somnolence
Quetiapine	50–300	1–2 weeks	Anxiety, GAD	Dizziness, extrapyramidal symptoms, increased diastolic blood pressure, dyslipidemia

Table 19.3 *(cont.)*

Drug	Recommended Dose for Adults (mg/day)	Treatment Response	Indications	Common Side Effects
Monoamine Oxidase Inhibitors				
Phenelzine	30–90	2–4 weeks	GAD, Panic disorder, SAD	Orthostatic hypotension, dizziness, headache

5-HT, 5-hydroxy tryptamine; *GAD,* generalized anxiety disorder; *GI,* gastrointestinal; *SAD,* social anxiety disorder. *Sources:* M. G. Craske, M. B. Stein, T. C. Eley, M. R. Milad, A. Holmes, R. M. Rapee, & H.-U. Wittchen, Anxiety disorders. *Nature Reviews Disease Primers,* **3** (2017) 1–19. https://doi.org/10.1038/nrdp.2017.24; D. J. Nutt, Overview of diagnosis and drug treatments of anxiety disorders. *CNS Spectrums,* **10** (2005) 49–56. https://doi .org/10.1017/s1092852900009901; A. Garakani, J. W. Murrough, R. C. Freire, R. P. Thom, K. Larkin, F. D. Buono, & D. V. Iosifescu, Pharmacotherapy of anxiety disorders: current and emerging treatment options. *Frontiers in Psychiatry,* **11** (2020) 595584. https://doi.org/10.3389/fpsyt.2020.595584; C. E. Griffin, A. M. Kaye, F. R. Bueno, & A. D. Kaye, Benzodiazepine pharmacology and central nervous system–mediated effects. *The Ochsner Journal,* **13** (2013) 214–223.

Table 19.4 Some of the psychotherapies most commonly utilized in the treatment of anxiety disorders

Psychotherapy Type	Population	Indication	Short Term / Long Term
Cognitive-behavioral therapy	Children, adolescents, adults	GAD, social phobia, specific phobia, panic disorder	Short term – 8-20 sessions
Psychodynamic therapy	Adults	GAD, panic disorder, social anxiety disorder, agoraphobia	Short term – 24 sessions + 3 intro sessions
Mindfulness and acceptance techniques	Adults	Mood disorders including anxiety disorders	Long term

GAD, Generalized anxiety disorder. *Sources:* M. G. Craske, M. B. Stein, T. C. Eley, M. R. Milad, A. Holmes, R. M. Rapee, & H.-U. Wittchen, Anxiety disorders. *Nature Reviews Disease Primers,* **3** (2017) 1–19. https://doi.org/10.1038/nrdp.2017.24; P. Giacobbe & A. Flint, Diagnosis and management of anxiety disorders. *Continuum (Minneapolis, Minn.),* **24** (2018) 893–919. https://doi .org/10.1212/CON.0000000000000607; M. E. Beutel, L. Greenberg, R. D. Lane, & C. Subic-Wrana, Treating anxiety disorders by emotion-focused psychodynamic psychotherapy (EFPP): an integrative, transdiagnostic approach. *Clinical Psychology & Psychotherapy,* **26** (2019) 1–13. https://doi.org/10.1002/cpp.2325; S. G. Hofmann, A. T. Sawyer, A. A. Witt, & D. Oh, The effect of mindfulness-based therapy on anxiety and depression: a meta-analytic review. *Journal of Consulting and Clinical Psychology,* **78** (2010) 169–183. https://doi.org/10.1037/a0018555.

capability to manage the situation. CBT works to solve these discrepancies through specific therapies [58]. One of the most common therapies is exposure to the feared stimuli in an environment that is otherwise safe (exposure therapy or desensitization). In this way the patient unlearns the anxiety associated with the stimuli. Other additional therapies include grounding techniques that help relax the patient [58]. Functional magnetic resonance imaging (fMRI) data collected during exposure to feared stimuli before and after psycho-therapy show that there is decreased activation in the right insula, the anterior cingulate cortex, and the dorsolateral prefrontal cortex. This leads to a suggestion that during therapy, there may be a normalization of the threat perceived by the feared stimuli, indicating the positive effects of psychotherapy in patients with anxiety disorders [62]. CBT has been shown to be highly effective, with decreased symptoms and increased quality of life, with several anxiety disorders compared to no treatment or placebo options including generalized anxiety disorder, social phobia, specific phobia, and panic disorder [63]. However, there are several barriers between patients and CBT that lead to lower numbers of patients receiving this kind of treatment. These barriers include lack of therapists, costs and time associated with CBT, and the general stigma of therapy. The advent of online therapy may be an important option for patients who struggle with these barriers [58].

Other methods of psychotherapy have less evidence to support their effectiveness in treating anxiety disorders but are still used by some. These include mindfulness and acceptance-based approaches in which the patient learns to accept their anxious feelings with meditation and breathing techniques [20]. Psychodynamic therapies focus on processing emotion to help the patient become aware of their emotional ties to anxiety and gain more control over them [64].

19.5.7 Other Treatments

Combination treatment of both psychotherapy and pharmacological treatments is often seen in patients. While there are a limited number of studies that explore this option, meta-analytic evidence has shown that combination treatment generally outperforms single-mode therapy [18].

Complementary and alternative medicine is also often used by many patients with anxiety disorders. These treatments include relaxation techniques, herbal medications, yoga and exercise, and acupuncture. While these treatments show potential to be used, they lack support by evidence and clinical trials [66].

19.5.8 Prevention

Prevention of anxiety disorders is an underexplored area of anxiety disorder research. Due to the early onset of anxiety disorders, most preventative efforts have been concentrated on children and adolescents. Universal measures of prevention that have been executed in research studies are often executed at the classroom level, comprising of teaching students low-level anxiety management skills. Although studies have shown limited but significant effects of universal measures, long-term results have yet to be verified [20].

Selective intervention targets populations that are more likely to develop an anxiety disorder later in life due to risk factors. One such program that is widely studied is the Cool Little Kids program, which targets preschool children who have an inhibited temperament and overprotective parents (two risk factors for preschool children). This program teaches the parents of these children methods to overcome their child's inhibited temperament and fears while they themselves learn how to be less overbearing. Studies showed that after follow-up of 1 year, there was a significant decrease in anxiety symptoms and no anxiety disorders in children who participated in the program [67].

Indicated intervention targets older children and adolescents who already exhibit signs of anxiety symptoms but don't meet criteria for an anxiety disorder. In this population, prevention consists of learning relaxation techniques and making anxiety management strategies. Analyses have shown limited but significant results for indicated intervention [20].

19.5.9 Ongoing Research

Newer studies are attempting to translate data from animal studies to humans using imaging techniques such as fMRI, although the current challenge is the paucity of these studies [46]. The aim of these studies is to delineate the neural circuitry involved in anxiety, which appears to be distinct from the fear model as previously hypothesized [68, 69]. Of particular interest recently is the BNST region, which could be a potential target for the treatment of anxiety disorders [70]. Although it is not currently first line, recent studies have also shown promising results in the neuromodulatory treatment of anxiety such as repetitive transcranial magnetic stimulation (rTMS) of dlPFC regions of the brain as well as deep brain stimulation of the BNST for refractory symptoms [71, 72].

Simultaneously, the search for novel pharmacological treatments for anxiety targeting various neurochemical systems such as the monoamine (psychedelics), glutamate, cannabinoid, cholinergic, and neuropeptide systems is currently underway [73, 74]. Of note, there has been a recent emphasis on the development of pharmacological drugs aimed at inducing neuroplasticity for a more sustained clinical effect versus acute anxiolytic properties. Newer studies are also attempting to study fear-potentiated responses in adolescence, an approach that could provide more insight into the developmental underpinnings of anxiety disorders [75, 76]. Due to the remarkable heterogeneity of anxiety disorders with overlapping symptomatology across various psychiatric and neurological conditions, it is imperative that future studies be aimed at understanding the neurobiological mechanisms underlying them. This would in turn aid in the development of more targeted interventions that would ultimately lead to greater success rates in the treatment of anxiety and its related disorders.

Conflict of Interest

Sudhakar Selvaraj is currently an employee of Intra-cellular Therapies, Inc. and holds share interests. He has received research support from Flow Neuroscience and is a principal or sub-investigator for clinical trials funded by Flow Neuroscience, Compass Pathways, LivaNova, and Janssen. He is also an associate professor of psychiatry (Adjunct) at UTHealth McGovern Medical School, Houston, TX, USA. Dr. Selvaraj has received consultant fee or honoraria from Worldwide Clinical Trials/Inversago, Vicore Pharma, British Medical Journal Publishing Group, and Psychiatry Education Forum LLC.

Funding

Dr. Sudhakar Selvaraj has received grants/research support from NIMH (1R21MH119441–01A1), NIMH (1R21MH129888–01A1), and NICHD (1R21HD106779–01A1).

Acknowledgment

The content of this study is solely the responsibility of the authors and does not necessarily represent the official views of the NIH, UTHealth, or Intra-cellular Therapies. The UTHealth institution and Intra-cellular Therapies played no role in the preparation, review, or approval of the book chapter and the decision to submit the chapter for publication.

References

1. A. J. Baxter, T. Vos, K. M. Scott, A. J. Ferrari, & H. A. Whiteford, The global burden of anxiety disorders in 2010. *Psychological Medicine*, **44** (2014) 2363–2374. https://doi.org/10.1017/S0033291713003243.

2. D. A. Revicki, K. Travers, K. W. Wyrwich, H. Svedsäter, J. Locklear, M. S. Mattera, D. V. Sheehan, & S. Montgomery, Humanistic and economic burden of generalized anxiety disorder in North America and Europe. *Journal of Affective Disorders*, **140** (2012) 103–112. https://doi.org/10.1016/j.jad.2011.11.014.

3. A. Konnopka & H. König, Economic burden of anxiety disorders: a systematic review and meta-analysis. *PharmacoEconomics*, **38** (2020) 25–37. https://doi.org/10.1007/s40273-019-00849-7.

4. J. Sareen, B. J. Cox, T. O. Afifi, R. de Graaf, G. J. G. Asmundson, M. ten Have, & M. B. Stein, Anxiety disorders and risk for suicidal ideation and suicide attempts: a population-based longitudinal study of adults. *Archives of General Psychiatry*, **62** (2005) 1249–1257. https://doi.org/10.1001/archpsyc.62.11.1249.

5. M.-A. Crocq, A history of anxiety: from Hippocrates to DSM. *Dialogues in Clinical Neuroscience*, **17** (2015) 319–325.

6. M.-A. Crocq, The history of generalized anxiety disorder as a diagnostic category. *Dialogues in Clinical Neuroscience*, **19** (2017) 107–116.

7. Anxiety Disorders. *Diagnostic and Statistical Manual of Mental Disorders* (American Psychiatric Association Publishing, 2022). https://doi.org/10.1176/appi.books.9780890425787.x05_Anxiety_Disorders.

8. R. C. Kessler, M. Angermeyer, J. C. Anthony, R. DE Graaf, K. Demyttenaere, I. Gasquet, G. DE Girolamo, S. Gluzman, O. Gureje, J. M. Haro, N. Kawakami, A. Karam, D. Levinson, M. E. Medina Mora, M. A. Oakley Browne, J. Posada-Villa, D. J. Stein, C. H. Adley Tsang, S. Aguilar-Gaxiola, J. Alonso, S. Lee, S. Heeringa, B.-E. Pennell, P. Berglund, M. J. Gruber, M. Petukhova, S. Chatterji, & T. B. Ustün, Lifetime prevalence and age-of-onset distributions of mental disorders in the World Health Organization's World Mental Health Survey Initiative. *World Psychiatry: Official Journal of the World Psychiatric Association (WPA)*, **6** (2007) 168–176.

9. A. J. Baxter, K. M. Scott, T. Vos, & H. A. Whiteford, Global prevalence of anxiety disorders: a systematic review and meta-regression. *Psychological Medicine*, **43** (2013) 897–910. https://doi.org/10.1017/S003329171200147X.

10. D. Silove, J. Alonso, E. Bromet, M. Gruber, N. Sampson, K. Scott, L. Andrade, C. Benjet, J. M. Caldas de Almeida, G. De Girolamo, P. de Jonge, K. Demyttenaere, F. Fiestas, S. Florescu, O. Gureje, Y. He, E. Karam, J.-P. Lepine, S. Murphy, J. Villa-Posada, Z. Zarkov, & R. C. Kessler, Pediatric-onset and adult-onset separation anxiety disorder across countries in the World Mental Health Survey. *American Journal of Psychiatry*, **172** (2015) 647–656. https://doi.org/10.1176/appi.ajp.2015.14091185.

11. R. L. Bergman, J. Piacentini, & J. T. McCracken, Prevalence and description of selective mutism in a school-based sample. *Journal of the American Academy of Child and Adolescent Psychiatry*, **41** (2002) 938–946. https://doi.org/10.1097/00004583-200208000-00012

12. W. W. Eaton, O. J. Bienvenu, & B. Miloyan, Specific phobias. *The Lancet. Psychiatry*, **5** (2018) 678–686. https://doi.org/10.1016/S2215-0366(18)30169-X.

13. M. B. Stein & D. J. Stein, Social anxiety disorder. *The Lancet*, **371** (2008) 1115–1125. https://doi.org/10.1016/S0140-6736(08)60488-2.

14. R. C. Kessler, W. T. Chiu, R. Jin, A. M. Ruscio, K. Shear, & E. E. Walters, The epidemiology of panic attacks, panic disorder, and agoraphobia in the National Comorbidity Survey replication. *Archives of General Psychiatry*, **63** (2006) 415–424.

https://doi.org/10.1001/archpsyc.63.4
.415.

15. K. Balaram & R. Marwaha, Agoraphobia. *StatPearls* (StatPearls Publishing, 2023).

16. R. B. Weisberg, Overview of generalized anxiety disorder. *The Journal of Clinical Psychiatry*, **70** (2009) 4.

17. M. K. Hofmeijer-Sevink, N. M. Batelaan, H. J. G. M. van Megen, B. W. Penninx, D. C. Cath, M. A. van den Hout, & A. J. L. M. van Balkom, Clinical relevance of comorbidity in anxiety disorders: a report from the Netherlands Study of Depression and Anxiety (NESDA). *Journal of Affective Disorders*, **137** (2012) 106–112. https://doi.org/10.1016/j.jad.2011.12.008.

18. B. W. Penninx, D. S. Pine, E. A. Holmes, & A. Reif, Anxiety disorders. *Lancet (London)*, **397** (2021) 914–927. https://doi.org/10.1016/S0140-6736(21)00359-7.

19. R. C. Kessler, A. M. Ruscio, K. Shear, & H.-U. Wittchen, Epidemiology of anxiety disorders. *Current Topics in Behavioral Neurosciences*, **2** (2010) 21–35.

20. M. G. Craske, M. B. Stein, T. C. Eley, M. R. Milad, A. Holmes, R. M. Rapee, & H.-U. Wittchen, Anxiety disorders. *Nature Reviews Disease Primers*, **3** (2017) 1–19. https://doi.org/10.1038/nrdp.2017.24.

21. J. M. de Lijster, B. Dierckx, E. M. W. J. Utens, F. C. Verhulst, C. Zieldorff, G. C. Dieleman, & J. S. Legerstee, The age of onset of anxiety disorders. *Canadian Journal of Psychiatry. Revue Canadienne De Psychiatrie*, **62** (2017) 237–246. https://doi.org/10.1177/0706743716640757.

22. C. P. McLean, A. Asnaani, B. T. Litz, & S. G. Hofmann, Gender differences in anxiety disorders: prevalence, course of illness, comorbidity and burden of illness. *Journal of Psychiatric Research*, **45** (2011) 1027–1035. https://doi.org/10.1016/j.jpsychires.2011.03.006.

23. R. Lieb, Anxiety disorders: clinical presentation and epidemiology. *Handbook of Experimental Pharmacology* (2005) 405–432. https://doi.org/10.1007/3-540-28082-0_14.

24. T. Michael, U. Zetsche, & J. Margraf, Epidemiology of anxiety disorders. *Psychiatry*, **6** (2007) 136–142. https://doi.org/10.1016/j.mppsy.2007.01.007.

25. S. M. Meier & J. Deckert, Genetics of anxiety disorders. *Current Psychiatry Reports*, **21** (2019) 16. https://doi.org/10.1007/s11920-019-1002-7.

26. D. F. Levey, J. Gelernter, R. Polimanti, H. Zhou, Z. Cheng, M. Aslan, R. Quaden, J. Concato, K. Radhakrishnan, J. Bryois, P. F. Sullivan, Million Veteran Program, & M. B. Stein, Reproducible genetic risk loci for anxiety: results from ~200,000 participants in the Million Veteran Program. *The American Journal of Psychiatry*, **177** (2020) 223–232. https://doi.org/10.1176/appi.ajp.2019.19030256.

27. S. Sharma, A. Powers, B. Bradley, & K. J. Ressler, Gene × environment determinants of stress- and anxiety-related disorders. *Annual Review of Psychology*, **67** (2016) 239–261. https://doi.org/10.1146/annurev-psych-122414-033408.

28. M. A. Schiele & K. Domschke, Epigenetics at the crossroads between genes, environment and resilience in anxiety disorders. *Genes, Brain and Behavior*, **17** (2018) e12423. https://doi.org/10.1111/gbb.12423.

29. J. E. LeDoux, Emotion circuits in the brain. *Annual Review of Neuroscience*, **23** (2000) 155–184. https://doi.org/10.1146/annurev.neuro.23.1.155.

30. D. Treit, C. Pesold, & S. Rotzinger, Dissociating the anti-fear effects of septal and amygdaloid lesions using two pharmacologically validated models of rat anxiety. *Behavioral Neuroscience*, **107** (1993) 770–785. https://doi.org/10.1037//0735-7044.107.5.770.

31. M. Davis, D. L. Walker, L. Miles, & C. Grillon, Phasic vs sustained fear in rats and humans: role of the extended amygdala in fear vs anxiety. *Neuropsychopharmacology*, **35** (2010) 105–135. https://doi.org/10.1038/npp.2009.109.

32. M. A. Lebow & A. Chen, Overshadowed by the amygdala: the bed nucleus of the stria terminalis emerges as key to psychiatric disorders. *Molecular Psychiatry*, **21** (2016) 450–463. https://doi.org/10.1038/mp.2016.1.

33. J. H. Jennings, D. R. Sparta, A. M. Stamatakis, R. L. Ung, K. E. Pleil, T. L. Kash, & G. D. Stuber, Distinct extended amygdala circuits for divergent motivational states. *Nature*, **496** (2013) 224–228. https://doi.org/10.1038/nature12041.

34. S.-Y. Kim, A. Adhikari, S. Y. Lee, J. H. Marshel, C. K. Kim, C. S. Mallory, M. Lo, S. Pak, J. Mattis, B. K. Lim, R. C. Malenka, M. R. Warden, R. Neve, K. M. Tye, & K. Deisseroth, Diverging neural pathways assemble a behavioural state from separable features in anxiety. *Nature*, **496** (2013) 219–223. https://doi.org/10.1038/nature12018.

35. O. J. Robinson, A. C. Pike, B. Cornwell, & C. Grillon, The translational neural circuitry of anxiety. *Journal of Neurology, Neurosurgery, and Psychiatry*, **90** (2019) 1353–1360. https://doi.org/10.1136/jnnp-2019-321400.

36. L. W. Swanson, A direct projection from Ammon's horn to prefrontal cortex in the rat. *Brain Research*, **217** (1981) 150–154. https://doi.org/10.1016/0006-8993(81)90192-x.

37. R. P. Vertes, Differential projections of the infralimbic and prelimbic cortex in the rat. *Synapse (New York)*, **51** (2004) 32–58. https://doi.org/10.1002/syn.10279.

38. S. J. Bishop, Trait anxiety and impoverished prefrontal control of attention. *Nature Neuroscience*, **12** (2009) 92–98. https://doi.org/10.1038/nn.2242.

39. N. L. Balderston, J. Liu, R. Roberson-Nay, M. Ernst, & C. Grillon, The relationship between dlPFC activity during unpredictable threat and CO_2-induced panic symptoms. *Translational Psychiatry*, **7** (2017) 1266. https://doi.org/10.1038/s41398-017-0006-5.

40. K. E. Vytal, C. Overstreet, D. R. Charney, O. J. Robinson, & C. Grillon, Sustained anxiety increases amygdala–dorsomedial prefrontal coupling: a mechanism for maintaining an anxious state in healthy adults. *Journal of Psychiatry & Neuroscience*, **39** (2014) 321–329. https://doi.org/10.1503/jpn.130145.

41. O. J. Robinson, D. R. Charney, C. Overstreet, K. Vytal, & C. Grillon, The adaptive threat bias in anxiety: amygdala-dorsomedial prefrontal cortex coupling and aversive amplification. *NeuroImage*, **60** (2012) 523–529. https://doi.org/10.1016/j.neuroimage.2011.11.096.

42. R. Kalisch & A. M. V. Gerlicher, Making a mountain out of a molehill: on the role of the rostral dorsal anterior cingulate and dorsomedial prefrontal cortex in conscious threat appraisal, catastrophizing, and worrying. *Neuroscience and Biobehavioral Reviews*, **42** (2014) 1–8. https://doi.org/10.1016/j.neubiorev.2014.02.002.

43. K. Hilbert, U. Lueken, & K. Beesdo-Baum, Neural structures, functioning and connectivity in generalized anxiety disorder and interaction with neuroendocrine systems: a systematic review. *Journal of Affective Disorders*, **158** (2014) 114–126. https://doi.org/10.1016/j.jad.2014.01.022.

44. D. P. M. Tromp, D. W. Grupe, D. J. Oathes, D. R. McFarlin, P. J. Hernandez, T. R. A. Kral, J. E. Lee, M. Adams, A. L. Alexander, & J. B. Nitschke, Reduced structural connectivity of a major frontolimbic pathway in generalized anxiety disorder. *Archives of General Psychiatry*, **69** (2012) 925–934. https://doi.org/10.1001/archgenpsychiatry.2011.2178.

45. J. Maslowsky, K. Mogg, B. P. Bradley, E. McClure-Tone, M. Ernst, D. S. Pine, & C. S. Monk, A preliminary investigation of neural correlates of treatment in adolescents with generalized anxiety disorder. *Journal of Child and Adolescent Psychopharmacology*, **20** (2010) 105–111. https://doi.org/10.1089/cap.2009.0049.

46. D. Madonna, G. Delvecchio, J. C. Soares, & P. Brambilla, Structural and functional neuroimaging studies in generalized

anxiety disorder: a SYI. *Brasileira De Psiquiatria (Sao Paulo, Brazil, 1999)*, **41** (2019) 336–362. https://doi.org/10.1590/1516-4446-2018-0108.

47. A. Harrewijn, E. M. Cardinale, N. A. Groenewold, J. M. Bas-Hoogendam, M. Aghajani, K. Hilbert, N. Cardoner, D. Porta-Casteràs, S. Gosnell, R. Salas, A. P. Jackowski, P. M. Pan, G. A. Salum, K. S. Blair, J. R. Blair, M. Z. Hammoud, M. R. Milad, K. L. Burkhouse, K. L. Phan, H. K. Schroeder, J. R. Strawn, K. Beesdo-Baum, N. Jahanshad, S. I. Thomopoulos, R. Buckner, J. A. Nielsen, J. W. Smoller, J. C. Soares, B. Mwangi, M. J. Wu, G. B. Zunta-Soares, M. Assaf, G. J. Diefenbach, P. Brambilla, E. Maggioni, D. Hofmann, T. Straube, C. Andreescu, R. Berta, E. Tamburo, R. B. Price, G. G. Manfro, F. Agosta, E. Canu, C. Cividini, M. Filippi, M. Kostić, A. Munjiza Jovanovic, B. A. V. Alberton, B. Benson, G. F. Freitag, C. A. Filippi, A. L. Gold, E. Leibenluft, G. V. Ringlein, K. E. Werwath, H. Zwiebel, A. Zugman, H. J. Grabe, S. Van der Auwera, K. Wittfeld, H. Völzke, R. Bülow, N. L. Balderston, M. Ernst, C. Grillon, L. R. Mujica-Parodi, H. van Nieuwenhuizen, H. D. Critchley, E. Makovac, M. Mancini, F. Meeten, C. Ottaviani, T. M. Ball, G. A. Fonzo, M. P. Paulus, M. B. Stein, R. E. Gur, R. C. Gur, A. N. Kaczkurkin, B. Larsen, T. D. Satterthwaite, J. Harper, M. Myers, M. T. Perino, C. M. Sylvester, Q. Yu, U. Lueken, D. J. Veltman, P. M. Thompson, D. J. Stein, N. J. A. Van der Wee, A. M. Winkler, & D. S. Pine, Cortical and subcortical brain structure in generalized anxiety disorder: findings from 28 research sites in the ENIGMA–Anxiety Working Group. *Translational Psychiatry*, **11** (2021). https://doi.org/10.1038/s41398-021-01622-1.

48. J. C. Wu, M. S. Buchsbaum, T. G. Hershey, E. Hazlett, N. Sicotte, & J. C. Johnson, PET in generalized anxiety disorder. *Biological Psychiatry*, **29** (1991) 1181–1199. https://doi.org/10.1016/0006-3223(91)90326-h.

49. E. Hernández, S. Lastra, M. Urbina, I. Carreira, & L. Lima, Serotonin, 5-hydroxyindoleacetic acid and serotonin transporter in blood peripheral lymphocytes of patients with generalized anxiety disorder. *International Immunopharmacology*, **2** (2002) 893–900. https://doi.org/10.1016/s1567-5769(02)00025-5.

50. G. Gerra, A. Zaimovic, U. Zambelli, M. Timpano, N. Reali, S. Bernasconi, & F. Brambilla, Neuroendocrine responses to psychological stress in adolescents with anxiety disorder. *Neuropsychobiology*, **42** (2000) 82–92. https://doi.org/10.1159/000026677.

51. N. Vogelzangs, A. T. F. Beekman, P. de Jonge, & B. W. J. H. Penninx, Anxiety disorders and inflammation in a large adult cohort. *Translational Psychiatry*, **3** (2013) e249. https://doi.org/10.1038/tp.2013.27.

52. H. Costello, R. L. Gould, E. Abrol, & R. Howard, Systematic review and meta-analysis of the association between peripheral inflammatory cytokines and generalised anxiety disorder. *BMJ Open*, **9** (2019) e027925. https://doi.org/10.1136/bmjopen-2018-027925.

53. O. J. Robinson, C. Overstreet, P. S. Allen, A. Letkiewicz, K. Vytal, D. S. Pine, & C. Grillon, The role of serotonin in the neurocircuitry of negative affective bias: serotonergic modulation of the dorsal medial prefrontal-amygdala "aversive amplification" circuit. *NeuroImage*, **78** (2013) 217–223. https://doi.org/10.1016/j.neuroimage.2013.03.075.

54. C. O. Carlisi & O. J. Robinson, The role of prefrontal–subcortical circuitry in negative bias in anxiety: translational, developmental and treatment perspectives. *Brain and Neuroscience Advances*, **2** (2018) 2398212818774223. https://doi.org/10.1177/2398212818774223.

55. C. Grillon, E. Hale, L. Lieberman, A. Davis, D. S. Pine, & M. Ernst, The CRH1 antagonist GSK561679 increases human fear but not anxiety as assessed by startle. *Neuropsychopharmacology*, **40** (2015) 1064–1071. https://doi.org/10.1038/npp.2014.316.

56. G. F. Koob & E. P. Zorrilla, Update on corticotropin-releasing factor pharmacotherapy for psychiatric disorders: a revisionist view. *Neuropsychopharmacology*, **37** (2012) 308–309. https://doi.org/10.1038/npp .2011.213.

57. S. Steudte, T. Stalder, L. Dettenborn, E. Klumbies, P. Foley, K. Beesdo-Baum, & C. Kirschbaum, Decreased hair cortisol concentrations in generalised anxiety disorder. *Psychiatry Research*, **186** (2011) 310–314. https://doi.org/10.1016/j .psychres.2010.09.002

58. P. Giacobbe & A. Flint, Diagnosis and management of anxiety disorders. *Continuum (Minneapolis, Minn.)*, **24** (2018) 893–919. https://doi.org/10.1212/ CON.0000000000000607.

59. D. J. Nutt, Overview of diagnosis and drug treatments of anxiety disorders. *CNS Spectrums*, **10** (2005) 49–56. https://doi .org/10.1017/s1092852900009901

60. A. Garakani, J. W. Murrough, R. C. Freire, R. P. Thom, K. Larkin, F. D. Buono, & D. V. Iosifescu, Pharmacotherapy of anxiety disorders: current and emerging treatment options. *Frontiers in Psychiatry*, **11** (2020) 595584. https://doi.org/10.3389/fpsyt.2020 .595584.

61. C. E. Griffin, A. M. Kaye, F. R. Bueno, & A. D. Kaye, Benzodiazepine pharmacology and central nervous system–mediated effects. *The Ochsner Journal*, **13** (2013) 214–223.

62. E. Schrammen, K. Roesmann, D. Rosenbaum, R. Redlich, J. Harenbrock, U. Dannlowski, & E. J. Leehr, Functional neural changes associated with psychotherapy in anxiety disorders: a meta-analysis of longitudinal fMRI studies. *Neuroscience and Biobehavioral Reviews*, **142** (2022) 104895. https://doi .org/10.1016/j.neubiorev.2022.104895.

63. B. O. Olatunji, J. M. Cisler, & B. J. Deacon, Efficacy of cognitive behavioral therapy for anxiety disorders: a review of meta-analytic findings. *The Psychiatric Clinics of North America*, **33** (2010)

557–577. https://doi.org/10.1016/j.psc .2010.04.002.

64. M. E. Beutel, L. Greenberg, R. D. Lane, & C. Subic-Wrana, Treating anxiety disorders by emotion-focused psychodynamic psychotherapy (EFPP): an integrative, transdiagnostic approach. *Clinical Psychology & Psychotherapy*, **26** (2019) 1–13. https://doi.org/10.1002/cpp .2325.

65. S. G. Hofmann, A. T. Sawyer, A. A. Witt, & D. Oh, The effect of mindfulness-based therapy on anxiety and depression: a meta-analytic review. *Journal of Consulting and Clinical Psychology*, **78** (2010) 169–183. https://doi.org/10.1037/ a0018555.

66. V. Trkulja & H. Barić, Current research on complementary and alternative medicine (CAM) in the treatment of anxiety disorders: an evidence-based review. *Advances in Experimental Medicine and Biology*, **1191** (2020) 415–449. https://doi.org/10.1007/978- 981-32-9705-0_22.

67. J. K. Bayer, L. A. Prendergast, A. Brown, L. Harris, L. Bretherton, H. Hiscock, R. Beatson, C. Mihalopoulos, & R. M. Rapee, Cool Little Kids translational trial to prevent internalising: two-year outcomes and prediction of parent engagement. *Child and Adolescent Mental Health*, **26** (2021) 211–219.

68. J. E. LeDoux & D. S. Pine, Using neuroscience to help understand fear and anxiety: a two-system framework. *American Journal of Psychiatry*, **173** (2016) 1083–1093. https://doi.org/10 .1176/appi.ajp.2016.16030353.

69. P. Tovote, J. P. Fadok, & A. Lüthi, Neuronal circuits for fear and anxiety. *Nature Reviews. Neuroscience*, **16** (2015) 317–331. https://doi.org/10.1038/ nrn3945.

70. S. N. Avery, J. A. Clauss, & J. U. Blackford, The human BNST: functional role in anxiety and addiction. *Neuropsychopharmacology*, **41** (2016) 126–141. https://doi.org/10.1038/npp .2015.185.

71. L. Luyten, S. Hendrickx, S. Raymaekers, L. Gabriëls, & B. Nuttin, Electrical stimulation in the bed nucleus of the stria terminalis alleviates severe obsessive-compulsive disorder. *Molecular Psychiatry*, **21** (2016) 1272–1280. https://doi.org/10.1038/mp.2015.124.

72. D. Dilkov, E. R. Hawken, E. Kaludiev, & R. Milev, Repetitive transcranial magnetic stimulation of the right dorsal lateral prefrontal cortex in the treatment of generalized anxiety disorder: a randomized, double-blind sham controlled clinical trial. *Progress in Neuro-Psychopharmacology & Biological Psychiatry*, **78** (2017) 61–65. https://doi.org/10.1016/j.pnpbp.2017.05.018.

73. N. Singewald, S. B. Sartori, A. Reif, & A. Holmes, Alleviating anxiety and taming trauma: novel pharmacotherapeutics for anxiety disorders and posttraumatic stress disorder. *Neuropharmacology*, **226** (2023) 109418. https://doi.org/10.1016/j.neuropharm.2023.109418.

74. S. B. Sartori & N. Singewald, Novel pharmacological targets in drug development for the treatment of anxiety and anxiety-related disorders. *Pharmacology & Therapeutics*, **204** (2019) 107402. https://doi.org/10.1016/j.pharmthera.2019.107402.

75. A. Schmitz, K. Merikangas, H. Swendsen, L. Cui, L. Heaton, & C. Grillon, Measuring anxious responses to predictable and unpredictable threat in children and adolescents. *Journal of Experimental Child Psychology*, **110** (2011) 159–170. https://doi.org/10.1016/j.jecp.2011.02.014.

76. J. C. Britton, C. Grillon, S. Lissek, M. A. Norcross, K. L. Szuhany, G. Chen, M. Ernst, E. E. Nelson, E. Leibenluft, T. Shechner, & D. S. Pine, Response to learned threat: an FMRI study in adolescent and adult anxiety. *The American Journal of Psychiatry*, **170** (2013) 1195–1204. https://doi.org/10.1176/appi.ajp.2013.12050651.

Chapter 20

Obsessive-Compulsive Disorder

Jordan T. Stiede, Emily R. Strouphauer, Erika S. Trent,
Sameer A. Sheth, Nisha Giridharan, Wayne K. Goodman,
Andrew D. Wiese, and Eric A. Storch

20.1 Introduction

Obsessive-compulsive disorder (OCD) is a neurobehavioral condition characterized by intrusive and recurrent thoughts, urges, or images (i.e., obsessions) and repetitive behaviors or mental acts (i.e., compulsions) aimed at reducing distress associated with such obsessions [1]. OCD is a heterogenous disorder with a wide range of clinical presentations that generally fall into one of several dimensions [2]. Adult lifetime prevalence is estimated at 1.5% in women and 1.0% in men [3]. Prevalence rates are higher in girls than boys starting at age 11 [4]. Among younger children, studies have found either higher prevalence rates in boys than girls [4] or no gender differences [5].

The onset of OCD demonstrates two peaks across the life span. On average, pediatric-onset OCD begins in preadolescence (i.e., 9–10 years ± 2.5 years) while adult-onset OCD begins in early adulthood (i.e., 22–24 years) [6]. After initial onset, OCD symptoms frequently follow a chronic course without treatment, and relapse is common; however, early intervention is linked to better long-term outcomes [2]. In the past several decades, advances in OCD research have improved its identification and treatment. This chapter provides an up-to-date overview of the clinical presentation of OCD and diagnostic considerations, pathophysiology, and evidence-based treatment approaches. We conclude with suggestions for future research directions.

20.2 Clinical Presentation/Diagnosis

A diagnosis of OCD requires the presence of obsessions or compulsions that are time consuming (i.e., over 1 hour a day), clinically distressing or functionally impairing, and are not better explained by other factors such as substance use, medical conditions, or another mental disorder [1]. Although the Diagnostic and Statistical Manual – 5th Edition (DSM-5) [1] does not require an individual to have both obsessions *and* compulsions, in practice it is extremely rare to have one without the other, and the content of obsessions and compulsions are usually functionally linked [7]. One notable change between the DSM-IV and DSM-5 is the reclassification of OCD from its previous category of "anxiety disorders" to a new category of "obsessive-compulsive and related disorders" (OCRDs). Accurate differential diagnosis between OCD and other OCRDs (i.e., trichotillomania, excoriation, hoarding, and body dysmorphic disorder) is important in selecting appropriate treatment approaches [2].

OCD is associated with diminished quality of life and significant impairment in multiple areas, including social, occupational, academic, and physical functioning [7]. Severe OCD symptoms, lower insight, and greater family accommodation of OCD behaviors (e.g., providing cleaning products to a patient with contamination OCD) are also linked to greater functional impairment [8]. Further, psychiatric comorbidities are common and are associated with increased impairment and poorer quality of life [9]. Given significant functional impairment associated with OCD, it is important that clinicians conduct an accurate assessment and provide evidence-based treatment for this condition.

20.3 Assessment

Assessment of OCD includes identifying an individual's specific obsessions and compulsions across different domains of OCD (e.g., contamination fears, taboo thoughts, fears of causing harm, need for symmetry or exactness, need to hoard; see Table 20.1) and assessing symptom severity. The Yale-Brown Obsessive-Compulsive Scales (First and Second editions; Y-BOCS-I and -II) [10, 11] and Children's Y-BOCS (CY-BOCS-I and -II) [12, 13] are the gold-standard clinician-administered instruments for assessing specific OCD symptoms and severity in adults and children, respectively. Validated self-report measures of OCD include the Florida Obsessive-Compulsive Inventory (FOCI) [14] and the Obsessive-Compulsive Inventory-Revised (OCI-R) [15]. Both have also been adapted for use with children (Child-FOCI [C-FOCI]; OCI-Children's Version [OCI-CV]) [16, 17]. While not as comprehensive as the (C)Y-BOCS, such self-report measures are brief and easy to administer and score.

20.4 Pathophysiology

Although the pathophysiology of OCD is not fully understood, several biological factors may contribute to its development. Genetics appear as likely contributors to this highly heritable condition, as documented by twin and family aggregation studies [18, 19]. A large-scale, multigenerational familial clustering investigation found that, among relatives of individuals with OCD, the risk of developing OCD increases proportionately to the degree of genetic relatedness [19]. Twin studies have consistently found higher concordance rates for OCD in monozygotic twins over dizygotic twins [20, 21], with overall OCD heritability estimated to be 48% [21].

OCD also involves abnormal neurotransmitter activity including serotonin, dopamine, and glutamate, and several genetic association studies in OCD have examined candidate genes corresponding to these neurotransmitters [18]. The most promising candidate gene, SLC1A1, encodes the neuronal glutamate transporter 3 (EAAT3). Variants in the SLC1A1 gene may underlie the generation of compulsive behavior in OCD [22]. However, supporting evidence is limited, and future research should continue to examine the association between EAAT3 polymorphisms and OCD symptomatology.

The pathophysiology of OCD is also often associated with neurobiological alterations. Structural and functional changes in cortico-striato-thalamo-cortical (CSTC) loops, including the basal ganglia, may influence brain circuitry associated with maladaptive habits and the loss of brain mechanisms implicated with inhibiting certain responses [23]. CSTC loops are involved in several cognitive and executive functions including learning and decision-making as well motor responses to emotional stimuli. OCD is thought to be related to an imbalance in direct and indirect pathways in the CSTC circuit, and excessive positive feedback through the direct pathway in OCD leads to hyperactivation of the orbitofrontal cortex and subsequent OCD symptomatology.

Table 20.1 Examples of common obsessions, compulsions, and avoidance behaviors in different dimensions of obsessive-compulsive disorder

OCD Dimension	Obsessions	Compulsions	Avoidance
Contamination	Concerns with germs Concerns with contaminants or chemicals Concerns of harming others by spreading germs or contaminants	Washing, bathing, or grooming Cleaning objects or pets	Avoidance of contact with contaminated objects or people
Unacceptable/ Taboo Thoughts	Concerns regarding one's sexual orientation or gender identity Concerns with sacrilege or blasphemy	Checking Mental rituals (e.g., repeated prayer, phrases) Religious rituals Superstitious rituals	Avoidance of activities, places, people that trigger obsessions
Harm/ Responsibility	Fears of harming self/ others out of carelessness Fears of being responsible for terrible events	Checking locks, appliances, switches Reassurance seeking Confessing	Avoidance of handling dangerous objects out of fear of harming others
Symmetry	Need for symmetry or exactness Bothered by things not being "just right" Need for perfection	Arranging Ordering Evening up Ritualistic repeating Counting	
Hoarding	Fears of losing objects, information, or people	Saving/collecting useless items Picking up objects Examining objects that leave possession Buying unneeded items Retaining information	Avoidance of shopping out of concern of buying unneeded items

20.5 Theoretical Models of Obsessive-Compulsive Disorder

The *cognitive model* of OCD proposes that obsessions are caused by maladaptive beliefs about intrusive thoughts [24]. Three maladaptive beliefs in OCD are: (1) *overestimation of threat* and *inflated responsibility* (i.e., belief that harm is likely and one is responsible for causing harm); (2) *overimportance* and *control of thoughts* (i.e., belief that all thoughts have significance and one has full control over their thoughts); and (3) *perfectionism* and *intolerance of uncertainty* (e.g., belief that things must be performed perfectly or known with certainty) [25].

These cognitive biases magnify the distress associated with intrusive thoughts, which drives individuals to avoid triggers or perform compulsions to neutralize the thought. Such avoidance and/or compulsions result in a missed opportunity to gather evidence that contradicts the belief, which reinforces the original belief, and thus maintains the disorder. For instance, an individual with obsessive fears about accidentally causing a fire overestimates the threat of a fire and perceives inflated responsibility; compulsively checking the stove robs them of the opportunity to see the minimal level of threat and responsibility, thereby reinforcing their original distorted belief (e.g., "Had I not checked the stove, I *would* have caused a fire."). While the cognitive model of OCD informs treatment by identifying cognitive biases that maintain OCD, recent research shows that not all individuals have such biases [7]. Thus, the role of behavioral learning in OCD also must be considered, as it is a core element of current psychotherapeutics for OCD.

The *behavioral model* of OCD proposes that OCD is developed and maintained through the learning principles of classical and operant conditioning. Through this lens, OCD develops following repeated pairing of a neutral stimulus (i.e., intrusive thoughts) and aversive stimulus (i.e., feared outcome), which results in the once-neutral stimulus eliciting a conditioned fear response (classical conditioning). Subsequently, OCD is maintained through operant conditioning [7]. When individuals experience obsessive thoughts, they experience increased anxiety or distress; when they perform the associated compulsion, anxiety or distress is alleviated. This short-term reduction in distress is negatively reinforcing; however, in the long term, this repeated process contributes to the maintenance of OCD [26]. ERP maps onto these learning principles. When a patient is repeatedly exposed to a conditioned stimulus (e.g., touching a doorknob in the case of contamination OCD) without engaging in the compulsion (e.g., handwashing), the conditioned association between obsessive stimuli and fear response is extinguished (i.e., habituation), and the negative reinforcement of the compulsive response is attenuated.

The *inhibitory model of learning* is a recent additional framework that explains the process of change in OCD during ERP [27]. This model argues that during ERP, individuals acquire new information that violates their originally held expectations about the associations between an OCD trigger and feared outcomes. Thus, rather than "unlearning" a fear, individuals learn new information through ERP that inhibits the original fear. The inhibitory model is empirically supported and has informed approaches to exposures that differ from habituation-based approaches [27].

20.6 Treatment for Obsessive-Compulsive Disorder

20.6.1 Core Treatment Elements of Cognitive-Behavioral Therapy

The following section reviews the core treatment elements of CBT for OCD, with an emphasis on ERP. Most randomized controlled trials (RCTs) incorporate CBT protocols that include 14–20 twice-weekly or weekly sessions. Although a session-by-session overview is beyond the scope of this chapter, a brief summary of the core components of treatment are described [28].

Information Gathering, Psychoeducation, Goal Setting. Through clinical interviewing, clinicians confirm a diagnosis of OCD. Specific obsessional content and corresponding compulsions are identified, along with avoidant behaviors, both overt and covert (mental rituals). Additionally, contextual factors contributing to symptoms are assessed, as symptoms may present differently across contexts. This may be aided by administration of the (C)Y-BOCS-I and -II to further understand patients' OCD symptoms and associated severity. Patient self-monitoring forms that track triggers, obsessions, and compulsions are also utilized, along with input from other informants such as partners and parents. Furthermore, clinicians discuss psychoeducation related to OCD, ERP treatment rationale, and components of treatment. Patients have the opportunity to ask questions about OCD symptoms and treatment course, and clinicians and patients develop treatment goals.

Exposure and Response Prevention (ERP). *In vivo* and imaginal exposures are used in session and assigned as homework, in collaboration with the patient. *In vivo* exposures allow patients to confront situations that lead to distress (e.g., touching a doorknob for contamination-related OCD), and imaginal exposures involve creating a detailed script or recording of a feared situation and vividly imagining the situation while repeatedly reading or listening to the content. Imaginal exposures are typically used when *in vivo* cannot ethically or logistically be performed, such as when obsessional concerns are specific to disease (e.g., HIV/AIDS).

In session, clinicians and patients collaboratively develop an exposure hierarchy, which consists of the patient's OCD-related triggers and feared situations arranged from least to most distressing on a subjective units of distress scale (SUDS) that ranges from 0 (no distress) to 100 (maximum distress). Patient-reported SUDS are monitored throughout the exposure, with habituation-based models suggesting that the exposure continues until patients indicate a 50% SUDS reduction from the peak SUDS value. Tracking SUDS allows clinicians to compare anticipated peak SUDS ratings to actual SUDS ratings and highlight the possible expectancy violation (e.g., something bad will happen). Further, it is imperative that patients resist rituals during and after the exposure, and clinicians should look for subtle safety behaviors, such as looking away from the feared stimulus or mental compulsions/avoidance. After exposure completion, patients' interpretation of distress reductions should be discussed, with the hope that new learning occurs as patients' expectations are violated.

Initial exposures should elicit little to moderate distress to allow for exposure completion without compulsions to facilitate mastery and confidence with the exposure process. Although exposures can be completed in a graduated fashion based on the hierarchy, rigid adherence to the originally outlined hierarchy is not expected. Flexible progression through exposures (i.e., choosing tasks that evoke different levels of distress) may enhance learning generalization [29]. Finally, exposure exercises should be assigned as homework to ensure practice and generalization to different settings.

Relapse Prevention. Throughout treatment, patients should become more active in designing in-session exposures and homework assignments, which will help them continue to apply ERP principles after treatment termination. Clinicians should encourage patients to engage in "situational exposures" as they naturally occur in the environment. Although symptoms often persist following treatment termination, a detailed relapse prevention plan that reviews key elements of treatment will help patients address remaining symptoms.

20.6.2 Research Support of Cognitive-Behavioral Therapy

CBT with ERP is the gold-standard treatment for children, adolescents, and adults with OCD, with empirical support from meta-analyses and systematic reviews of RCTs

[30–33]. In adults, a recent meta-analysis demonstrated large effect sizes of ERP compared to waitlist (Hedges' $g = 1.31$) and placebo controls (Hedges' $g = 1.33$) [31]. ERP was also significantly more effective than antidepressant medication (Hedges' $g = .55$), and the addition of ERP to antidepressant medication led to greater effects than the use of medication alone. Further, approximately 65% of patients responded to ERP treatment as evidenced by percent reduction on the YBOCS and Clinical Global Impression-Improvement (CGI-I) scale ratings [31].

In youth, a recent meta-analysis showed that ERP is more effective than placebo (Hedges' $g = .93$) and waitlist controls (Hedges' $g = 1.53$) [32]. Several trials have also demonstrated the superiority of ERP to active treatment comparisons, such as psychoeducation and relaxation training, in both young children (5–8 years old) [34, 35] and school-age children to adolescents [36]. Further, meta-analyses have estimated ERP treatment response rates at 68–70% in children and adolescents [32, 37], which is similar to the response rate of ERP plus serotonin reuptake inhibitors (SRIs; 66%) and significantly higher than SRIs alone (49%) [32].

Additionally, leading health care organizations, including the American Psychological Association Society of Clinical Psychology, Society of Clinical Child and Adolescent Psychology, and National Institute for Health and Care Excellence (NICE), identify CBT with ERP as an optimal treatment option and first-line psychotherapeutic intervention for OCD [38–40].

Despite the robust evidence base for ERP, many patients with OCD do not receive this intervention because of therapist misconceptions related to the safety of the approach, patient inability to tolerate exposures, and the belief that ERP is not needed for effective OCD treatment [41]. Yet, in a survey of approximately 300 clinicians that use ERP, Schneider et al. found a near-zero (less than 0.01% per patient) chance of serious negative consequences during exposures, with no adverse events related to patients acting on intrusive thoughts [42]. Further, recent meta-analyses have shown that ERP attrition rates are similar to or lower than those of other interventions for OCD (e.g., pharmacological treatment, cognitive therapy) [43, 44]. In addition, perceived limitations of ERP have led to the examination of third-wave CBT approaches for OCD (e.g., acceptance and commitment therapy, mindfulness-based cognitive therapy). These third-wave approaches focus on the function of intrusive thoughts beyond their content and incorporate transdiagnostic skills, such as mindfulness and values-based action. However, a narrative review of RCTs testing third-wave CBT interventions for OCD found that these approaches are only effective insofar as they include ERP [45]. Other literature has also shown that exposures are the key ingredient of CBT for OCD, regardless of the theoretical model (i.e., habituation or inhibitory learning) used to conceptualize the condition [46].

20.6.3 Pharmacological Treatment

Selective serotonin reuptake inhibitors (SSRIs) are the mainstay for pharmacological management of OCD due to their proven efficacy and benign side effect profile. The US Food and Drug Administration (FDA) has approved several SSRIs for the treatment of OCD, including fluoxetine, fluvoxamine, sertraline, and paroxetine, though only fluoxetine, fluvoxamine, and sertraline are FDA approved for children and adolescents [47]. Two other off-label SSRIs commonly used to treat OCD are citalopram and escitalopram

[48]. Generally, SSRIs are efficacious in treating OCD at higher doses with an adequate therapeutic trial of 8–12 weeks [47]. Therapeutic dosages of each SSRI differ based on pharmacologic potency, patient metabolism, and OCD severity. Usual target dosages are 20mg/day of escitalopram, 40–60 mg/day of fluoxetine, paroxetine, or citalopram, and 200mg/day of fluvoxamine or sertraline, but dosages may be titrated upward until adequate response is achieved, with trial data suggesting a dose-dependent treatment response [48].

Clomipramine, a tricyclic antidepressant (TCA), was the first pharmacological agent with proven efficacy for OCD, though its use has been widely replaced by SSRIs due to its more problematic side effect and safety profile [49]. Once symptom improvement on a stable medication regimen has been achieved, continuation of treatment is typically advised to prevent OCD relapse [49]. However, a recent RCT found that among SSRI-medicated adults with OCD who responded well to ERP treatment, SSRI discontinuation resulted in noninferior outcomes in terms of OCD symptom recurrence compared to adults who continued their SSRI [50].

20.6.4 Deep Transcranial Magnetic Stimulation

Deep transcranial magnetic stimulation (DTMS) has demonstrated initial efficacy in OCD treatment. DTMS is a noninvasive procedure involving electromagnetic pulses emitted from an external device to the brain through coils of wire placed on the scalp. The induced magnetic field depolarizes neurons and modulates the underlying cortical activity. Elaborate coil winding patterns ('H coils') or double-cone configurations enable significantly greater field penetration depth compared to repetitive transcranial magnetic stimulation [51]. While DTMS has demonstrated efficacy relative to sham treatment, treatment effects were modest, and the intervention protocol may be burdensome [52].

20.6.5 Neurosurgery

Surgical options for adults with severe, treatment-refractory OCD include stereotactic ablation and deep brain stimulation (DBS). Ablative procedures for OCD were the earliest to emerge and involve creating lesions of target brain regions thought to be involved in the pathophysiology of OCD, including the anterior limb of the internal capsule and the anterior cingulate. Years of experience from lesioning ultimately led to the development of DBS, which involves surgical implantation of electrodes into similar target areas within the CSTC network. DBS may be advantageous to ablative procedures for OCD due to its reversibility and adjustability [53]. However, patients must tolerate chronic implantation of a medical device and be able to attend regular programming visits with a psychiatrist. DBS is an effective treatment option and has shown response rates of approximately 66% in adults with severe OCD [54]. Studies suggest that DBS for OCD is more cost effective than treatment as usual in up to 87% of cases, indicating that the initial expense may be offset by reduced health care consumption over time [55]. Additional research is needed to determine the ethical implications of using DBS in adolescents with severe OCD who have not responded to CBT or medication. In a recent survey in which parents were presented with vignettes of adolescents with treatment-resistant OCD, Storch et al. found that parents were willing to consider DBS as a possible treatment option in the presence of refractory status [56].

20.7 Conclusion

OCD is a heterogenous condition that occurs with relative frequency. Adults and youth with OCD often experience significant functional impairment, which can lead to decreased quality of life [7]. CBT, with an emphasis on ERP, and SSRIs are well-established treatment options that can help alleviate OCD symptoms and related impairment. It is imperative that future efforts continue to focus on disseminating and training clinicians in ERP across a variety of settings and disciplines, which will increase patient access to care and decrease negative perceptions of ERP. More studies on the use of telehealth and other innovative ways to deliver CBT, such as internet-based self-help programs, could also improve access and efficiency of treatment. Further, future research on moderators that impact the effects of ERP for adults and youth with OCD may inform clinical decision-making to improve treatment outcomes. DTMS has also demonstrated modest efficacy, but findings should be replicated, especially when compared to similarly intensive treatment protocols (e.g., daily ERP sessions). Finally, deep brain stimulation has emerged as a robust intervention for those with refractory OCD.

References

1. American Psychiatric Association. *Diagnostic and Statistical Manual of Mental Disorders.* American Psychiatric Publishing; 2013.

2. N. A. Fineberg, E. Hollander, S. Pallanti, et al. Clinical advances in obsessive-compulsive disorder: a position statement by the International College of Obsessive-Compulsive Spectrum Disorders. *International Clinical Psychopharmacology* 2020; **35**: 173–193.

3. E. Fawcett, H. Power, J. Fawcett. Women are at greater risk of OCD than men: a meta-analytic review of OCD prevalence worldwide. *The Journal of Clinical Psychiatry* 2020; **81**: 13075.

4. P. G. Alvarenga, R. C. Cesar, J. F. Leckman, et al. Obsessive-compulsive symptom dimensions in a population-based, cross-sectional sample of school-aged children. *Journal of Psychiatric Research* 2015; **62**: 108–114.

5. S. Dalsgaard, E. Thorsteinsson, B. B. Trabjerg, et al. Incidence rates and cumulative incidences of the full spectrum of diagnosed mental disorders in childhood and adolescence *JAMA Psychiatry* 2020; **77**: 155–164.

6. D. A. Geller, S. Homayoun, G. Johnson. Developmental considerations in obsessive compulsive disorder: comparing pediatric and adult-onset cases. *Frontiers in Psychiatry* 2021; **12**: 1–15.

7. Y. Markarian, M. J. Larson, M. A. Aldea, et al. Multiple pathways to functional impairment in obsessive-compulsive disorder. *Clinical Psychology Review* 2010; **30**: 78–88.

8. E. A. Storch, M. J. Larson, J. Muroff, et al. Predictors of functional impairment in pediatric obsessive-compulsive disorder. *Journal of Anxiety Disorders* 2010; **24**: 275–283.

9. J. D. Huppert, H. B. Simpson, K. J. Nissenson. Quality of life and functional impairment in obsessive-compulsive disorder: a comparison of patients with and without comorbidity, patients in remission, and healthy controls. *Depression and Anxiety* 2009; **26**: 39–45.

10. W. K. Goodman, L. H. Price, S. A. Rasmussen, et al. The Yale-Brown Obsessive Compulsive Scale: I. Development, use, and reliability. *Archives of General Psychiatry* 1989; **46**: 1006–1011.

11. E. A. Storch, S. A. Rasmussen, L. H. Price, et al. Development and psychometric evaluation of the Yale–Brown Obsessive-Compulsive Scale – Second Edition. *Psychological Assessment* 2010; **22**: 223–232.

12. L. Scahill, M. A. Riddle, M. McSwiggin-Hardin, et al. Children's Yale-Brown Obsessive Compulsive Scale: reliability and validity. *Journal of the American Academy of Child & Adolescent Psychiatry* 1997; **36**: 844–852.

13. E. A. Storch, J. F. McGuire, M. S. Wu, et al. Development and psychometric evaluation of the Children's Yale-Brown Obsessive-Compulsive Scale Second Edition. *Journal of the American Academy of Child & Adolescent Psychiatry* 2019; **58**: 92–98.

14. E. A. Storch, D. Bagner, L. J. Merlo, et al. Florida obsessive-compulsive inventory: development, reliability, and validity. *Journal of Clinical Psychology* 2007; **63**: 851–859.

15. E. B. Foa, J. D. Huppert, S. Leiberg, et al. The Obsessive-Compulsive Inventory: development and validation of a short version. *Psychological Assessment.* 2002; **14**: 485–496.

16. E. A. Storch, M. Khanna, L. J. Merlo, et al. Children's Florida Obsessive Compulsive Inventory: psychometric properties and feasibility of a self-report measure of obsessive-compulsive symptoms in youth. *Child Psychiatry and Human Development* 2009; **40**: 467–483.

17. A. Abramovitch, J. S. Abramowitz, D. McKay, et al. The OCI-CV-R: a revision of the Obsessive-Compulsive Inventory – Child Version. *Journal of Anxiety Disorders* 2022; **86**: 102532.

18. W. K. Goodman, E. A. Storch, S. A. Sheth. Harmonizing the neurobiology and treatment of obsessive-compulsive disorder. *The American Journal of Psychiatry* 2021; **178**: 17–29.

19. D. Mataix-Cols, M. Boman, B. Monzani, et al. Population-based, multigenerational family clustering study of obsessive-compulsive disorder. *JAMA Psychiatry* 2013; **70**: 709–717.

20. H. A. Browne, S. L. Gair, J. M. Scharf, D. E. Grice. Genetics of obsessive-compulsive disorder and related disorders. *Psychiatric Clinics of North America.* 2014; **37**: 319–335.

21. B. Monzani, F. Rijsdijk, J. Harris, D. Mataix-Cols. The structure of genetic and environmental risk factors for dimensional representations of DSM-5 obsessive-compulsive spectrum disorders. *JAMA Psychiatry.* 2014; **71**: 182–189.

22. A. P. Escobar, J. R. Wendland, A. E. Chávez, P. R. Moya. The neuronal glutamate transporter EAAT3 in obsessive-compulsive disorder. *Frontiers in Pharmacology* 2019; **10**: 1362.

23. J. E. Grant, and S. R. Chamberlain. Exploring the neurobiology of OCD: clinical implications. *Psychiatry Times* 2020. Available at: www.psychiatrictimes.com/view/exploring-neurobiology-ocd-clinical-implications.

24. S. Rachman. A Cognitive Theory of Obsessions. In E. Sanavio, ed., *Behavior and Cognitive Therapy Today.* Elsevier; 1998:209–222.

25. Group OCCW, et al. Psychometric validation of the obsessive belief questionnaire and interpretation of intrusions inventory – part 2: factor analyses and testing of a brief version. *Behaviour Research and Therapy* 2005; **43**: 1527–1542.

26. S. Spencer, J. T. Stiede, A. Wiese, W. Goodman, A. Guzick, E. A. Storch. Cognitive-behavioral therapy for obsessive-compulsive disorder. *Psychiatric Clinics* 2022; **46**: 167–180.

27. J. F. McGuire and E. A. Storch. An inhibitory learning approach to cognitive-behavioral therapy for children and adolescents. *Cognitive and Behavioral Practice.* 2019; **26**: 214–224.

28. E. B. Foa, E. Yadin, T. K. Lichner. *Exposure and Response (Ritual) Prevention for Obsessive-Compulsive Disorder: Therapist Guide,* 2nd ed. Oxford University Press; 2012.

29. M. G. Craske, B. Liao, L. Brown, B. Vervliet. Role of inhibition in exposure therapy. *Journal of Experimental Psychopathology* 2012; **3**: 322–345.

30. B. O. Olatunji, M. L. Davis, M. B. Powers, J. A. J. Smits. Cognitive-behavioral therapy for obsessive-compulsive

disorder: a meta-analysis of treatment outcome and moderators. *Journal of Psychiatric Research* 2013; **47**: 33–41.

31. L. G. Öst, A. Havnen, B. Hansen, G. Kvale. Cognitive behavioral treatments of obsessive–compulsive disorder: a systematic review and meta-analysis of studies published 1993–2014. *Clinical Psychology Review* 2015; **40**: 156–169.

32. L. G. Öst, E. N. Riise, G. J. Wergeland, B. Hansen, G. Kvale. Cognitive behavioral and pharmacological treatments of OCD in children: a systematic review and meta-analysis. *Journal of Anxiety Disorders* 2016; **43**: 58–69.

33. C. F. Uhre, V. F. Uhre, N. N. Lønfeldt, et al. Systematic review and meta-analysis: cognitive-behavioral therapy for obsessive-compulsive disorder in children and adolescents. *Journal of the American Academy of Child & Adolescent Psychiatry* 2020; **59**: 64–77.

34. J. B. Freeman, A. M. Garcia, L. Coyne, et al. Early childhood OCD: preliminary findings from a family-based cognitive-behavioral approach. *Journal of the American Academy of Child & Adolescent Psychiatry* 2008; **47**: 593–602.

35. J. Freeman, J. Sapyta, A. Garcia, et al. Family-based treatment of early childhood obsessive-compulsive disorder: the Pediatric Obsessive-Compulsive Disorder Treatment Study for Young Children (POTS Jr) – a randomized clinical trial. *JAMA Psychiatry* 2014; **71**: 689–698.

36. J. Piacentini, R. L. Bergman, S. Chang, et al. Controlled comparison of family cognitive behavioral therapy and psychoeducation/relaxation training for child obsessive-compulsive disorder. *Journal of the American Academy of Child & Adolescent Psychiatry* 2011; **50**: 1149–1161.

37. J. F. McGuire, J. Piacentini, A. B. Lewin, E. A. Brennan, T. K. Murphy, E. A. Storch. A meta-analysis of cognitive behavior therapy and medication for child obsessive–compulsive disorder: moderators of treatment efficacy,

response, and remission. *Depression and Anxiety* 2015; **32**: 580–593.

38. D. Tolin, T. Melnyk, B. Marx; Society of Clinical Psychology, American Psychological Association. Exposure and response prevention for obsessive-compulsive disorder: empirically supported treatment report. 2015.

39. J. Freeman, K. Benito, J. Herren, et al. Evidence base update of psychosocial treatments for pediatric obsessive-compulsive disorder: evaluating, improving, and transporting what works. *Journal of Clinical Child and Adolescent Psychology.* 2018; **47**: 669–698.

40. National Institute for Health and Care Excellence. *Obsessive-Compulsive Disorder: Evidence Update.* The British Psychological Society and The Royal College of Psychiatrists; 2013.

41. B. J. Deacon, N. R. Farrell, J. J. Kemp, et al. Assessing therapist reservations about exposure therapy for anxiety disorders: the Therapist Beliefs about Exposure Scale. *Journal of Anxiety Disorders* 2013; **27**: 772–780.

42. S. C. Schneider, L. Knott, S. L. Cepeda, et al. Serious negative consequences associated with exposure and response prevention for obsessive-compulsive disorder: a survey of therapist attitudes and experiences. *Depression and Anxiety.* 2020; **37**: 418–428.

43. C. Johnco, J. F. McGuire, T. Roper, E. A. Storch. A meta-analysis of dropout rates from exposure with response prevention and pharmacological treatment for youth with obsessive compulsive disorder. *Depression and Anxiety* 2020; **37**: 407–417.

44. C. W. Ong, J. W. Clyde, E. J. Bluett, M. E. Levin, M. P. Twohig. Dropout rates in exposure with response prevention for obsessive-compulsive disorder: what do the data really say? *Journal of Anxiety Disorders* 2016; **40**: 8–17.

45. E. S. Trent, A. G. Guzick, A. G. Viana, E. A. Storch. Third-wave cognitive behavioral therapy for obsessive compulsive disorder? *Advances in*

Psychiatry and Behavioral Health 2021; **1**: 37–51.

46. J. S. Abramowitz and J. J. Arch. Strategies for improving long-term outcomes in cognitive behavioral therapy for obsessive-compulsive disorder: insights from learning theory. *Cognitive and Behavioral Practice* 2014; **21**: 20–31.

47. L. Koran, G. Hanna, E. Hollander, et al. Practice guideline for the treatment of patients with obsessive-compulsive disorder. *The American Journal of Psychiatry* 2007; **164**: 5–53.

48. M. Lambert. APA releases guidelines on treating obsessive-compulsive disorder. *American Family Physician* 2008; **78**: 131–135.

49. C. Pittenger and M. H. Bloch. Pharmacological treatment of obsessive-compulsive disorder. *Psychiatric Clinics of North America* 2014; **37**: 375–391.

50. E. B. Foa, H. B. Simpson, T. Gallagher, et al. Maintenance of wellness in patients with obsessive-compulsive disorder who discontinue medication after exposure/response prevention augmentation: a randomized clinical trial. *JAMA Psychiatry* 2022; **79**: 193.

51. A. G. McCathern, D. S. Mathai, R. Y. Cho, W. K. Goodman, E. A. Storch. Deep transcranial magnetic stimulation for obsessive compulsive disorder. *Expert Review of Neurotherapeutics* 2020; **20**: 1029–1036.

52. L. Carmi, U. Alyagon, N. Barnea-Ygael, et al. Clinical and electrophysiological outcomes of deep TMS over the medial prefrontal and anterior cingulate cortices in OCD patients. *Brain Stimulation* 2018; **11**: 158–165.

53. C. Borders, F. Hsu, A. J. Sweidan, E. S. Matei, R. G. Bota. Deep brain stimulation for obsessive compulsive disorder: a review of results by anatomical target. *Mental Illness.* 2018; **10**: 7900.

54. R. Gadot, R. Najera, S. Hirani, et al. Efficacy of deep brain stimulation for treatment-resistant obsessive-compulsive disorder: systematic review and meta-analysis. *Journal of Neurology, Neurosurgery & Psychiatry* 2022; **93**: 1166–1173.

55. R. Najera, S. Gregory, B. Shofty, et al. Cost-effectiveness analysis of radiosurgical capsulotomy versus treatment as usual for treatment-resistant obsessive-compulsive disorder. *Journal of Neurosurgery* 2022; **138**: 347–357.

56. E. A. Storch, S. L. Cepeda, E. Lee, et al. Parental attitudes toward deep brain stimulation in adolescents with treatment-resistant conditions. *Journal of Child and Adolescent Psychopharmacology* 2020; **30**: 97–103.

Posttraumatic Stress Disorder
An Update on Diagnosis, Etiology, and Treatment

John M. Bouras

21.1 Introduction

Stress can be defined as a state of worry or mental tension caused by a difficult situation [1]. Stress is a natural human response to challenges and threats we face in our lives. Everyone experiences stress to some degree. When individuals are exposed to extremely threatening or horrific (traumatic) events, they may develop a syndrome of physiological and psychological symptoms referred to as posttraumatic stress disorder (PTSD).

Even though more than half of the general population experiences a traumatic event in their lifetime, approximately 6.8% of people will ultimately develop PTSD [2–4]. Prevalence rates of PTSD in the United States are 3.5%, whereas in Europe, Asia, Africa, or Latin America they are between 0.5% to 1%. In the United States, we see higher rates of PTSD among nonwhite ethnic groups (US Latinos, African Americans, Native American/Alaska Natives), women (twice as much as men), rape survivors, veterans, and first responders. Comorbidities with other psychiatric disorders seem to be "the norm" with over 80% of participants with lifetime PTSD in the United States National Co-morbidity survey having at least one other disorder [5].

21.1.1 Risk Factors in Development of Posttraumatic Stress Disorder

Not all individuals exposed to a traumatic event necessarily develop PTSD. Some predictions could be made based on the presence of certain risk factors [2, 6, 7]. Individuals who are more vulnerable are the ones with past personal or family history of trauma, prior psychiatric condition, female gender, and psychosocial (lower socioeconomic status, lack of education, minority status) as well as personality features where the individual's locus of control is primarily based on external factors. The nature of the traumatic event is also important, as the higher the perceived life threat, trauma severity, interpersonal violence, and emotions/dissociation evoked, the higher the likelihood to develop PTSD. Moral injury, defined as failing to prevent or bearing witness to acts that transgress deeply held moral beliefs, is an emerging concept, which was observed with health care workers during early days of the COVID-19 pandemic. What happens in the aftermath of trauma is also important, as subsequent life stress and perceived lack of social support are associated with higher PTSD rates.

PTSD is usually exacerbated by delays in seeking and receiving treatment. According the 2005 National Comorbidity Survey study [8], only 7.1% of PTSD patients made contact for treatment within 1 year of onset of PTSD symptoms, whereas the cumulative lifetime probability of treatment contact was 65.3%.

21.2 Clinical Presentation/Diagnosis

There have been several terms (*nostalgia, soldier's heart, shell shock, battle fatigue, combat fatigue, gross stress reaction, post-Vietnam syndrome*) used to describe accounts of what we now call PTSD [9, 10]. The first Diagnostic and Statistical Manual of Mental Disorders (DSM-I) introduced the term "Gross Stress Reaction." It was in 1980, with the third edition of the Diagnostic and Statistical Manual of Mental Disorders, that the term *posttraumatic stress disorder* (PTSD) was introduced under the section of anxiety disorders [11]. The 5th edition of Diagnostic and Statistical Manual for Mental disorders modified the criteria and moved the diagnosis under the Trauma and Stressor Related section [12].

21.2.1 DSM-5 Criteria

Diagnosing PTSD requires having a preceding traumatic exposure or event, a minimum of six symptoms from four symptom clusters (see Table 21.1) that last at least for 1 month, and result in significant distress in functioning [12].

The individual may have directly experienced the traumatic event, witnessed it happening to others, or learned about it happening to a close family member or friend. Repeated exposure to horrific details of trauma, such as seen with deployed military personnel, first responders, and health care workers, may result in PTSD. A minimum of one symptom is required from each of the symptom clusters of intrusion and avoidance; a minimum of two symptoms are required from each of the symptom clusters of negative alterations in cognition and mood, and hyperarousal/hyperactivity (see Table 21.1).

21.2.2 Children Less Than 6 Years Old

Children 6 years and younger may experience PTSD symptoms slightly differently. For example, symptoms may be reexperienced through play that refers directly or symbolically to the trauma, whereas mood changes may be the primary manifestation of the negative alterations in mood and cognition because of developmental limitations in expressing thoughts and feelings.

21.2.3 Specifiers

An individual meeting the criteria for PTSD may also meet the criteria for specifiers. If the full criteria of PTSD are not met until at least 6 months after the event, then a specifier "with delayed expression" is added. If there are symptoms of depersonalization or derealization in response to the stressor, then a specifier "with dissociative symptoms" is added.

21.2.4 ICD-11 Criteria

The PTSD criteria are slightly different in the ICD-11 [13], where only three core elements are required for diagnosis: (1) reexperiencing the traumatic event, as evidenced by intrusive memories, flashbacks, and/or nightmares; (2) avoidance of traumatic reminders, as evidenced by the avoidance of internal and/or external stimuli; and (3) a persistent sense of threat, evidenced by hypervigilance and increased startle. Also, a

Table 21.1 PTSD symptoms by symptom cluster, simplified. (See DSM-5 for exact wording of symptoms.)

		Symptom Clusters		
	Intrusion	**Avoidance**	**Negative Alterations in Mood and Cognition**	**Hyperarousal/ Hyperreactivity**
Number of Symptoms	≥ 1 symptom	≥ 1 symptom	≥ 2 symptoms	≥ 2 symptoms
Symptoms	• Has distressing memories • Has distressing dreams • Has flashbacks • Develops intense/ prolonged psychological distress upon cues of trauma • Marked physiological reactions upon cues	• Avoids distressing memories, thoughts, feelings related to trauma • Avoids external reminders related to trauma	• Unable to remember important aspects of event • Sees self negatively, lack of trust • Blame oneself for traumatic event • Experiences fear, horror, anger, guilt, or shame • Not participating in significant activities as much • Feeling detached or estranged • Unable to experience happiness, loving feelings, satisfaction	• Irritable and angry leading to aggression (verbal, physical) • Self-destructive and reckless • Hypervigilant • Easily startles • Cannot focus • Problems with sleep

diagnosis of *Complex PTSD* (CPTSD) may be made if the individual meets criteria for PTSD and three additional features related to *disturbances in self-organization* (DSO). These include (1) affective dysregulation (e.g., trouble calming down, numbing); (2) negative self-concept (e.g., worthlessness); and (3) disturbed relationships (e.g., difficulty feeling close to others).

21.2.5 Clinical Approach

A careful psychiatric interview may help clarify the differential diagnoses as well as any comorbidities. Consider a diagnosis of adjustment disorder or major depressive disorder (if the traumatic event was not life threatening or there are no other PTSD criteria); acute stress disorder (if duration of symptoms are less than 1 month); generalized or panic disorder or obsessive compulsive disorder (if experienced symptoms are not related to the experienced traumatic event); personality disorder (if there were interpersonal difficulties before the traumatic event); dissociative disorders (especially with amnesia, identity disorder, and derealization/depersonalization disorder), functional neurological disorder (if symptoms prior to exposure to traumatic event); psychotic disorders (if there are hallucinations or other perceptual disturbances); and traumatic brain injury (if there is persistent disorientation and confusion). It is important to treat both PTSD and all comorbidities.

21.3 Pathophysiology and Pathogenesis

The neurobiology of PTSD is complex involving structural, hormonal, and chemical changes in brain neural networks.

21.3.1 Neuroanatomic

Brain circuits associated with adaptation to stress and fear conditioning have been shown to be structurally altered in patients with PTSD [14–16]. According to structural and functional brain imaging studies, patients with PTSD show hyperactive amygdala function. As amygdala usually helps assess the importance of sensory information and prompts for appropriate response, increased amygdala activity leads to an exaggerated fear response. At the same time, the ventromedial prefrontal cortex (vmPFC) is smaller and hypoactive. This results in decreased inhibitory control on the amygdala (and its stress response), which leads to attentional bias toward threat cues. The hippocampus is also smaller, making it less effective in its role of fear extinction and conditioning.

21.3.2 Neuroendocrine

A predominant feature of PTSD is dysregulation of the glucocorticoid signaling in the hypothalamic–pituitary–adrenal (HPA) axis [17]. Humans, like other mammals, respond to stress by secretion of corticotropin-releasing hormone (CRH) by nerve cells in the hypothalamus, which stimulates the anterior pituitary to release adrenocorticotropin hormone (ACTH), which further stimulates the adrenal gland to release glucocorticoids such as cortisol. Cortisol in turn inhibits further production of CRH via a negative feedback loop and reduces the noradrenergic stress response.

In PTSD, cortisol levels are paradoxically low. This causes reduced negative feedback to the hypothalamus, leading to elevated CRH levels and increased adrenergic response.

CRH receptors in the pituitary are downregulated, leading to a blunted ACTH response and decreased cortisol release. Studies with low-dose dexamethasone suppression testing suggest that low cortisol levels in PTSD are the result of increased negative feedback sensitivity to the HPA axis.

21.3.3 Neurochemical

Altered regulation of catecholamines, serotonin, amino acid, and peptides has been seen in PTSD patients [17, 18]. Increased adrenergic tone results in elevated norepinephrine (NE) levels, which may account for PTSD symptoms such as hyperarousal, exaggerated startle response, and increased encoding of fear memories. Altered serotonin (5-HT) neurotransmission has been implicated in PTSD, suggesting a role in PTSD symptoms such as hypervigilance, increased startle response, impulsivity, and intrusive memories. Gamma-aminobutyric acid (GABA) levels are decreased, whereas glutamate levels are increased. This leads to less disinhibition of physiological responses to stress and increased risk for dissociation symptoms, respectively. Neuropeptide Y (NPY) levels are lower in PTSD patients, resulting in decreased anxiolytic and stress-buffering properties, as well as contribution to noradrenergic hyperactivity in PTSD patients [19].

21.3.4 Genetic

We are in the early stages of trying to fully understand the relationship of genetic variations and their role in modifying risk factors for the development of PTSD [20, 21]. Several studies have looked at NPY, corticotropin-releasing hormone receptor (CRHR1) gene, brain-derived neurotrophic factor (BDNF), variants of serotonin (5-HT) transporter gene (SLC6A4), and catechol-o-methyltransferase (COMT) gene and their association with PTSD. Further studies may lead to the potential of clinical therapeutic interventions in the future.

21.4 Treatment and Management

The current evidence-based options for PTSD include psychotherapy and pharmacotherapy interventions. It was thought that psychological debriefing may help prevent PTSD. Several studies have shown that not only it had no benefit [22], but some individuals fared worse [23], especially the ones who are more traumatized. Instead, providing information, emotional support, and practical assistance is recommended and encouraged.

21.4.1 Psychotherapy

Most treatment guidelines recommend trauma-focused psychotherapy as a first-line treatment for PTSD [24]. They directly address memories, thoughts, and feelings associated with the traumatic event. Cognitive-behavioral therapy (CBT) that is trauma-focused has been extensively studied in the treatment of PTSD [25, 26]. Prolonged exposure (PE) is utilized to block the avoidance response and to extinguish the fear response. It incorporates safety information, so that the patient learns to differentiate the traumatic event from the current context. Cognitive processing therapy helps patients challenge their overgeneralized beliefs by instilling trust, safety, control, and improved self-esteem. Narrative exposure therapy and written exposure therapy have shown some evidence to support their use in treatment [27, 28]. Eye movement desensitization and reprocessing therapy, where patients develop a mental image of the traumatic event while tracking a bilateral stimulus, has been efficacious, but it has been criticized for not being consistent with the current understanding of the neurobiological processes involved in PTSD [29, 30].

21.4.2 Pharmacotherapy

Selective serotonin reuptake inhibitors (SSRIs) and serotonin-norepinephrine reuptake inhibitors (SNRIs) have shown benefits in the treatment of PTSD [31], with small effect size [32]. Paroxetine, fluoxetine, and venlafaxine have the most robust evidence, although sertraline, duloxetine, and desvenlafaxine are acceptable alternatives [30]. There is limited effect of these medications on insomnia, hyperarousal, or other PTSD-specific symptoms [33, 34].

Prazosin has been used as an augmenting agent to target PTSD-associated nightmares and hyperarousal response [30]. Mirtazapine has some evidence for augmentation response to SSRI/SNRI and insomnia. Trazodone is frequently used for sleep anecdotally, even though there is not much scientific evidence supporting its use. Atypical antipsychotics such as quetiapine and risperidone may be used to treat patients with PTSD, but they should be used with caution given their broad side effect profile [35, 36]. Other medications that have shown limited to no benefit are risperidone, topiramate, and pregabalin. Benzodiazepine medications are not recommended for the treatment of PTSD due to their strong sedative, addictive, and dissociative properties. The dissociation and hypnotic sedation foster trauma reliving intrusive symptoms, which in turn worsens avoidant symptoms of PTSD. There is research looking into the use of ketamine and repetitive transcranial stimulation in treatment of PTSD, but so far there is not adequate evidence for generalized use [37, 38].

References

1. World Health Organization. What Is Stress? 2023. www.who.int/news-room/questions-and-answers/item/stress#:~:text=Stress%20can%20be%20defined%20as,experiences%20stress%20to%20some%20degree (accessed September 7, 2023).

2. R. C. Kessler, S. Aguilar-Gaxiola, J. Alonso, et al. Trauma and PTSD in the WHO World Mental Health Surveys. *European Journal of Psychotraumatology*, 8 (2017) 1353383. https://doi.org/10.1080/20008198.2017.1353383.

3. R. C. Kessler, P. Berglund, O. Demler, R. Jin, K. R. Merikangas, & E. E. Walters, Lifetime prevalence and age-of-onset distributions of DSM-IV disorders in the National Comorbidity Survey Replication. *Archives of General Psychiatry*, 62 (2005) 593–602. https://doi.org/10.1001/archpsyc.62.6.593.

4. R. C. Kessler, W. T. Chiu, O. Demler, K. R. Merikangas, & E. E. Walters, Prevalence, severity, and comorbidity of 12-month DSM-IV disorders in the National Comorbidity Survey Replication. *Archives of General Psychiatry*, 62 (2005) 617–627. https://doi.org/10.1001/archpsyc.62.6.617.

5. R. C. Kessler, A. Sonnega, E. Bromet, M. Hughes, & C. B. Nelson, Posttraumatic stress disorder in the National Comorbidity Survey. *Archives of General Psychiatry*, 52 (1995) 1048–1060. https://doi.org/10.1001/archpsyc.1995.03950240066012.

6. C. R. Brewin, B. Andrews, & J. D. Valentine, Meta-analysis of risk factors for posttraumatic stress disorder in trauma-exposed adults. *Journal of Consulting and Clinical Psychology*, 68 (2000) 748–766. https://doi.org/10.1037//0022-006x.68.5.748.

7. E. J. Ozer, S. R. Best, T. L. Lipsey, & D. S. Weiss, Predictors of posttraumatic stress disorder and symptoms in adults: a meta-analysis. *Psychological Bulletin*, **129** (2003) 52–73. https://doi.org/10.1037/0033-2909.129.1.52.

8. P. S. Wang, P. Berglund, M. Olfson, H. A. Pincus, K. B. Wells, & R. C. Kessler, Failure and delay in initial treatment contact after first onset of mental disorders in the National Comorbidity Survey replication. *Archives of General Psychiatry*, **62** (2005) 603–613. https://doi.org/10.1001/archpsyc.62.6.603.

9. C. S. Myers, A Contribution to the Study of Shell Shock.: Being an Account of Three Cases of Loss of Memory, Vision, Smell, and Taste, Admitted into the Duchess of Westminster's War Hospital, Le Touquet. *The Lancet*, **185** (1915) 316–320. https://doi.org/10.1016/S0140-6736(00)52916-X.

10. R. J. Daly, Samuel Pepys and post-traumatic stress disorder. *The British Journal of Psychiatry: The Journal of Mental Science*, **143** (1983) 64–68. https://doi.org/10.1192/bjp.143.1.64.

11. R. E. Kendell, Diagnostic and Statistical Manual of Mental Disorders, 3rd ed., revised (DSM-III-R). *American Journal of Psychiatry*, **145** (1988) 1301–1302. https://doi.org/10.1176/ajp.145.10.1301.

12. Diagnostic and Statistical Manual of Mental Disorders. *DSM Library* (n.d.). https://dsm.psychiatryonline.org/doi/book/10.1176/appi.books.9780890425787 (accessed September 7, 2023).

13. ICD-11 for Mortality and Morbidity Statistics. (n.d.). https://icd.who.int/browse11/l-m/en#/http://id.who.int/icd/entity/2070699808 (accessed September 7, 2023).

14. M. Koenigs & J. Grafman, Post-traumatic stress disorder: the role of medial prefrontal cortex and amygdala. *The Neuroscientist*, **15** (2009) 540–548. https://doi.org/10.1177/1073858409333072.

15. S. J. H. van Rooij, M. Kennis, R. Sjouwerman, et al. Smaller hippocampal volume as a vulnerability factor for the persistence of post-traumatic stress disorder. *Psychological Medicine*, **45** (2015) 2737–2746. https://doi.org/10.1017/S0033291715000707.

16. J. D. Bremner, P. Randall, T. M. Scott, R. A. Bronen, J. P. Seibyl, S. M. Southwick, R. C. Delaney, G. McCarthy, D. S. Charney, & R. B. Innis, MRI-based measurement of hippocampal volume in patients with combat-related posttraumatic stress disorder. *The American Journal of Psychiatry*, **152** (1995) 973–981.

17. J. E. Sherin & C. B. Nemeroff, Post-traumatic stress disorder: the neurobiological impact of psychological trauma. *Dialogues in Clinical Neuroscience*, **13** (2011) 263–278.

18. K. J. Ressler & C. B. Nemeroff, Role of serotonergic and noradrenergic systems in the pathophysiology of depression and anxiety disorders. *Depression and Anxiety*, **12** Suppl 1 (2000) 2–19. https://doi.org/10.1002/1520-6394(2000)12:1+<2::AID-DA2>3.0.CO;2-4.

19. A. M. Rasmusson, R. L. Hauger, C. A. Morgan, J. D. Bremner, D. S. Charney, & S. M. Southwick, Low baseline and yohimbine-stimulated plasma neuropeptide Y (NPY) levels in combat-related PTSD. *Biological Psychiatry*, **47** (2000) 526–539. https://doi.org/10.1016/s0006-3223(99)00185-7.

20. R. R. Souza, L. J. Noble, & C. K. McIntyre, Using the single prolonged stress model to examine the pathophysiology of PTSD. *Frontiers in Pharmacology*, **8** (2017) 615.

21. B. Togay & R. S. El-Mallakh, Posttraumatic stress disorder: from pathophysiology to pharmacology. *Current Psychiatry*, **19** (2020) 33–39. www.mdedge.com/psychiatry/article/221338/ptsd/posttraumatic-stress-disorder-pathophysiology-pharmacology (accessed September 7, 2023).

22. S. C. Rose, J. Bisson, R. Churchill, & S. Wessely, Psychological debriefing for preventing post traumatic stress disorder (PTSD). *Cochrane Database of Systematic Reviews* (2002). https://doi.org/10.1002/14651858.CD000560.

23. M. Sijbrandij, M. Olff, J. B. Reitsma, I. V. E. Carlier, & B. P. R. Gersons, Emotional or educational debriefing after psychological trauma: randomised controlled trial. *The British Journal of Psychiatry: The Journal of Mental Science*, **189** (2006) 150–155. https://doi.org/10 .1192/bjp.bp.105.021121.

24. J. C. Morganstein, G. H. Wynn, & J. C. West, Post-traumatic stress disorder: update on diagnosis and treatment. *BJPsych Advances*, **27** (2021) 184–186. https://doi.org/10.1192/bja.2021.13.

25. A. Ehlers, D. M. Clark, A. Hackmann, F. McManus, M. Fennell, C. Herbert, & R. Mayou, A randomized controlled trial of cognitive therapy, a self-help booklet, and repeated assessments as early interventions for posttraumatic stress disorder. *Archives of General Psychiatry*, **60** (2003) 1024–1032. https://doi.org/10 .1001/archpsyc.60.10.1024.

26. J. I. Bisson, J. P. Shepherd, D. Joy, R. Probert, & R. G. Newcombe, Early cognitive-behavioural therapy for post-traumatic stress symptoms after physical injury: randomised controlled trial. *The British Journal of Psychiatry: The Journal of Mental Science*, **184** (2004) 63–69. https://doi.org/10.1192/bjp.184.1.63.

27. H. Stenmark, C. Catani, F. Neuner, T. Elbert, & A. Holen, Treating PTSD in refugees and asylum seekers within the general health care system: a randomized controlled multicenter study. *Behaviour Research and Therapy*, **51** (2013) 641–647. https://doi.org/10.1016/j.brat .2013.07.002.

28. D. M. Sloan, B. P. Marx, P. A. Resick, S. Young-McCaughan, K. A. Dondanville, J. Mintz, B. T. Litz, & A. L. Peterson, Study design comparing written exposure therapy to cognitive processing therapy for PTSD among military service members: a noninferiority trial. *Contemporary Clinical Trials Communications*, **17** (2019) 100507. https://doi.org/10.1016/j.conctc.2019 .100507.

29. J. I. Bisson, L. Berliner, M. Cloitre, D. Forbes, T. K. Jensen, C. Lewis, C. M. Monson, M. Olff, S. Pilling, D. S. Riggs, N. P. Roberts, & F. Shapiro, The International Society for Traumatic Stress Studies new guidelines for the prevention and treatment of posttraumatic stress disorder: methodology and development process. *Journal of Traumatic Stress*, **32** (2019) 475–483. https://doi.org/10.1002/ jts.22421.

30. C. Schrader & A. Ross, A review of PTSD and current treatment strategies. *Missouri Medicine*, **118** (2021) 546–551.

31. J. C. Morganstein, G. H. Wynn, & J. C. West, Post-traumatic stress disorder: update on diagnosis and treatment. *BJPsych Advances*, **27** (2021) 184–186. https://doi.org/10.1192/bja.2021.13.

32. M. Hoskins, J. Pearce, A. Bethell, L. Dankova, C. Barbui, W. A. Tol, M. van Ommeren, J. de Jong, S. Seedat, H. Chen, & J. I. Bisson, Pharmacotherapy for post-traumatic stress disorder: systematic review and meta-analysis. *The British Journal of Psychiatry*, **206** (2015) 93–100. https://doi.org/10.1192/bjp.bp.114.148551.

33. K. Brady, T. Pearlstein, G. M. Asnis, D. Baker, B. Rothbaum, C. R. Sikes, & G. M. Farfel, Efficacy and safety of sertraline treatment of posttraumatic stress disorder: a randomized controlled trial. *JAMA*, **283** (2000) 1837–1844. https://doi .org/10.1001/jama.283.14.1837.

34. J. R. T. Davidson, L. R. Landerman, G. M. Farfel, & C. M. Clary, Characterizing the effects of sertraline in post-traumatic stress disorder. *Psychological Medicine*, **32** (2002) 661–670. https://doi.org/10.1017/ s0033291702005469.

35. G. Villarreal, M. B. Hamner, J. M. Cañive, S. Robert, L. A. Calais, V. Durklaski, Y. Zhai, & C. Qualls, Efficacy of quetiapine monotherapy in posttraumatic stress disorder: a randomized, placebo-controlled trial. *The American Journal of Psychiatry*, **173** (2016) 1205–1212. https:// doi.org/10.1176/appi.ajp.2016.15070967.

36. J. H. Krystal, R. A. Rosenheck, J. A. Cramer, J. C. Vessicchio, K. M. Jones, J. E. Vertrees, R. A. Horney, G. D. Huang, C. Stock, & Veterans Affairs Cooperative Study No. 504 Group, Adjunctive

risperidone treatment for antidepressant-resistant symptoms of chronic military service-related PTSD: a randomized trial. *JAMA*, **306** (2011) 493–502. https://doi.org/10.1001/jama.2011.1080.

37. A. E. Philipp-Muller, C. J. Stephenson, E. Moghimi, A. H. Shirazi, R. Milev, G. Vazquez, T. Reshetukha, & N. Alavi, Combining ketamine and psychotherapy for the treatment of posttraumatic stress disorder: a systematic review and meta-analysis. *The Journal of Clinical Psychiatry*, **84** (2023) 22br14564. https://doi.org/10.4088/JCP.22br14564.

38. F. A. Kozel, M. A. Motes, N. Didehbani, B. DeLaRosa, C. Bass, C. D. Schraufnagel, P. Jones, C. R. Morgan, J. S. Spence, M. A. Kraut, & J. Hart, Repetitive TMS to augment cognitive processing therapy in combat veterans of recent conflicts with PTSD: a randomized clinical trial. *Journal of Affective Disorders*, **229** (2018) 506–514. https://doi.org/10.1016/j.jad.2017.12.046.

Borderline Personality Disorder

Marcos S. Croci, Marcelo J. A. A. Brañas, Stephen Conway, Julia Jurist, and Lois W. Choi-Kain

22.1 Introduction

Following a systematic review by John Gunderson [1], borderline personality disorder (BPD) was introduced in the third edition of the Diagnostic and Statistical Manual of Mental Disorders (DSM-III) in 1980. BPD symptoms, which include emotional and behavioral dysregulation, can be reliably identified and grouped in a coherent nosological entity beginning in early adolescence (12 years old and onward), with a prevalence of 2.7% in adults [2, 3]. Its clinical picture is often accompanied by various comorbidities and an elevated risk of suicide, posing a significant challenge for clinicians and a high burden for individuals, families, and health care systems [4].

The perception of BPD has shifted from stigmatized and untreatable to one with more scientific clarity and a better prognosis. Longitudinal studies have shown high symptomatic remission (about 85%) and low recurrence (about 15%) in 10 years [5]. While specialized treatments may be necessary for a minority of cases, there is a shortage of care for BPD, and generalist approaches, which rely on basic principles of care, have been shown to be comparable in treating the disorder [6].

With 22% of psychiatric inpatients and 12% of outpatients meeting the criteria for BPD [7], clinicians need to know about its underlying mechanisms, presentations, and treatment. In this chapter, we will provide an overview of the latest knowledge to assist clinicians in the identification and basic clinical management of BPD.

22.2 Clinical Presentation/Diagnosis

22.2.1 Descriptive Psychopathology/Phenomenology

BPD is a disorder marked by instability in self-image and interpersonal relationships [8]. The features of BPD fall within four domains of psychopathology: interpersonal instability (unstable relationships, abandonment fears), emotional dysregulation (affective/mood lability, anger, feelings of emptiness), behavioral dysregulation (impulsivity, chronic suicidal or self-harming behaviors), and cognitive and/or self-disturbance (transient psychotic-like symptoms including paranoid ideations or dissociative symptoms, identity disturbance) [9]. The symptoms of BPD are generally precipitated by interpersonal events, such as a real or perceived rejection, or life stressors, although some patients may have difficulty making this connection due to the rapid shifts in their emotional experiences and poor reflective ability. Clinicians and family members are frequently emotionally impacted by dysphoric mood and self-destructive behavior commonly seen in individuals with BPD. Therefore, psychoeducation and communication skills are essential to effectively support individuals with this condition.

22.2.2 Clinical Assessment

The assessment of BPD is conducted through a clinical interview. Patients often initially present for the treatment of a mood, anxiety, trauma-related, eating, or substance use disorders, or during a significantly destabilizing life stressor or crisis. In the emergency department or inpatient psychiatric hospital setting, self-harm and suicidality are the most common presentation.

In assessment, the clinician aims to understand the patient's inner experience, self-understanding, and interpersonal functioning, focusing on establishing which features are present and constitute a pervasive and inflexible pattern [10]. Collateral information from a family member, significant other, or friend who knows the patient well is of great utility in the clinical assessment.

There are several instruments for diagnosing BPD. The Structured Clinical Interview for DSM-IV Axis II disorders (SCID-II) is a semistructured interview for diagnosing all personality disorders. The Childhood Interview for DSM-IV Borderline Personality Disorder (CI-BPD) is a diagnostic intrument for adolescent BPD. Lastly, two commonly used self-report instruments for symptom tracking and screening are the Borderline Symptom List (BSL) and the McLean Screening Instrument for BPD (MSI-BPD), respectively [9].

22.2.3 DSM and ICD Diagnosis

Currently, there are two primary forms of classification systems for personality disorders. The categorical model describes clinical syndromes based on the grouping of symptoms, as in the DSM-5-TR, section II, where an individual is diagnosed with BPD if they meet the diagnostic threshold of five out of the nine symptoms/criteria [10] (see Table 22.1). In contrast, dimensional models evaluate individuals based on a continuum of specific traits (e.g., extroversion-introversion dimension) or personality functioning (self and interpersonal). The Alternative Model for Personality Disorders (AMPD) in section III of DSM-5-TR retained a categorical approach but combined it with a dimensional one (i.e., hybrid model). The World Health Organization International Classification of Diseases (ICD-11) fully employed the dimensional and excluded all categorical classifications [11].

In both the AMPD and ICD-11, personality functioning is assessed first (Criterion A), evaluating self (i.e., identity and self-direction) and interpersonal functioning (i.e., empathy and intimacy). Secondly, trait characteristics are identified, such as negative affectivity, detachment, antagonism/dissociality, disinhibition, and psychoticism [7]. In the ICD-11 system, psychoticism was replaced by the trait anankastia (obsessive-compulsive personality). In the AMPD, clinicians can still diagnose BPD, while in the ICD-11, clinicians identifying BPD symptoms will code more generally as a personality disorder with the option of a borderline pattern [11].

22.2.4 Comorbidity/Co-occurrence and Differential Diagnosis

Co-occurring disorders are common, such as anxiety (88%), major depressive (61–83%), substance use (64%), post-traumatic stress (PTSD) (30.2%), attention deficit and

Table 22.1 DSM-5-TR borderline personality disorder diagnostic criteria [10].

A pervasive pattern of instability of interpersonal relationships, self-image, and affects, and marked impulsivity, beginning by early adulthood and present in a variety of contexts, as indicated by five (or more) of the following:

Frantic efforts to avoid real or imagined abandonment. (Note: Do not include suicidal or self-mutilating behavior covered in Criterion 5.)

A pattern of unstable and intense interpersonal relationships characterized by alternating between extremes of idealization and devaluation.

Identity disturbance: markedly and persistently unstable self-image or sense of self.

Impulsivity in at least two areas that are potentially self-damaging (e.g., spending, sex, substance abuse, reckless driving, binge eating). (Note: Do not include suicidal or self-mutilating behavior covered in Criterion 5.)

Recurrent suicidal behavior, gestures, or threats, or self-mutilating behavior.

Affective instability due to a marked reactivity of mood (e.g., intense episodic dysphoria, irritability, or anxiety usually lasting a few hours and only rarely more than a few days).

Chronic feelings of emptiness.

Inappropriate, intense anger or difficulty controlling anger (e.g., frequent displays of temper, constant anger, recurrent physical fights).

Transient, stress-related paranoid ideation or severe dissociative symptoms.

hyperactivity (33.7%), eating (53%), bipolar spectrum (10–20%), or other personality disorders [4, 9, 12]. Given the overlapping symptomatology among BPD and many other psychiatric disorders, patients are sometimes misdiagnosed with another psychiatric disorder(s) when a diagnosis of BPD better explains the core psychopathology. It is essential to consider a broad differential diagnosis. See Table 22.2.

22.3 Course

BPD typically emerges during adolescence and young adulthood, with evidence showing that the disorder in adolescents is valid and similar to adult BPD [6]. BPD traits exhibit a normative increase from early to mid-adolescence and a subsequent decrease in early adulthood. However, there is a group that deviates from the norm and develops BPD as adults [13].

Certain prognostic factors, such as absence of childhood sexual abuse, more education, stable work history, lack of anxious cluster personality disorder, low neuroticism, and high agreeableness, may predict more favorable outcomes for patients with BPD [14, 15]. Acute symptoms, such as self-harm, remit relatively quickly compared to temperamental symptoms such as depression, anger, emptiness, and loneliness [16]. Although many patients with BPD achieve remission (i.e., no longer meeting BPD criteria for at least 2 years), only 40–60% reach functional recovery (i.e., 2-year symptomatic remission associated with at least one meaningful relationship with a friend or partner and the ability to work or study full time) [14, 17].

Table 22.2 Main aspects of differential diagnosis in BPD symptoms [4, 9, 12].

Disorder	Features
Major Depression	• BPD is characterized by unstable affect that lasts hours to days, while distinct major depression has a persistent depressive syndrome, including alteration of appetite and sleep. • Subjective experience of depression is related to feelings of failure and guilt, while in BPD anger, loneliness and emptiness are prominent.
Bipolar Disorder	• BPD unstable affects are triggered by interpersonal events, while in BD are usually autonomous mood alterations. • BD has manic/hypomanic episodes, not present in BPD psychopathology.
Anxiety Disorders	• BPD anxiety is prompted by interpersonal events and context. • In BPD there are ruminations related to other people's feelings and thinking (hypermentalizing).
Substance Use Disorders	• Substance use in BPD has primarily emotional regulation and interpersonal function. • More common as intermittent substance use.
Eating Disorders	• Nonspecified ED are the most common in BPD and usually increase during stressful periods.
Psychotic Disorders	• Psychotic symptoms in BPD are transient and stress related.
Complex PTSD	• Identity diffusion and rejection sensitivity are more characteristic of BPD, while in Complex PTSD there is a prominent negative sense of self.
Antisocial Personality Disorder	• Traits of callousness and persistent compromised affective empathy are present in ASPD.
Narcissistic Personality Disorder	• Emotional reactivity triggered by self-esteem threat • Traits of grandiosity, vulnerable self-esteem

22.4 Pathophysiology

BPD results from the complex interplay between genetic and environmental factors. Innate biological features (e.g., temperament, genetics) and early life adversity (e.g., maltreatment, neglect) predispose individuals to be more vulnerable to stress, which can further alter gene expression and brain development [18]. This interactive process contributes to the development of self and interpersonal instability. In this section, we will review these mechanisms, as well as neural circuitry alterations in BPD.

22.4.1 Environmental/Genetic Factors and Hormonal Alterations

BPD has a heritability of approximately 40–60% [19]. Childhood adversity, such as physical and sexual abuse, is also a significant risk factor for BPD [20]. Early BPD symptoms, such as temperamental sensitivity and irritability, predict adverse parental responses such as decreased affection as well as inconsistent or aversive behavior. These responses challenge the development of emotional and social skills, contributing to the emergence of BPD in adolescence and adulthood [9]. Insecure, disorganized attachment to the primary caregiver can impair self-control and increase stress reactivity, and is predictive of borderline symptoms [21]. Comorbid psychopathology in adolescence and young adulthood, such as depression, anxiety, substance use, conduct, oppositional defiant, attention deficit/hyperactivity disorders, and self-harm, also increase the risk for BPD [13].

BPD is a disorder of stress sensitivity. Dysfunction in the hypothalamic–pituitary–adrenal (HPA) axis, has been found in stress-sensitive populations [22]. Early adversity correlates with HPA hyperactivity and mediates alterations in neural circuitry, particularly in the limbic system (e.g., amygdala and hippocampus), which are responsible for threat detection [23]. Oxytocin – a hormone associated with parent–child interactions that counteract stress responses in social contexts – is decreased in adults with BPD, especially in those with disorganized attachment and a history of maltreatment [24]. Taken together, social threat detection systems are hyperreactive and not counterbalanced by soothing biological mechanisms in BPD, which contributes to the interpersonal hypersensitivity and emotion dysregulation seen clinically.

22.4.2 Neural Circuitry

Alterations in several brain circuits have been identified in BPD phenotypes: interpersonal instability, cognitive and self-disturbance, emotional dysregulation, and behavioral disinhibition [9].

Higher bottom-up activation (i.e., emotional processing involving the amygdala, hippocampus, insula, and rostral anterior cingulate cortex [ACC]) and lower top-down regulation (i.e., involving prefrontal cortex [PFC] and dorsal ACC) are associated with emotional dysregulation, marked by hypervigilance to social threats [9]. Studies have shown greater and persistent amygdala activation in response to angry faces and negative emotional stimuli tasks, respectively [23, 25]. Additionally, difficulty identifying and changing negative cognitions (i.e., cognitive reappraisal) were associated with lower PFC activation in BPD [9]. Promisingly, preliminary findings, such as lower amygdala activation for negative emotional images after DBT, suggest that some prefrontal-limbic dysfunction could be improved with treatment [26].

Impulsivity has also been associated with neuroimaging findings in BPD. Difficulties in anticipating negative outcomes and inhibiting motor responses in affective tasks were associated with activation in the ventral striatum and the PFC, respectively [26, 27]. Additionally, brain regions related to subjective appraisal of pain, such as the posterior insula, and its functional relationships with other brain areas (e.g., dorsolateral prefrontal cortex) are altered in BPD [29], which may explain the use of self-injurious behaviors as stress relief.

Alterations in the connectivity between prefrontal regions that overlap with the default mode network – involved in identifying and understanding the mental state of both the self and others (i.e., mentalizing) and autobiographical memory – and the limbic system are associated with the interpersonal instability phenotype [9]. Difficulty shifting attention away from social information (emotional scenes) during a pragmatic neurocognitive task was correlated with a higher coupling of the medial PFC and amygdala for BPD subjects [30]. And enhanced activation in the default mode network is associated with unstable self and social representations [31]. These findings provide insight into the mechanisms driving patients with BPD's difficulties with understanding themselves and others.

22.5 Treatment/Management

BPD was once considered untreatable and used as a label for troublesome and "treatment-resistant patients." The symptoms of BPD make it challenging to treat the disorder without an approach that is tailored to its features. Empirical findings from randomized controlled trials (RCTs) of psychosocial treatments designed for BPD have shown improvement in suicidality, self-harm, BPD symptoms, and psychosocial function [4]. Psychoeducation is a key component of treatment; clinicians treating BPD should inform patients of their diagnosis and provide information, including symptoms and treatment plan [9].

22.5.1 Evidence-Based Therapies

Psychotherapies are the most effective treatment for BPD. The most well-known specialized treatments are dialectical behavior therapy (DBT), mentalization-based treatment (MBT), and transference-focused psychotherapy (TFP) [32–34]. Other specialized treatments with positive results on RCTs are schema-focused therapy [35] and systems training for emotional predictability and problem-solving (STEPPS) [36, 37]. Across these effective treatment approaches that lead to improvement of BPD, there are common factors operating on underlying BPD psychopathology. These include a well-defined treatment framework, a model to understand the patient's symptoms, focus on affect and management of arousal, emphasis on treatment relationship, an active therapist, exploratory interventions, and change-oriented interventions [38, 39].

Specialized treatments are not widely available in most health care systems due to their cost, intensiveness, and lack of trained clinicians; the supply does not meet the demand [40]. However, well-informed and generalist approaches have been developed and shown comparable efficacy with specialized psychotherapies. These treatments include general or good psychiatric management (GPM), which was as effective as DBT in the largest RCT for BPD patients [35], and structured clinical management [41, 42]. Generalist approaches incorporate common factors mentioned prior so any clinician can help patients with BPD more effectively.

Treatment adaptations for adolescents have been found to be effective in randomized controlled trials (RCTs) [43]. The goal of early intervention is for teenagers to return to the typical developmental track and prevent them from becoming chronic patients commonly seen in psychiatric units [44].

See Table 22.3 for more information about the major treatments, DBT, MBT, TFP, and GPM.

22.5.2 Acute Management of Suicidality and Self-Harming Behavior

Suicidality and self-harm are core features of BPD [12]. Most treatments provide a framework to help patients address those behaviors proactively, such as teaching coping skills and joint crisis planning. It is common for patients to present to general clinicians in mental health settings in acute crises, and therefore essential for professionals to

Table 22.3 Main characteristics of evidence-based treatments for BPD [6, 32, 33, 41].

	DBT	MBT	TFP	GPM
Theory	Biosocial theory	Attachment and theory of mind	Objects Relations	Eclectic model (medical and psychological)
BPD Development	Emotional vulnerable temperament interacts with invalidating environment: reinforcing emotional dysregulation	Insecure attachment and epistemic mistrust stem from suboptimal early caregiver–child relationships	Negative temperamental disposition associated with early adversity	Genetically based interpersonal hypersensitivity causing mismatch between patient and environment
BPD Model	Emotion dysregulation drives nonadaptive behaviors	Capacity of mentalizing impaired, particularly in interpersonal context	Split object relations causing identity diffusion and unstable relationships	Interpersonal hypersensitivity drives BPD symptoms, such as self-harm and anxiety
Primary Therapy Function	Learn skills to manage emotions and behavior	Enhance mentalizing capacity	Integrate objects relations	Attainment stable function in life (job, nonromantic relationships)
Typical Structure	Individual therapy, skills groups, phone coaching	Individual therapy, MBT group, psychoeducation group	Twice a week individual therapy	Flexible; main clinician once a week if useful; split treatments (groups, family, psychopharmacology) as needed
Evidence	***	**	*	*

understand these behaviors. Clinicians should review the prompting events prior to the episode, assess the behavior's dangerousness (e.g., differentiate lethal intent from nonsuicidal self-injury), and perform suicide risk assessment [42]. Simultaneously, clinicians should maintain a supportive stance. Keeping crisis management in the outpatient setting is preferred. If inpatient hospitalization is necessary, it should be short, with a focus on solving the problems prompting hospitalization and active post-discharge planning to address the risk of future crises [45]. Sedative medications such as low-potency antipsychotics or antihistamines can be prescribed in the short term and then discontinued., [46]. Psychoeducation about BPD and its symptoms, emphasizing its treatability, is also beneficial in these situations.

22.5.3 Psychopharmacological Treatments

It is common for patients with BPD to receive multiple medications, despite the lack of evidence supporting their use [47]. One study showed that 90% are at least taking one medication, with 80% and 54% prescription rates for two and three drugs, respectively [48]. Therefore, several treatment guidelines do not recommend medications besides for treating co-occurring disorders (e.g., selective serotonin reuptake inhibitors [SSRIs] for depression) or short-term crisis interventions [4]. In the context of co-occurring disorders, psychopharmacotherapy is used adjunctively for their treatment, but expectations that pharmacology will solve the problems of BPD are not supported by the literature [45].

If medication is considered, clinicians and patients should select a symptom target and collaboratively monitor side effects and responses. If the drug is not helpful, it should be tapered off. Antipsychotics are the most studied class, with effects mainly on cognitive-perceptual symptoms but also on impulsive/aggressive behaviors and affective instability [49]. Mood stabilizers have been used for targeting affective instability, but more recent evidence has shown no difference with the placebo group [50]. Antidepressants, such as SSRIs, do not yield consistent improvements in treating BPD despite being widely prescribed due to the high prevalence of anxiety and depression in this group [49]. Benzodiazepines and other hypnotics are relatively contraindicated due to their disinhibiting effects and abuse potential [42].

22.5.4 Management of Complex Comorbidity

When there are co-occurring disorders, an important decision is which disorder to prioritize, which may impact medication prescription. Major depressive disorder, bulimia, anxiety symptoms, intermittent substance use, and adult-onset PTSD usually remit with BPD's remission improvement. Therefore, BPD should be prioritized in those scenarios [9]. There are also instances where comorbidity should take priority over BPD, either because there is an acute medical risk (e.g., severe eating disorders such as anorexia) or because the condition will impede effective psychotherapy for BPD (e.g., antisocial personality disorder, complex PTSD, mania or hypomania in bipolar disorder, severe substance use disorder) [4]. Distinct major depressive episodes, especially with clear neurovegetative symptoms, should be treated concurrently with antidepressants [42].

22.6 Conclusion

Borderline personality disorder is a serious and prevalent mental health condition characterized by interpersonal hypersensivity, emotion dysregulaton and impulsivity.

Psychotherapy is the most effective form of treatment and pharmacotherapy is reserved mostly for co-ocurring disorders. Because of the discrepancy between the rate of remission and recovery, treatments can be improved by focusing on psychosocial functioning to improve long-term prognosis. Well-informed generalist approaches can help non-specialist clinicians manage most patients with BPD.

References

1. J. G. Gunderson and M. T. Singer. Defining borderline patients: an overview. *Am J Psychiatry*. 1975;**132**:1–10.

2. M. C. Zanarini, J. Horwood, D. Wolke, et al. Prevalence of DSM-IV borderline personality disorder in two community samples: 6,330 English 11-year-olds and 34,653 American adults. *J Personal Disord*. 2011;**25**:607–619.

3. T. J. Trull, S. Jahng, R. L. Tomko, et al. Revised NESARC personality disorder diagnoses: gender, prevalence, and comorbidity with substance dependence disorders. *J Personal Disord*. 2010;**24**:412–426.

4. M. Bohus, J. Stoffers-Winterling, C. Sharp, et al. Borderline personality disorder. *Lancet (London)*. 2021;**398**:1528–1540.

5. J. G. Gunderson. Clinical practice: borderline personality disorder. *N Engl J Med*. 2011;**364**:2037–2042.

6. L. W. Choi-Kain, E. B. Albert, and J. G. Gunderson. Evidence-based treatments for borderline personality disorder: implementation, integration, and stepped care. *Harv Rev Psychiatry*. 2016;**24**:342–356.

7. C. Sharp. Personality disorders. *N Engl J Med*. 2022;**387**:916–923.

8. F. Leichsenring, N. Heim, F. Leweke, et al. Borderline personality disorder. *JAMA*. 2023;**329**:670–679.

9. J. G. Gunderson, S. C. Herpertz, A. E. Skodol, et al. Borderline personality disorder. *Nat Rev Dis Primer*. 2018;**4**:18029.

10. American Psychiatric Association. *Diagnostic and Statistical Manual of Mental Disorders: DSM-5*. 5th ed. American Psychiatric Association; 2013.

11. B. Bach and M. B. First. Application of the ICD-11 classification of personality disorders. *BMC Psychiatry*. 2018;**18**:351. Available from: https://bmcpsychiatry.biomedcentral.com/articles/10.1186/s12888-018-1908-3.

12. J. G. Gunderson and P. S. Links. *Borderline Personality Disorder: A Clinical Guide*. 2nd ed. American Psychiatric Publishing; 2008.

13. A. M. Chanen and M. Kaess. Developmental pathways to borderline personality disorder. *Curr Psychiatry Rep*. 2012;**14**:45–53.

14. J. G. Gunderson. Ten-year course of borderline personality disorder: psychopathology and function from the collaborative longitudinal personality disorders study. *Arch Gen Psychiatry*. 2011;**68**:827. Available from: http://archpsyc.jamanetwork.com/article.aspx?doi=10.1001/archgenpsychiatry.2011.37.

15. M. C. Zanarini, F. R. Frankenburg, J. Hennen, et al. Prediction of the 10-year course of borderline personality disorder. *Am J Psychiatry*. 2006;**163**:827–832. Available from: http://psychiatryonline.org/doi/abs/10.1176/ajp.2006.163.5.827.

16. M. C. Zanarini, F. R. Frankenburg, D. B. Reich, et al. Fluidity of the subsyndromal phenomenology of borderline personality disorder over 16 years of prospective follow-up. *Am J Psychiatry*. 2016;**173**:688–694. Available from: http://ajp.psychiatryonline.org/doi/10.1176/appi.ajp.2015.15081045.

17. M. C. Zanarini, F. R. Frankenburg, D. B. Reich, et al. Attainment and stability of sustained symptomatic remission and recovery among patients with borderline personality disorder and axis ii comparison subjects: a 16-year prospective follow-up study. *Am*

J Psychiatry. 2012;**169**:476–483. Available from: http://psychiatryonline.org/doi/abs/10.1176/appi.ajp.2011.11101550.

18. N. Cattane, R. Rossi, M. Lanfredi, et al. Borderline personality disorder and childhood trauma: exploring the affected biological systems and mechanisms. *BMC Psychiatry*. 2017;**17**:221.

19. S. Torgersen, S. Lygren, P. A. Oien, et al. A twin study of personality disorders. *Compr. Psychiatry* 2000;**41**:416–425.

20. J. Ibrahim, N. Cosgrave, M. Woolgar. Childhood maltreatment and its link to borderline personality disorder features in children: a systematic review approach. *Clin Child Psychol Psychiatry*. 2017;**23**:57–76.

21. P. Fonagy and A. Bateman. The development of borderline personality disorder: a mentalizing model. *J Personal Disord*. 2008;**22**:4–21.

22. E. R. de Kloet, M. Joëls, F. Holsboer. Stress and the brain: from adaptation to disease. *Nat Rev Neurosci*. 2005;**6**:463–475.

23. L. Schulze, C. Schmahl, I. Niedtfeld. Neural correlates of disturbed emotion processing in borderline personality disorder: a multimodal meta-analysis. *Biol Psychiatry*. 2016;**79**:97–106.

24. K. Bertsch, M. Gamer, B. Schmidt, et al. Oxytocin and reduction of social threat hypersensitivity in women with borderline personality disorder. *Am J Psychiatry*. 2013;**170**:1169–1177.

25. N. H. Donegan, C. A. Sanislow, H. P. Blumberg, et al. Amygdala hyperreactivity in borderline personality disorder: implications for emotional dysregulation. *Biol Psychiatry* 2003;**54**:1284–1293.

26. M. C. Herbort, J. Soch, T. Wüstenberg, et al. A negative relationship between ventral striatal loss anticipation response and impulsivity in borderline personality disorder. *NeuroImage Clin*. 2016;**12**:724–736.

27. P. H. Soloff, R. White, A. Omari, et al. Affective context interferes with brain responses during cognitive processing in borderline personality disorder: fMRI evidence. *Psychiatry Res*. 2015;**233**:23–35.

28. I. Niedtfeld, R. Schmitt, D. Winter, et al. Pain-mediated affect regulation is reduced after dialectical behavior therapy in borderline personality disorder: a longitudinal fMRI study. *Soc Cogn Affect Neurosci*. 2017;**12**:739–747.

29. I. Niedtfeld, P. Kirsch, L. Schulze, et al. Functional connectivity of pain- mediated affect regulation in borderline personality disorder. *PLoS ONE*. 2012;**7**:e33293.

30. A. Krause-Utz, B. M. Elzinga, N. Y. L. Oei, et al. Amygdala and dorsal anterior cingulate connectivity during an emotional working memory task in borderline personality disorder patients with interpersonal trauma history. *Front Hum Neurosci*. 2014;**8**:848.

31. J. E. Beeney, M. N. Hallquist, W. D. Ellison, et al. Self-other disturbance in borderline personality disorder: neural, self-report, and performance-based evidence. *Personal Disord*. 2016;**7**:28–39.

32. F. E. Yeomans, J. F. Clarkin, O. F. Kernberg. *Transference-Focused Psychotherapy for Borderline Personality Disorder: A Clinical Guide*. American Psychiatric Publishing; 2015.

33. M. Linehan. *Cognitive-Behavioral Treatment of Borderline Personality Disorder*. Guilford Press; 1993.

34. A. Bateman and P. Fonagy. *Mentalization-Based Treatment for Personality Disorders: A Practical Guide*. Oxford University Press; 2016.

35. S. F. McMain, P. S. Links, W. H. Gnam, et al. A randomized trial of dialectical behavior therapy versus general psychiatric management for borderline personality disorder. *Am J Psychiatry*. 2009;**166**:1365–1374. Available from: http://psychiatryonline.org/doi/abs/10.1176/appi.ajp.2009.09010039.

36. N. Blum, D. St. John, B. Pfohl, et al. Systems Training for Emotional Predictability and Problem Solving (STEPPS) for outpatients with borderline personality disorder: a randomized controlled trial and 1-year follow-up. *Am*

J Psychiatry. 2008;**165**:468–478. Available from: http://psychiatryonline.org/doi/abs/10.1176/appi.ajp.2007.07071079.

37. J. E. Young, J. S. Klosko, M. E. Weishaar. *Schema Therapy: A Practitioner's Guide.* Guilford; 2007.

38. A. Bateman, C. Campbell, P. Luyten, et al. A mentalization-based approach to common factors in the treatment of borderline personality disorder. *Current Opinion in Psychology.* 2018;**21**:44–49.

39. I. Weinberg, E. Ronningstam, M. J. Goldblatt, et al. Common factors in empirically supported treatments of borderline personality disorder. *Curr Psychiatry Reports.* 2010;**13**(1):60–68.

40. E. A. Iliakis, A. K. I. Sonley, G. S. Ilagan, et al. Treatment of borderline personality disorder: is supply adequate to meet public health needs? *Psychiatr Serv.* 2019;**70**(9):772–781.

41. A. Bateman and R. Krawitz. *Borderline Personality Disorder: An Evidence-Based Guide for Generalist Mental Health Professionals.* Oxford University Press; 2013.

42. J. G. Gunderson and P. S. Links. *Handbook of Good Psychiatric Management for Borderline Personality Disorder.* American Psychiatric Publishing; 2014.

43. T. I. Rossouw and P. Fonagy. Mentalization-based treatment for self-harm in adolescents: a randomized controlled trial. *J Am Acad Child Adolesc Psychiatry.* 2012;**51**:1304–1313.e3. Available from: https://linkinghub.elsevier.com/retrieve/pii/S0890856712007368.

44. L. W. Choi-Kain and C. Sharp. *Handbook of Good Psychiatric Management for*

Adolescents with Borderline Personality Disorder. American Psychiatric Association Publishing, 2021.

45. L. W. Choi-Kain and J. G. Gunderson. *Applications of Good Psychiatric Management for Borderline Personality Disorder: A Practical Guide.* American Psychiatric Association Publishing, 2019.

46. National Collaborating Centre for Mental Health. *Borderline Personality Disorder: Treatment and Management.* British Psychological Society; 2009.

47. J. Stoffers-Winterling, O. J. Storebø, K. Lieb. Pharmacotherapy for borderline personality disorder: an update of published, unpublished and ongoing studies. *Curr Psychiatry Rep.* 2020;**22**:37. Available from: https://link.springer.com/10.1007/s11920-020-01164-1.

48. R. Bridler, A. Häberle, S. T. Müller, et al. Psychopharmacological treatment of 2195 in-patients with borderline personality disorder: a comparison with other psychiatric disorders. *Europ Neuropsychopharmacol.* 2015;**25**:763–772.

49. K. Lieb, B. Völlm, G. Rücker, et al. Pharmacotherapy for borderline personality disorder: Cochrane systematic review of randomised trials. *Br J Psychiatry.* 2010;**196**:4–12. Available from: www.cambridge.org/core/product/identifier/S0007125000008035/type/journal_article.

50. M. J. Crawford, R. Sanatinia, B. Barrett, et al. The clinical effectiveness and cost-effectiveness of lamotrigine in borderline personality disorder: a randomized placebo-controlled trial. *Am J Psychiatry.* 2018;**175**:756–764. Available from: http://ajp.psychiatryonline.org/doi/10.1176/appi.ajp.2018.17091006.

Antisocial Personality Disorder

Morgan T. Deal and Juan J. Sosa

23.1 Introduction

Antisocial behaviors are described as actions that violate societal norms with disregard for the rights of others. Antisocial behaviors have been described in the literature as early as the 18th century [1]. Over time, antisocial behaviors were conceptualized into what is known today as antisocial personality disorder (ASPD). ASPD was the first formally recognized personality disorder described in the American Psychiatric Association's Diagnostic and Statistical Manual (DSM) of Mental Disorders in 1952. The first edition of the DSM described antisocial behaviors as a *sociopathic personality disturbance.* This was the basis for developing ASPD criteria published in future editions of the DSM [1]. Researchers and scholars have debated the relationship between psychopathy and ASPD; sometimes, the terms are used interchangeably [2]. Psychopathy is not recognized as part of the DSM-5-TR diagnostic criteria for ASPD, although it shares many of the same characteristics (e.g., deceitfulness and engaging in unlawful acts). However, the qualitative features in psychopathy are considered in the context of specific interpersonal and affective features (e.g., callousness, glibness, grandiosity, shallow affect) apparent in persons with psychopathy. Therefore, ASPD and psychopathy are currently considered two distinct but overlapping entities. Critics of the DSM have voiced concerns over the utility of a qualitative (or observational) approach to conceptualizing personality disorders, including ASPD. The DSM-5 provided an alternative dimensional-qualitative hybrid model that conceptualizes personality disorders as impairments in personality functioning and specific pathological personality traits [3].

Epidemiological data have been measured in general and specific populations (e.g., clinical and high-risk settings). General population studies report the prevalence rate of ASPD to be between 0.2% to 3.3% [4]. These studies have relied primarily on gathering specific qualitative data points (i.e., unlaw acts or violation of societal norms) to report the prevalence rate given the increased reliability and measurability of those data points compared to more dimensional ASPD features (i.e., deceitfulness or impulsivity) [5]. Various assessment instruments have been used, which may account for the variability of prevalence rates. More recent studies have focused on clinically relevant populations, such as those with comorbid substance use disorders. Recent data from the National Epidemiologic Survey on Alcohol and Related Conditions (NESARC-III) used DSM-5 criteria as its primary diagnostic tool and yielded a prevalence rate of 4.3% [6]. ASPD rates were highest in younger male adults living in rural areas. The overall rate was higher in males compared to females. A high rate of comorbid alcohol use disorder (68%) in individuals with ASPD was reported. Elevated rates of mood and anxiety disorders and medical comorbidities (e.g., infectious and heart diseases) were found in individuals with ASPD. Epidemiological studies in prisons showed a prevalence of 70% [7]. These studies also revealed similar rates of comorbid substance use and other psychiatric disorders, as seen in other studies. Subjects from low socioeconomic backgrounds were found to have higher rates of ASPD. However, it is unclear to what degree the rates in socially disadvantaged populations conflate antisocial behavior used as a survival strategy in challenging environments with antisocial behaviors due to ASPD.

23.2 Clinical Presentation/Diagnosis

ASPD is characterized by a pervasive pattern of repeated disregard for and violation of others' rights. To meet the criteria for ASPD, the DSM5-TR specifies that an individual must be at least 18 years old and exhibit two or more of the following:

1. Failure to conform to social norms
2. Deceitfulness
3. Impulsivity or failure to plan ahead
4. Irritability or aggressiveness
5. Reckless disregard for the safety of self or others
6. Consistent irresponsibility
7. Lack of remorse

Evidence of the onset of conduct disorder must be present before age 15 years. Antisocial behavior cannot occur exclusively during schizophrenia or bipolar disorder [3]. Diagnosing ASPD is often challenging because these individuals present with numerous complaints and may be deceiving. The following vignette is an example of a patient with ASPD presenting to an emergency department.

> Anthony is a 38-year-old incarcerated man with a history of alcohol, methamphetamine, and benzodiazepine abuse who presented to the emergency department after an alleged suicide attempt. Before a formal assessment, he is heard screaming at nurses and demanding a sandwich. He tells the on-call resident that he will kill himself if he is not prescribed a benzodiazepine for anxiety. Anthony becomes hostile and threatening toward the on-call resident and declines to speak with the attending. He states that he would rather sleep. Collateral information obtained from the accompanying correctional officers reveals several concerning behaviors in prison, including diverting prescribed medications, stealing items from cellmates, obtaining contraband, and reporting suicidal ideation unless given his own cell. Anthony is later observed laughing and joking while making inappropriate sexual comments toward female nurses.

The vignette illustrates many symptoms consistent with an ASPD diagnosis. Anthony is incarcerated (implying failure to conform to social norms), demonstrates irritability and aggressiveness toward medical staff, and exhibits deceitfulness (e.g., reporting suicidal ideation while demanding controlled substances). Collateral information from the correctional officers provided additional supporting data on failure to conform to social norms (e.g., obtaining contraband in prison and stealing from other inmates). Reviewing available written records and getting additional collateral information are beneficial in determining whether Anthony meets the remaining criteria for ASPD, because people with ASPD may not be forthcoming with their symptoms and often lack awareness about how their behaviors impact others. Examples of antisocial behaviors that may implicate an ASPD diagnosis and warrant further investigation include repeated criminal behaviors (regardless of whether the person is arrested), malingering symptoms, using aliases, failure to maintain consistent employment, repeated acts of violence, and substance misuse [3].

23.3 Pathophysiology

An exact etiology for ASPD has not been confirmed, but decades of research suggest a multifaceted and complex disease process. Early studies showed the progression of antisocial behaviors from childhood to adulthood. The earlier antisocial behaviors were exhibited in childhood (before age 15), the increased likelihood of exhibiting these behaviors into adulthood [8]. Additional studies showed that ASPD runs in families, and a primary risk factor for engaging in antisocial behaviors is being from a family with a history of committing antisocial acts [9, 10]. Another factor to consider within the context of twin and adoption studies is the substantial assortative mating observed with the studied population. Studies have shown that men and women who are more likely to engage in antisocial behaviors are more likely to have children with each other, which has implications for the intergenerational transmission of genetic risk factors associated with ASPD [11]. Parents exhibiting antisocial behaviors also have more children on average than their non-antisocial counterparts [9, 10].

Twin and adoption studies help us understand the genetic and environmental factors that may contribute to ASPD. When two monozygotic twin pairs are more similar than dizygotic twins, we can infer that those genetic factors contribute to a trait. If the similarity is more significant in a pair of dizygotic twins, we can infer that environmental factors rather than shared genetic information contributed to a shared trait. Adoption studies allow us to compare the similarity of biological relative dyads (e.g., biological parent–adoptee) who share 50% of their genetic information and 0% of their environment with the similarity of the nonbiological relative dyads (e.g., adoptive parent–adoptees). The adoptive parent–adoptee pairs share their environment and no genetic information, which allows us to make inferences about the influence of genetic factors versus environmental factors that can influence antisocial behavior disorders. These twin and adoption studies have revealed that genetic and environmental factors contribute to antisocial behavior and that the importance of those factors shifts from childhood into adulthood. Environmental factors appear to contribute more during childhood, and genetic factors during adulthood [12]. The genes associated with conduct disorders remain constant despite the environment, so the genetic risk factor for ASPD remains stable across the life span. The genetic risk for antisocial behaviors is associated with greater exposure to a high-risk environment and a greater sensitivity to the risks in those environments.

Like other psychiatric disorders, serotonergic pathways are disrupted in those with ASPD. It has been hypothesized that these genetic variations in MAOA and SLC6A4 genes (serotonergic pathways) lead to the development of symptoms commonly seen in those with ASPD. However, changes in these genes have been implicated in the development of similar symptoms in other conditions besides ASPD. Epigenetics has shown us that these genetic variations and environmental factors (e.g., adverse childhood experiences) impact the development or progression of ASPD [13]. Imaging studies (e.g., structural MRI, SPECT) have been completed to investigate and compare structural and morphological variations within brains that may be associated with ASPD. Imaging studies have localized structural changes in individuals with ASPD in the striatum and medial prefrontal cortex [14, 15].

Neither psychosocial nor biological factors alone have been identified as the primary etiology of antisocial behaviors. Instead, there is a complex etiology that involves genetic and environmental factors and how the two influence each other. Any child exposed to psychosocial risk factors (e.g., maltreatment/abuse, dysfunctional family, poverty) may have an increased risk for antisocial behaviors when exposed to these factors. Still, a child with a genetic predisposition exposed to these risk factors is likelier to develop ASPD. Even though there has been no identified primary etiology for ASPD, there has been robust research on the pathophysiology of ASPD compared to any other disorder [16]. Conduct disorders are the second-most studied disorder among the medical or psychological traits or disorders analyzed in twin studies.

23.4 Treatment/Management

Individuals with ASPD present a challenge for health care providers because of their complex clinical presentation, high comorbidity of medical and mental disorders, and increased utilization of health care resources [17]. There are currently no medications licensed explicitly for ASPD treatment. Low-quality available data on the pharmacological and psychological interventions for ASPD further complicate treatment decision-making [18, 19]. Many pharmacological studies evaluated manifestations of ASPD, particularly impulsive aggression, and included other psychiatric diagnoses [20–23]. Studies that feature individuals diagnosed with ASPD have relatively small sample sizes [19, 24, 25]. Table 23.1 summarizes the classes of medications prescribed off-label for ASPD and their effects. Based on current evidence, the routine prescribing of medications is not recommended for individuals with ASPD unless the medicines are intended to treat psychiatric comorbidities such as depression, anxiety, and substance abuse [26]. It is essential that clinicians consider the side effects risk, the potential for medication misuse, and treatment nonadherence when determining whether to prescribe psychotropic medications for patients with ASPD.

Research has refuted prior conventional wisdom that persons with ASPD do not benefit from psychotherapy or that psychotherapy somehow worsens ASPD [18, 27].

Table 23.1 Summary of the effects of medication classes prescribed off-label for individuals with ASPD.

Medication Class	Effects
Antidepressants	Fluoxetine reduced aggression in patients with cluster B personality disorders [20].
Mood stabilizers/ Antiepileptics	Divalproex sodium improved self-reported impulse control and self-restraint in patients with conduct disorder [21]. Phenytoin, lithium, and carbamazepine/oxcarbazepine are associated with reduced aggressive behavior in patients with histories of intermittent explosive disorder and impulsive aggression [22].
Atypical Antipsychotics	Quetiapine reduced impulsivity, aggressiveness, and irritability in patients with ASPD [24]. Clozapine reduced anger and violent incidents in patients with ASPD and psychopathic traits [25].

Studies have demonstrated that individuals diagnosed with ASPD can benefit from therapeutic community treatment and may abstain from substance use after receiving treatment with cognitive-behavioral therapy and contingency management [28, 29]. Considering the current evidence, it is reasonable to offer psychotherapy to individuals with ASPD to treat psychiatric comorbidities [26]. Managing patients with ASPD can feel daunting and engender countertransference reactions in treating clinicians because these individuals often lack insight, have difficulty building trusting relationships, and may outright reject treatment. Common countertransference reactions include fear of harm, helplessness, rejection, and hatred [30]. Clinicians must be aware of their countertransference and safety when managing individuals with ASPD. Treatment ideally should be provided in outpatient settings during regular working hours when staff is available to assist in the event of a violent outburst or emergency. Knowing the practice-specific safety protocols (e.g., how to activate panic alarms or whether security personnel is available to provide supervision) is practical. Clinicians can consider sitting near the door and leaving it open to allow for monitoring. During interviews, it is essential to be mindful of the patient's violence history and watch their reactions closely. Clinicians may benefit from addressing the patient using a neutral, respectful tone free of moral judgment [31].

After determining that an individual meets the criteria for ASPD, clinicians can educate patients about the diagnosis straightforwardly. They may also consider presenting the patient with DSM5-TR diagnostic criteria. Some persons with ASPD may benefit from an explanation of the roles of their developmental history and earlier adverse experiences in developing antisocial behaviors. People with ASPD can be admitted to an inpatient facility (if warranted) for further management of specific indications, including substance detoxification, suicidal ideation with plan and intent, mania, and psychosis [31]. Because individuals with ASPD are at higher risk for traumatic injury, suicide attempts, hepatitis, and HIV, it is prudent that clinicians evaluate for medical comorbidities and refer them for treatment when appropriate [17, 32]. Overall, ASPD is a complex personality disorder that requires tremendous effort from treating clinicians. Clinicians can successfully manage individuals with ASPD if they remain aware of the unique challenges of these patients while thoughtfully applying available research.

References

1. P. Tyrer, A. I. Farman, A. Zahmatkesh, R. Sanatinia. Classification and Definition of Antisocial Personality Disorder. In: D. W. Black, N. J. Kolla, eds. *Textbook of Antisocial Personality Disorder*. American Psychiatric Pub; 2022:4–8.

2. J. R. P. Ogloff. Psychopathy/antisocial personality disorder conundrum. *The Australian and New Zealand Journal of Psychiatry*. 2006;40(6–7):519–528.

3. American Psychiatric Association. *Diagnostic and statistical manual of mental disorders: DSM-5-TR. Fifth edition, text revision.* APA Publshing; 2022.

4. P. Moran. The epidemiology of antisocial personality disorder. *Social Psychiatry and Psychiatric Epidemiology*. 1999;34 (5):231–242.

5. R. Goldstein. Epidemiology of Antisocial Personality Disorder. In D. W. Black, N. J. Kolla, eds. *Textbook of Antisocial Personality Disorder*. American Psychiatric Publishers; 2022:30–32.

6. R. B. Goldstein, S. P. Chou, T. D. Saha, S. M. Smith, J. Jung, H. Zhang, et al. The epidemiology of antisocial behavioral syndromes in adulthood: results from the

National Epidemiologic Survey on Alcohol and Related Conditions–III. *The Journal of Clinical Psychiatry.* 2017;**78**(1):90–98.

7. S. Virdi, R. L Trestman. Personality Disorders. In R. L. Trestman, K. L. Appelbaum, J. L. Metzner, eds. *Oxford Textbook of Correctional Psychiatry.* Oxford University Press; 2015:196–197.

8. D. W. Black, R. B. Goldstein. Natural History and Course of Antisocial Personality Disorder. In D. W. Black, N. J. Kolla, eds. *Textbook of Antisocial Personality Disorder.* American Psychiatric Publishers; 2022:104–105.

9. D. P. Farrington, G. C. Barnes, S. Lambert. The concentration of offending in families. *Legal and Criminological Psychology.* 1996;**1**(1):47–63.

10. T. Frisell, P. Lichtenstein, N. Långström. Violent crime runs in families: a total population study of 12.5 million individuals. *Psychological Medicine.* 2010;**41**(1):97–105.

11. W. S. Slutske, C. N. Davis. Family, Twin, and Adoption Studies in Antisocial Personality Disorder and Antisocial Behavior. In D. W. Black, N .J. Kolla, eds. *Textbook of Antisocial Personality Disorder.* American Psychiatric Publishers; 2022:120–127.

12. S. H. Rhee, I. D. Waldman. Genetic and environmental influences on antisocial behavior: a meta-analysis of twin and adoption studies. *Psychological Bulletin.* 2002;**128**(3):490–529.

13. N. Weder, B. Z. Yang, H. Douglas-Palumberi, J. Massey, J. H. Krystal, J. Gelernter, et al. MAOA genotype, maltreatment, and aggressive behavior: the changing impact of genotype at varying levels of trauma. *Biological Psychiatry.* 2009;**65**(5):417–424.

14. R. J. Blar. Functional MRI Studies of Antisocial Personality Disorder. In D. W. Black, N. J. Kolla, eds. *Textbook of Antisocial Personality Disorder.* American Psychiatric Publishers; 2022:269–275.

15. N. J. Kolla, S. Houle. SPECT and PET Studies of Antisocial Personality Disorder

and Aggression. In D. W. Black, N. J. Kolla, eds. *Textbook of Antisocial Personality Disorder.* American Psychiatric Publishers; 2022:292–295.

16. T. J. Polderman, B. Benyamin, C. A. de Leeuw, P. F. Sullivan, A. van Bochoven, P. M. Visscher, et al. Meta-analysis of the heritability of human traits based on fifty years of twin studies. *Nature Genetics.* 2015;**47**(7):702–709.

17. D. W. Black. The natural history of antisocial personality disorder. *Canadian Journal of Psychiatry.* 2015;**60**(7):309–314.

18. S. Gibbon, N. R. Khalifa., N. H.-Y. Cheung, B. A. Völlm, L. McCarthy. Psychological interventions for antisocial personality disorder. *Cochrane Database of Systematic Reviews.* 2020;**2020**(9): CD007668.

19. N. R. Khalifa, S. Gibbon, B. A. Völlm, N. H.-Y. Cheung, L. McCarthy. Pharmacological interventions for antisocial personality disorder. *Cochrane Database of Systematic Reviews.* 2020;**2020**(9):CD007667.

20. E. F. Coccaro, R. J. Kavoussi. Fluoxetine and impulsive aggressive behavior in personality-disordered subjects. *The Journal of the American Medical Association.* 1998;**279**(17):1330J.

21. H. Steiner, M.L. Petersen, K. Saxena, S. Ford, Z. Matthews. Divalproex sodium for the treatment of conduct disorder: a randomized controlled clinical trial. *The Journal of Clinical Psychiatry.* 2003;**64**(10):1183–1191.

22. R. M. Jones, J. Arlidge, R. Gillham, S. Reagu, M. van den Bree, P. J. Taylor. Efficacy of mood stabilisers in the treatment of impulsive or repetitive aggression: systematic review and meta-analysis. *British Journal of Psychiatry.* 2011;**198**(2):93–98.

23. L. H. Ripoll, J. Triebwasser, L. J. Siever. Evidence-based pharmacotherapy for personality disorders. *The International Journal of Neuropsychopharmacology.* 2011;**14**(9):1257–1288.

24. C. Walker, J. Thomas, T. S. Allen. Treating impulsivity, irritability, and aggression of antisocial personality disorder with quetiapine. *International Journal of Offender Therapy and Comparative Criminology.* 2003;**47** (5):556–567.

25. D. Brown, F. Larkin, S. Sengupta, J. L. Romero-Ureclay, C. C. Ross, N. Gupta, M. Vinestock, M. Das. Clozapine: an effective treatment for seriously violent and psychopathic men with antisocial personality disorder in a UK high-security hospital. *CNS Spectrums.* 2014;**19** (5):391–402.

26. National Collaborating Centre for Mental Health (UK). *Antisocial Personality Disorder: Treatment, Management, and Prevention.* British Psychological Society; 2010.

27. K. D'Silva, C. Duggan, L. McCarthy. Does treatment really make psychopaths worse? A review of the evidence. *Journal of Personality Disorders.* 2004;**18** (2):163–177.

28. N. P. Messina, E. D. Wish, J. A. Hoffman, S. Nemes. Antisocial personality disorder and TC treatment outcomes. *The American Journal of Drug and Alcohol Abuse.* 2002;**28**(2):197–212.

29. N. Messina, D. Farabee, R. Rawson. Treatment responsivity of cocaine-dependent patients with antisocial personality disorder to cognitive-behavioral and contingency management interventions. *Journal of Consulting and Clinical Psychology.* 2003;**71** (2):320–329.

30. L. H. Strasburger. The Treatment of Antisocial Syndromes: The Therapist's Feelings. In: J. R. Meloy., ed. *The Mark of Cain: Psychoanalytic Insight and the Psychopath.* Analytic Press; 2001:301–308.

31. D. W. Black. Treatment Issues with Antisocial Personality Disorder. In D. W. Black, N. J. Kolla, eds. *Textbook of Antisocial Personality Disorder.* American Psychiatric Publishers; 2022:399–401.

32. R. K. Brooner, L. Greenfield, C. W. Schmidt, G. E. Bigelow. Antisocial personality disorder and HIV infection among intravenous drug abusers. *The American Journal of Psychiatry.* 1993;**150** (1):53–58.

Chapter

24

Other Personality Disorders

Maria Carolina Pedalino Pinheiro and Carolina Olmos

24.1 Introduction

Personality disorders play a major role in today's psychiatric clinical practice. To understand what a personality disorder is, it is first necessary to conceptualize what personality is. Personality consists of enduring patterns of thoughts, perceptions, and relationships with oneself and the environment. Such characteristics are repeated throughout different social and personal contexts.

Personality disorder arises when emotions, thoughts, impulsivity, and especially interpersonal behavior deviate markedly from the expectations of the individual's culture. Furthermore, when personality traits are inflexible and maladaptive in a wide range of situations, causing significant distress and impairment in social functioning, both in the private sphere and in the public sphere, the diagnosis of personality disorder becomes feasible.

Such characteristics may begin in childhood and/or adolescence and tend to remain stable over time, causing suffering and maladjustment to those individuals and often to those closest to them. Personality disorders are a group of disorders with diverse and complex psychiatric conditions that still need to be better understood across multiple dimensions: genetic, neurobiological, pharmacological, and psychodynamic. Given the impact that the presence of a personality disorder may have on patients' treatment response and in their interaction with the treatment team, a good understanding of these conditions is critical to preserve the doctor–patient relationship and improve patient's outcomes.

The worldwide prevalence of personality disorders in the general population is estimated at 11%, while among psychiatric patients it is about 40% [1]. These presentations are quite homogenous within each of the 11 diagnostic categories. Other comorbid psychiatric diagnosis, including substance abuse disorder and depression, are more prevalent in these patients, and this is often associated with a worse prognosis and increased suicide rates, as well as family issues and other social problems [2].

24.2 Presentation/Clinical Diagnosis

The consistent presence of certain behaviors and traits beginning in childhood, accentuated in adolescence, and continuing into adulthood is particularly suggestive of a personality disorder. The diagnosis of personality disorder is made when there are serious disturbances in the individual's character, constitution, and behavioral tendencies not directly as a result of another disease, injury, or other brain disorder. These disorders usually comprise several elements of the personality and are usually accompanied by personal distress and social disorganization evident by adolescence and persisting lastingly into adulthood.

Two sets of criteria are used to diagnose a personality disorder in the DSM-5-TR. The first set describes general features of a personality disorder, while the second describes specific features of each type of personality disorder.

The general characteristics of a personality disorder according to the DSM-5-TR are:

A. An enduring pattern of inner experience and behavior that deviates markedly from the expectations of the individual's culture. This pattern is manifested in two (or more) of the following areas:

- Cognition (i.e., ways of perceiving and interpreting self, other people, and events)
- Affectivity (i.e., the range, intensity, lability, and appropriateness of emotional response)
- Interpersonal functioning
- Impulse control

B. The enduring pattern is inflexible and pervasive across a broad range of personal and social situations.
C. The enduring pattern leads to clinically significant distress or impairment in social, occupational, and/or other important areas of functioning.
D. The pattern is stable and of long duration, and its onset can be traced back at least to adolescence or early adulthood.
E. The enduring pattern is not better explained as a manifestation or consequence of another mental disorder.
F. The enduring pattern is not attributable to the physiological effects of a substance (e.g., a drug of abuse, a medication) or another medical condition (e.g., head trauma) [3].

As for the specific types of personality disorders, the DSM-5-TR categorizes them into three clusters or groups, based on similarities in their descriptions.

We would also like to point out the relevance of considering the patient's cultural, ethnic, and social background when assessing for a personality disorder. Some of the core aspects of personality, such as emotional regulation or interpersonal functioning, and their appropriateness are strongly influenced by culture. A clinician should be aware how certain behavioral patterns that could appear rigid or dysfunctional may instead result from an adaptative response to a cultural constraint [3].

Cluster A encompasses paranoid, schizoid, and schizotypal personality disorders. Individuals with these conditions are perceived as eccentric and strange.

Cluster B is composed of antisocial, histrionic, narcissistic, and borderline personality disorders. Affected individuals are often emotional, erratic, and/or dramatic. Antisocial and borderline personality disorders are not discussed in this chapter. They will be addressed in specific chapters of this book.

Cluster C includes avoidant, obsessive-compulsive, and dependent personality disorders. Individuals with these disorders often appear anxious and fearful.

24.3 Cluster A

24.3.1 Paranoid Personality Disorder

This disorder is characterized by pervasive distrust or suspiciousness of others to the point that their motives are interpreted as malevolent. Prevalence is estimated to be between 2.3% and 4.4%, and it is more common in males [4, 5].

There are few studies on what treatments work best for affected individuals, given the nature of the disorder. Cognitive-behavioral therapy and psychodynamic therapy have been recommended, though no formal trials have been done [6].

24.3.2 Schizoid Personality Disorder

This disorder is characterized by a pervasive pattern of detachment from social relationships and a restricted range of expression of emotions in interpersonal settings that begins by early adulthood. These individuals often appear to be socially isolated or "loners," with no desire for intimacy.

Prevalence is estimated to be between 3.1% and 4.9%. More commonly diagnosed in males (may cause more impairment for males than females). Higher risk in relatives of individuals with schizophrenia or schizotypal personality disorder [4, 5].

Psychotherapies such as cognitive-behavioral therapy and psychodynamic therapy can be effective. Patients with schizoid personality can be introspective and over time may be able to build trust with a therapist to reveal schizoid fantasies [7].

24.3.3 Schizotypal Personality Disorder

This disorder is characterized by pervasive patterns of "strange" or "odd" behavior, appearance, and/or thinking. These peculiarities are not so severe as to warrant a diagnosis of schizophrenia, and there is no history of psychotic episodes. Individuals will often have ideas of reference but not to a delusional level. Symptoms may first appear in childhood, when the individual has peculiar thoughts, unusual language, and/or bizarre fantasies.

Prevalence ranges from 0.6 to 4.6%. Per DSM-5-TR, it is slightly more common in males than in females. There may be a more elevated risk for suicide in schizotypal personality disorder patients. It is more prevalent among first-degree biological relatives of individuals with schizophrenia [8].

Treatment is primarily with psychotherapy such as cognitive-behavioral therapy and psychodynamic psychotherapy. Clinicians should deal sensitively with these patients, especially regarding their peculiar thinking patterns and beliefs. Medications should be limited in use, as the evidence of their efficacy is lacking. Antipsychotics can be used together with psychotherapy when patients present illusions, ideas of reference, and other symptoms [9]. Some small studies have suggested the use of antipsychotics such as risperidone may be useful in reducing symptom severity [10].

24.4 Cluster B

24.4.1 Histrionic Personality Disorder

Affected individuals tend to be flamboyant, attention seeking, and demonstrate an excessive emotionality. Emotions are shallow and shift rapidly. Typically, they are attractive and seductive and, like narcissistic persons, overly concerned with their appearance. Individuals often use their physical appearance to draw the attention of others and may behave in a sexually provocative manner. They tend to exaggerate and dramatize their emotions, which otherwise lack depth. Prevalence is estimated to be 1.8%. It is more commonly diagnosed in females than in males [4, 5]. Psychotherapy is the treatment of choice, with a particular focus on the therapeutic alliance [11].

24.4.2 Narcissistic Personality Disorder

This is a personality disorder where individuals have a grandiose sense of their own self-importance but are also extremely sensitive to criticism due to their almost invariably very fragile self-esteem. They have little ability to empathize with others and are more concerned about appearance than substance. It is characterized by arrogance, grandiosity, a constant and excessive need for admiration, and a tendency to exploit others. Individuals with this condition often have a sense of excessive entitlement and may demand special treatment.

Prevalence estimates range between about 1% [12] to 6.2% in community samples [13]. Males account for 50% to 75% of diagnoses [3]. The manifestations and traits of narcissism may initially come to clinical attention or present exacerbation during challenging or unexpected life experiences or crises such as divorces, loss of employment, or bankruptcies. It is also noteworthy that these individuals have increased difficulties with aging, since they place high value in beauty, strength, and youthful attributes [3, 9].

Narcissistic personality disorder is a stable pattern, not shifting much over time, and there is very little evidence for working treatments with long-term results [14]. The treatment of this disorder is very difficult, since to make progress patients would need to renounce their narcissism [9]. Some studies mention the utility of treatments focusing on specific behavioral changes; however, the patient would still remain with its core characteristics. There is no evidence of successful treatment to the point of improving significantly their interpersonal relationships.

Higher-functioning narcissistic personalities may benefit from psychodynamic psychotherapy. Individual psychotherapy is viewed by many as the basic treatment of choice. However, some clinicians suggest a group therapy setting so patients can learn how to share with others and potentially develop a more empathic response [9].

24.5 Cluster C

24.5.1 Obsessive-Compulsive Personality Disorder

OCPD is a personality disorder where individuals may be perfectionistic, inflexible, and unable to express warm, tender feelings. There can be preoccupation with trivial details and rules as well as difficulty adapting to changes in routine. Obsessive-compulsive disorder is a separate disorder that involves irresistible obsessions and compulsions and is not the same as OCPD. OCPD is one of the most prevalent personality disorders, with an estimated prevalence ranging from 2.1% to 7.9%. Males are diagnosed twice as much as females. There is an association between this personality disorder and depression, bipolar disorder, and eating disorders (in particular with anorexia nervosa) [15]. Cognitive-behavioral therapy is the best validated treatment of OCPD [16].

24.5.2 Avoidant Personality Disorder

Affected individuals are timid and shy. Uncomfortable and afraid of rejection or criticism, they avoid social contact. They are self-critical and have low self-esteem. If given strong guarantees of uncritical acceptance, they may make friends and participate in social gatherings. Unlike individuals with schizoid personality disorder, they desire having friends. Estimated prevalence is 2.4%. Males and females are diagnosed equally [4, 5]. Psychotherapies such as cognitive-behavioral therapy and psychodynamic therapy can be effective. Therapists should encourage gradual exposures into the world and stay aware of threats to the patient's self-esteem [17].

24.5.3 Dependent Personality Disorder

This disorder is characterized by clingy and submissive behavior. Individuals are passive and allow others to direct their lives. Other people such as spouses or parents make all major life decisions, including where to live and what type of employment to obtain. These patients fear separation and tend to be indecisive and unable to take the initiative. They are often preoccupied with the thought of being left to fend for themselves and want others to assume responsibility for all major decision-making. Fearing abandonment, they have difficulty expressing disagreement. Prevalence estimates range from 0.49% to 0.6%. Males and females are generally diagnosed equally. History of chronic illness in childhood or separation anxiety disorder is a risk factor for developing dependent personality disorder [3–5].

Psychotherapy tends to be successful for these patients. Cognitive-behavioral therapy, assertiveness training, and group and family therapy were used in the past with good results. With the support of their therapist in insight-oriented therapies, patients can become more assertive, independent, and self-reliant [9]. Psychotherapy aims to support individuals in achieving self-reliance, while cognitive-behavioral therapy can assist in confronting negative thoughts and fostering self-sufficient behaviors.

24.6 Treatment of Personality Disorders

Whenever the treatment of complex psychiatric conditions is considered, a treatment plan should be developed, discussed, and modified over time. That includes information from the patient and other people involved in their support. Such a treatment plan should include psychotherapy, psychopharmacology, and psychoeducation, as well as the treatment of comorbidities. In times of crisis, the need for day treatment or brief hospitalization should be considered.

Psychotherapy has been the therapeutic intervention of choice for most personality disorders. Pharmacological treatment is usually auxiliary and focused on symptoms. Despite the high prevalence of personality disorders, there is limited knowledge about evidence-based psychopharmacological treatments. To date, drug treatment strategies have been much more commonly studied in three personality disorders: borderline, schizotypal, and avoidant personality [18].

Although there are no specific drugs for the treatment of personality disorders, clinical practice is largely guided by expert opinion and experience, which support the effectiveness of low-dose antipsychotics and mood stabilizers when applied to behavioral difficulties that interfere with performance, for example impulsivity, self-destructiveness and anger management, among others [19].

Pharmacological treatment in personality disorders can be separated by specific symptom domains, namely:

- Perceptual cognitive symptoms, such as hallucinatory symptoms or paranoid ideation, usually linked to stressful situations. In these cases, antipsychotic drugs are usually used in low doses [19].
- Symptoms of impulsivity and lack of behavioral control, such as self-mutilation, compulsions, or interpersonal conflicts. In these cases, the use of mood stabilizers is recommended [19]. In the specific case of recurrent self-injury, the use of omega-3 fatty acids as an adjunct to a mood stabilizer has been indicated, given its profile of benign side effects and preliminary evidence suggesting efficacy [20].
- Symptoms of affective dysregulation, such as affective lability, depressed mood, disproportionate anger, and pathological anxiety. Some meta-analysis studies have shown that mood stabilizers and low-dose antipsychotic drugs are more effective than antidepressants for treating affective dysregulation in this population [19].

On the other hand, certain medications should be avoided or considered only as a last resort:

- Medications that can be fatal in overdose, such as tricyclic antidepressants.
- Medications that can cause dependency over time, such as benzodiazepines and opioids.
- Medicating whenever there is a mood swing, as mood swings can occur frequently and with rapid onset.

It is important to note that, compared to the general population, many patients with personality disorders are more susceptible to side effects, tend to take more medications than prescribed, and are at greater risk of concomitant use of medications with illicit drugs and alcohol [1].

As for the therapeutic bond, it is fundamental to initially evaluate the personality type and general characteristics of the individual. Individuals with personality disorders can manifest a disturbed pattern in interpersonal relationships that can be deleterious in the therapeutic setting if they are not approached with skill by the clinician.

Some general characteristics of the psychotherapeutic support of each of the clusters can be useful. Individuals with Cluster A personality disorders – that is, schizotypal, schizoid, or paranoid – commonly do not seek treatment promptly unless they are experiencing an acute issue such as a depressive episode or substance use. These patients may have great difficulty establishing a therapeutic relationship. Individuals from Cluster B, including narcissistic, borderline, histrionic, and antisocial personality disorders, are typically associated with repeatedly testing and pushing the limits of the therapeutic relationship. Clinicians must be very careful to manage alliance breakdowns and avoid crossing appropriate boundaries in the quest to build a relationship. Individuals in Cluster C – that is, dependent, avoidant, and obsessive-compulsive personalities – tend to be more willing/able to assume responsibility for their issues and, therefore, more engaged in therapeutic processes [21].

One important distinction an experienced clinician should be able to make is between personality traits or styles and personality disorders. All individuals have distinctive personality patterns or traits, but they do not usually warrant a diagnosis of personality disorder. Inexperienced evaluators commonly overdiagnose patients with personality disorders. The features that differentiate pathological traits from normal traits are maladaptiveness and inflexibility, causing impaired functionality. Personality, as discussed in this chapter, is a pervasive and enduring aspect of the patient. However, patients are, most of the time, assessed during crisis situations, when certain personality traits might temporarily become more prominent and less adaptive. Therefore, the distinction between personality disorder and personality traits may be particularly challenging in a cross-sectional assessment [1].

References

1. A. E. Skodol, J. M. Oldham, *The American Psychiatric Association Publishing Textbook of Personality Disorders*, 3rd ed. (American Psychiatric Publishing, 2021).

2. T. A. Widiger, *The Oxford Handbook of Personality Disorders* (Oxford University Press, 2012).

3. American Psychiatric Association, *Diagnostic and Statistical Manual of Mental Disorders: DSM-5-TR*, 5th edition, text revision (American Psychiatric Association Publishing, 2022).

4. M. F. Lenzenweger, M. C. Lane, A. W. Loranger, R. C. Kessler, DSM-IV personality disorders in the national comorbidity survey replication. *Biological Psychiatry*, **62** (2007), 553–564. https://doi.org/10.1016/j.biopsych.2006.09.019.

5. D. S. Hasin, B. F. Grant, The National Epidemiologic Survey on Alcohol and Related Conditions (NESARC) waves 1 and 2. review and summary of findings. *Social Psychiatry and Psychiatric Epidemiology*, **50** (2015), 1609–1640. https://doi.org/10.1007/s00127-015-1088-0.

6. R. J. Lee, Mistrustful and misunderstood: a review of paranoid personality disorder. *Current Behavioral Neuroscience Reports*, **4** (2017), 151–165. https://doi.org/10.1007/s40473-017-0116-7.

7. W. D. Blackmon, Dungeons and Dragons: the use of a fantasy game in the psychotherapeutic treatment of a young adult. *American Journal of Psychotherapy*, **48** (1994), 624–632. https://doi.org/10.1176/appi.psychotherapy.1994.48.4.624.

8. T. Teraishi, H. Hori, D. Sasayama, J. Matsuo, S. Ogawa, I. Ishida, A. Nagashima, Y. Kinoshita, M. Ota, K. Hattori, H. Kunugi, Relationship between lifetime suicide attempts and schizotypal traits in patients with schizophrenia. *PLoS ONE*, **9** (2014), e107739. https://doi.org/10.1371/journal.pone.0107739.

9. R. Boland, M. Verduin, P. Ruiz, *Kaplan and Sadock's Synopsis of Psychiatry*, 12th ed. (Wolters Kluwer Health, 2021).

10. K. D. Jakobsen, E. Skyum, N. Hashemi, O. Schjerning, A. Fink-Jensen, J. Nielsen, Antipsychotic treatment of schizotypy and schizotypal personality disorder: a systematic review. *Journal of Psychopharmacology (Oxford, England)*, **31** (2017), 397–405. https://doi.org/10.1177/0269881117695879.

11. D. S. Bender, The therapeutic alliance in the treatment of personality disorders. *Journal of Psychiatric Practice*, **11** (2005), 73–87. https://doi.org/10.1097/00131746-200503000-00002.

12. N. Dhawan, M. E. Kunik, J. Oldham, J. Coverdale, Prevalence and treatment of narcissistic personality disorder in the community: a systematic review. *Comprehensive Psychiatry*, **51** (2010), 333–339. https://doi.org/10.1016/j.comppsych.2009.09.003.

13. F. S. Stinson, D. A. Dawson, B. F. Grant, R. B. Goldstein, S. P. Chou, H. Boji, S. M. Smith, W. J. Ruan, A. J. Pulay, T. D. Saha, R. P. Pickering, Prevalence, correlates, disability, and comorbidity of DSM-iv narcissistic personality disorder: results from the wave 2 National Epidemiologic Survey on Alcohol and Related Conditions. *Journal of Clinical Psychiatry*, **69** (2008), 1033–1045. https://doi.org/10.4088/JCP.v69n0701.

14. A. Vater, K. Ritter, S. Strunz, E. F. Ronningstam, B. Renneberg, S. Roepke, Stability of narcissistic personality disorder: tracking categorical and dimensional rating systems over a two-year period. *Personality Disorders*, **5** (2014), 305–313. https://doi.org/10.1037/per0000058.

15. S. Young, P. Rhodes, S. Touyz, P. Hay, The relationship between obsessive-compulsive personality disorder traits, obsessive-compulsive disorder and excessive exercise in patients with anorexia nervosa: a systematic review. *Journal of Eating Disorders*, **1** (2013), 16. https://doi.org/10.1186/2050-2974-1-16.

16. A. Diedrich, U. Voderholzer, Obsessive-compulsive personality disorder: a current review. *Current Psychiatry Reports*, **17** (2015), 2. https://doi.org/10.1007/s11920-014-0547-8.

17. A. Weinbrecht, L. Schulze, J. Boettcher, B. Renneberg, Avoidant personality disorder: a current review. *Current Psychiatry Reports*, **18** (2016), 29. https://doi.org/10.1007/s11920-016-0665-6.

18. S. C. Herpertz, M. Zanarini, C. S. Schulz, L. Siever, K. Lieb, H.-J. Möller. D, WFSBP Task Force on Personality, World Federation of Societies of Biological Psychiatry (WFSBP), Guidelines for biological treatment of personality disorders. *The World Journal of Biological Psychiatry*, **8** (2007), 212–244. https://doi.org/10.1080/15622970701685224.

19. T. Ingenhoven, P. Lafay, T. Rinne, J. Passchier, H. Duivenvoorden, Effectiveness of pharmacotherapy for severe personality disorders: meta-analyses of randomized controlled trials. *Journal of Clinical Psychiatry*, **71** (2010), 14–25. https://doi.org/10.4088/JCP.08r04526gre.

20. D. M. Karaszewska, T. Ingenhoven, R. J. T. Mocking, Marine omega-3 fatty acid supplementation for borderline personality disorder: a meta-analysis. *Journal of Clinical Psychiatry*, **82** (2021). https://doi.org/10.4088/JCP.20r13613.

21. V. Lingiardi, L. Filippucci, R. Baiocco, Therapeutic alliance evaluation in personality disorders psychotherapy. *Psychotherapy Research*, **15** (2005), 45–53. https://doi.org/10.1080/10503300512331327047.

Eating Disorders

Carrie J. McAdams

25.1 Introduction

Estimates are that 28.8 million individuals in the United States will be affected by an eating disorder (ED) during their lifetime [1]. EDs lead to increased health services and medical costs and reduce quality of life, but less than a quarter of patients receive treatment specifically for the ED [2, 3]. Further, although disordered eating symptoms improve acutely with treatments [4, 5], relapse should be anticipated, as maintaining recovery takes years [6, 7]. Increasing the number of clinicians comfortable and educated in the treatment of EDs is essential to meet these needs and has the potential to reduce the morbidity and mortality associated with EDs.

DSM-5 describes four main feeding and eating disorders: anorexia nervosa (AN), avoidant restrictive food intake disorder (ARFID), bulimia nervosa (BN), and binge-eating disorder (BED) [8]. Two additional diagnostic categories are unspecified feeding and eating disorders and other specified feeding and eating disorders (OSFED). OSFED includes five examples of subsyndromal eating disorders: atypical AN, subthreshold BN, subthreshold BED disorder, purging disorder, and night eating. Pica and rumination disorder are two feeding disorders outside the scope of this chapter.

EDs occur across all ages, genders, races, ethnicities, and socioeconomic groups [1, 9, 10]. In the largest US study of adults using standardized diagnostic interviews, lifetime prevalence of AN, BN, and BED was, respectively, 0.9%, 2.0%, and 3.7% in females and 0.6%, 0.1%, and 2.5% in males, and median age of onset for AN and BN was 18 years and for BED 21 years [1]. Estimates of prevalence of ARFID in children ranges from 1% to 3% [11, 12].

EDs are complex multifactorial disorders with biological, psychological, social, and environmental determinants intermingling to influence illness onset and maintenance. Many genes increase risk for development of EDs [13–15]. Genetic risks for AN include genes related to metabolic, anthropomorphic, and psychiatric traits [14]. Malnutrition alters the brain, both thinning the cortex [16] and changing neurotransmitter binding [17]. Because changes in eating behaviors and nutritional state affect physiology, EDs can also alter metabolic, endocrine, immune, and gastrointestinal functioning. Changes in the gut may also change the brain [18]. Sociocultural risk factors also influence the development of EDs. Culturally, the introduction of cable television to the Fijiian islands was associated with the development of compensatory purging behaviors in adolescent girls [19]. Socially, The Body Project can reduce the incidence of EDs, using a cognitive dissonance intervention targeting overvaluation of the thin ideal [20].

In Figure 25.1, domains important to consider when constructing a case formulation for an individual with an ED are stacked into a precarious tower, symbolizing their

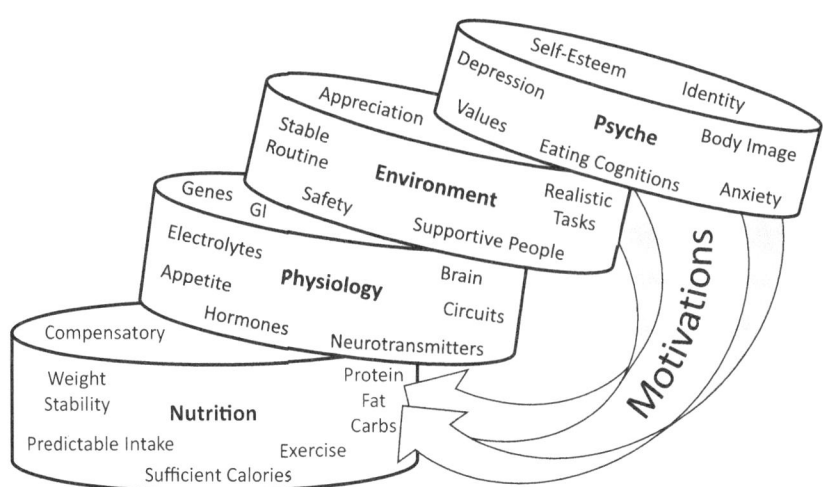

Figure 25.1 Both development and treatment of an eating disorder are complex. Here, a tower of disks symbolizes the importance of both internal (Physiology, Psyche) and external (Nutrition, Environment) components in both illness (collapsing) and recovery (stabilized). Motivations, both to engage in disordered eating as well as to recover, commonly come from the environment and psyche. Some potential concepts and factors to consider for individual case and treatment formulations are detailed within each disk.

interrelatedness and dependence. Both eating (Nutrition) and social experiences (Environment) alter both medical health (Physiology) and psychological state (Psyche). Motivations to both stay ill and engage in disordered eating as well as to recover are influenced both by social environment and by psychological and physiological state.

25.2 Diagnosis and Assessment

Combinations of behavioral and cognitive symptoms related to eating, body state, and self-evaluation define the specific DSM-5 EDs [8]. Unique for psychiatric diagnoses, the inability to meet energy requirements is also part of the criteria for AN, ARFID, and atypical AN. For ARFID, this is described as persistent failure to meet nutritional and/or energy needs; for AN and atypical AN, this is described as restriction of energy intake, but only in AN does it lead to significantly low body weight. Medical complications and psychopathology can be comparable to or even more severe in atypical AN than in classic AN [21].

Disordered eating behaviors fall into three main categories: restrictive eating, binge-eating, and compensatory behaviors. *Restrictive eating* refers to limiting food intake to levels lower than optimal for one's energy requirements. Restrictive food intake in AN, atypical AN, and BN is attributed to concerns about body shape and weight. In children with ARFID, restrictive eating may be related to a lack of interest in eating or food, avoidance based on the sensory characteristics of food, or concerns about aversive consequences of eating [22, 23].

Binge-eating refers to consumption of an unusually large amount of food in a discrete period while experiencing a sense of loss of control. Objective binge-eating episodes involve a calorie consumption that would be viewed by most people as more food than expected (an entire pizza or box of cereal), while a subjective binge-eating episode involves a similar sense of loss of control but with the amount of food that would not typically be viewed as excessive (two pieces of pizza or two donuts or cookies). Binge-eating episodes are also associated with the following symptoms: rapid eating, eating in secret, eating alone, feeling disgusted about the episode, feelings of shame. Binge-eating episodes weekly without compensatory episodes and three of those associated symptoms are defining of BED.

Compensatory behaviors refer to both nonpurging (e.g., prolonged fasting, compulsive exercise) and purging (e.g., vomiting, laxatives, diuretics) behaviors that are designed to avoid weight gain or to alleviate guilt associated with eating. Compensatory behaviors occur in relation to binge episodes in BN but can also occur following consumption of a normal or reduced amount of food in purging disorder, AN, and atypical AN. Weekly episodes of binge-eating in conjunction with compensatory behaviors are the behaviors defining of BN, while compensatory behaviors without binge episodes are defining of purging disorder. Concerning findings for compulsive exercise include continuing to exercise when injured or in bad weather, failing to take regular rest days, or experiencing distress if unable to engage in exercise.

Cognitive symptoms of EDs include ruminations related to both food and eating (e.g., calorie tracking) and one's body features (e.g., reflection in mirrors, weight). Cognitive ruminations about food, calories, weight, and shape are concerning when they impede other important activities. This can be detected by asking the patients about how much time they are engaged in cognitions on a typical day or if such thoughts interfere with other desired or required activities. Feeling like one's weight and shape are defining one's self-worth (e.g., overvaluation of body shape) is a cognitive symptom common to AN, atypical AN, and BN, can occur in BED [24], but is exclusionary for ARFID. Focusing on one's appearance or weight can be a maladaptive coping mechanism to manage negative emotions [25].

Specific changes in emotional state are not a defining characteristic of EDs, but many emotional changes can occur during an ED. Anxiety and fears related to eating are common, including such issues as food anxiety, tension around food, fears about body sensations in response to eating, anxiety about eating in social situations, and a fear of judgment about weight gain [26]. Patients may also present with a chief complaint that appears unrelated to EDs, but the problem may be a consequence of disordered eating, such as fatigue or constipation. Anxiety, depression, and difficulties concentrating are all distressing, ego-dystonic problems, while restrictive eating and overexercise are ego-syntonic. Starvation is associated not only with body preoccupations (an ED cognition) but also with anhedonia, sleep disturbances, appetite dysregulation, concentration, and energy changes [27] – symptoms also present in mood disorders. Energy and attention problems occur in response to low blood sugar [28] but could also be part of attention deficit/hyperactivity disorder (ADHD). EDs are frequently comorbid with mood, anxiety, ADHD, and substance use disorders [29–34]. Timelines examining both psychopathology symptoms in conjunction with eating and weight changes can be helpful to determine if comorbidity or a time-limited consequence of the ED.

Screening for EDs can be helpful in primary care, as medical comorbidities may be a presenting complaint, such as weight changes, infertility, cardiovascular problems, or bone health. Both the SCOFF [35] and Screen for Disordered Eating [36] have high sensitivity and specificity. Asking patients to recall their food consumption from the previous day is another screening approach, providing an overview of food content and eating patterns, and assessing for use of hunger and satiety cues. These conversations allow education about the need for energy, fat, and protein for optimal mental and physical health and can identify individual challenges related to appetite, restriction, overeating, compensatory behaviors, and comorbidities.

A medical examination is recommended for all ED patients both to ensure medical stability and to establish the appropriate level of care [37, 38]. Medical stability can be affected by disordered eating, changing both resting and orthostatic vital signs, including temperature, blood pressure, heart rate, weight, and growth. Both underweight and weight-suppressed patients may have bradycardia or hypotension [39, 40]. An electrocardiogram is recommended in patients with AN, severe purging behavior, and to assess QTc interval for medications [38].

Recommended laboratory assessments are a complete blood panel with differential and metabolic panel (electrolytes, liver enzymes, and renal function) as well as magnesium and phosphorus [38]. Electrolyte abnormalities, including hypokalemic alkalosis, are common in individuals with purging behaviors. Hypoglycemia, low levels of estrogen or testosterone, abnormal levels thyroid hormone and growth hormone, and hypersecretion of corticotrophin-releasing hormone are common [41]. Blood tests in restricting EDs can also be normal even when a patient is at risk of severe complications, and assessments should be performed in collaboration with a physician with experience in case of extreme AN (BMI < 15) due to the high-risk of life-threatening complications [42]. Refeeding syndrome is defined by acute changes in electrolytes, thiamine, and organ dysfunction following initiation of nutritional rehabilitation of malnourished patients; close medical monitoring of patients at risk for refeeding syndrome is essential [43].

25.3 Treatment

25.3.1 Building an Alliance

Eating disorders can be affected every time a patient with disordered eating interacts with a clinician. The anticipation of shame and the fear of the judgment can result in individuals avoiding medical attention [44] or not reporting serious symptoms [45]. Stigmatizing experiences when seeking treatment for one's ED is negatively associated with recovery from EDs [46]. Psychological features common in EDs, including shame [47], perfectionism [48], negative self-worth [49], difficulties with attachment [50], and processing social stimuli [51], increase the risk of physician–patient interactions having negative emotional and behavioral consequences. Being met with care and consideration during treatment improves both patient satisfaction about managing their EDs and outcomes [52]. Effective physician–patient communication is essential in treatment of EDs, such as practicing active listening, offering emotional support, encouraging patients to ask questions, and being willing to share in decision-making.

25.3.2 Teamwork and Levels of Care

Treatment of an ED is complex, as factors both internal to a patient (physiology and psyche) and external (nutrition and environment) are relevant to both illness and recovery (Figure 25.1). These factors interact with each other in complex ways. For example, nutrition can have both acute (blood sugar) and chronic (infertility) impacts on physiological state. Similarly, social environment can impact psychological state both acutely (a loss creating sadness) or in a chronic manner (repeated failures leading to low self-esteem). An integrated treatment team is recommended, as recovery depends on coordination and changes in multiple areas [53]. Treatment teams are often composed of a primary care physician (PCP), psychiatrist, dietician, therapist, as well as family and friends. Regular communication among team members ensures accountability for behavioral changes, reduces risk of splitting, and assures consensus regarding treatment goals. Frequency of appointments with different team members is determined by psychopathology severity and extent of medical complications. PCPs provide ongoing recovery support and monitoring for signs of relapse after treatments with other team members conclude. Motivation for recovery should be reinforced and supported by all the clinicians, as well as the supportive people in each patient's life.

As patients present with a wide range of symptom severity, treatment occurs across a spectrum of intensity from medical hospitalization to outpatient providers to self-help. Inpatient treatment should be reserved for medically compromised patients. General medical wards are necessary if cardiac monitoring, intravenous infusions, or frequent lab monitoring are indicated based on medical state [38]. Rapid weight regain is associated with better outcomes in AN [54] but can require more intensive medical support [41]. Psychiatric inpatient and residential programs provide round-the-clock supervision while imposing a regular schedule and eating routine – interventions that may be necessary to break disordered eating patterns or manage comorbid psychiatric symptoms. Partial day and intensive outpatient programs offer meal support and therapy. ED behaviors usually diminish rapidly within these highly structured treatment settings, but ED cognitions can persist for years. Importantly, most ED treatment will be occurring in the outpatient setting, as reaching and sustaining recovery takes years [6, 7].

Working with the patient to identify their motivation for recovery is a constant component of treatment influenced internally by the patient as well as externally by the clinical team and social environment (Figure 25.1). This includes encouraging the patient build an identity apart from the ED and identify a social environment that can support their recovery [55, 56]. Motivation should be continually nurtured and amplified to counter both disordered eating cognitions and behaviors. Many individuals with EDs have insight and want to change their disordered eating, but some pursue treatment only at the urging of others, such as parents, pediatricians, teachers, and friends. In severe cases with malnourishment, motivation for recovery may be absent. For these patients, nutritional rehabilitation and attainment of medical stability should be prioritized before focusing on psychosocial components. Patients mandated to treatment for EDs usually have more medical severity at baseline and may take longer to treat, but their outcomes are similar to those who attend voluntarily making mandated treatment appropriate for some cases [57]. As recovery progresses, discussing how disordered eating cognitions and behaviors impact the individual's health and life goals can improve insight and support development of internal motivating factors for recovery.

25.3.3 Medical Nutrition Therapy

Medical nutrition therapy involves establishing a regular eating pattern with meals and snacks of predictable amounts of food at regular times. Dieticians, family, and friends may help outsource decision-making about frequency and content of meals. Success in changing symptoms is reinforcing, so setting small but realistic and attainable goals is desired. Altering behavioral patterns is often more effective than concentrating on cessation of pathological behaviors. People with binge-spectrum EDs often succeed at adding snacks and balancing nutrients in meals, while restrictive ED patients do well with gradually increasing their eating frequency and food quantity. In underweight individuals, supplementation with high-calorie protein shakes may help, as titration up to 3,000–4,000 kcal per day is typically required. Patients with purging behaviors find smaller meals can reduce triggers related to fullness, and waiting a length of time after eating before engaging in compensatory behaviors can break binge-purge cycles. Ensuring protein, carbohydrates, and fats are in meals and snacks slows digestion, stabilizes blood sugars, and increases satiety.

Both clinicians and patients benefit by recognizing that changing disordered eating behaviors is usually challenging, regardless of the type of behavior (restriction, compensatory, or binge-eating). Explaining that many routine behaviors are not always conscious decisions at initial intake is important. This can help alleviate the tendency to engage in self-blaming ruminations if the patient feels unable to change a behavior. Restrictive eating can become more of an unconscious habit as illness duration persists [58]. Disordered eating behaviors often start during periods of significant life stress as a maladaptive coping mechanism but can persist after stressors resolve in part due to the impact of altered nutrition on physiology and psyche.

The circadian clock is closely tied to eating and feeding behaviors. A normal sleep–wake cycle consists of approximately 16 hours of daytime wakefulness and 8 hours of nighttime sleep. Light therapy, an evidence-based treatment for depression, is an effective technique for managing appetite dysregulation in relation to mood [59, 60]. Pilot studies also suggest improvement in ED symptoms [61, 62]. Use of a light therapy lamp can be a more feasible early behavioral change for patients than changing long-standing disordered eating patterns, and helping patients recognize that they can succeed with behavioral changes is essential to overall treatment.

25.3.4 Psychotherapy

Psychotherapy is the mainstay of treatment for EDs, supporting patients in modifying behaviors and cognitions and regulating emotions. Therapy can improve insight about psychological and environmental triggers of disordered eating behaviors and change core beliefs about oneself, one's appearance, and self-worth. The therapist is often the most frequently seen clinician on the team and provides accountability about disordered eating behaviors while also serving as a supportive person in the patient's life. Many modalities of therapy have shown benefits, including but not limited to cognitive-behavioral therapies, family therapies, interpersonal psychotherapy, exposure-response prevention therapies, dialectical-behavioral therapies, and specialist supportive clinical management.

Family-based therapy (FBT) for AN and BN is the first choice for children, adolescents, and emerging adults [63]. Family therapy involves helping parents learn to create a safe and predictable structure and moves decision-making about eating from the child to the parents, minimizing blame related to disordered eating and maximizing emotional support for the child [64]. FBT is currently being studied for ARFID [65], with some pilot cases completed [66, 67].

Enhanced cognitive-behavioral therapy for EDs is considered the first-line treatment for adults and an alternative to family-based therapy for adolescents for both AN and

BN. The first eight sessions focus on establishing a regular eating pattern, then progresses to cognitive and emotional challenges: body image, dietary restraint, and mood triggers. This treatment has large effect sizes in binge-spectrum eating disorders (both BN and BED) in both adults and adolescents but less robust data for underweight individuals [68, 69]. Improvement by the eighth session is suggestive of a better long-term outcome for adults in a transdiagnostic sample of EDs [70], and may be an appropriate time to reassess the potential need for a higher level of care. Cognitive-behavioral therapy for ARFID encourages underweight patients to eat larger volumes of preferred foods initially during nutritional rehabilitation, and then introduces variety with in-session exposures [71].

Outcomes do not vary significantly across different types of psychological therapies in AN and BN [72–74]. For BED, both cognitive-behavioral therapy and structured self-help are effective in reducing symptoms [75]. Finally, virtual options are now improving access to therapies specific for EDs [76].

25.3.5 Pharmacology

Pharmacotherapy is adjunctive to psychotherapy in EDs, with only two medications with specific US Food and Drug Administration (FDA) approval. Treatment of comorbidities, such as anxiety, mood, and substance use disorders, can benefit from appropriate psyc hopharmacological treatments. However, psychoactive medications often impact appetite, and gastrointestinal function and absorption may differ with eating patterns.

Limited evidence supports psychoactive medications for AN and ARFID, possibly because brain changes and alterations in gastrointestinal function may compromise psychopharmacologic effects when individuals are malnourished [77]. Olanzapine, when compared to placebo, showed a modest increase in weight gain in outpatient adults with long illness duration of AN [78]. However, when prescribed in conjunction with structured psychotherapeutic interventions, olanzapine did not increase weight gain, but did improve psychological symptoms [79–81]. Aripiprazole has been studied in open-label studies in adolescents and young adults, with modest improvements in weight gain [82]. In case studies of ARFID, olanzapine use was associated with reduced anxiety, improved eating behaviors, and weight restoration [67]. Second-generation atypical antipsychotics should be reserved for patients with high illness severity.

The two medications approved by the FDA are for binge-spectrum EDs: fluoxetine and lisdexamfetamine. Fluoxetine (60 mg/day) provides a short-term improvement in symptoms for BN [83]. Lisdexamfetamine dimesylate (50 and 70 mg) reduced the number of binge-eating days per week in adults diagnosed with BED [84]. Although FDA approval has not been obtained, a meta-analysis suggests symptom improvement in binge-spectrum eating disorders for all second-generation antidepressants as well as topiramate [85]. Naltrexone has shown benefits in reducing binge-episodes in adolescents [86] and in adults with both depression and binge-eating [87].

25.4 Conclusion

EDs are challenging illnesses to treat and can persist for many years. It is imperative for this not to be viewed as a reflection of the patient's lack of desire to improve but rather the inherent difficulties in treating multifaceted disorders. Making and sustaining behavioral changes are difficult for people. Clinicians working with patients with EDs must reinforce and amplify any motivations that the patients have to provide hope for recovery. This can require constructing a nurturing environment where even the smallest of positive changes is championed but also providing objective feedback to help patients visualize progress toward their goal. Working with patients with EDs is challenging, as the disordered cycle can be difficult to alter, but also rewarding, as complete recovery is achievable.

References

1. Hudson JI, Hiripi E, Pope Jr. HG, Kessler RC. The prevalence and correlates of eating disorders in the National Comorbidity Survey Replication. *Biological Psychiatry*. 2007;61(3):348–358. doi: S0006-3223(06)00474-4 [pii] 10 .1016/j.biopsych.2006.03.040.

2. Striegel Weissman R, Rosselli F. Reducing the burden of suffering from eating disorders: unmet treatment needs, cost of illness, and the quest for cost-effectiveness. *Behaviour Research and Therapy*. 2017;88:49–64. doi: 10.1016/j .brat.2016.09.006.

3. Hay P, Mitchison D, Collado AEL, Gonzalez-Chica DA, Stocks N, Touyz S. Burden and health-related quality of life of eating disorders, including avoidant/ restrictive food intake disorder (ARFID), in the Australian population. *Journal of Eating Disorders*. 2017;5:21. doi: 10.1186/ s40337-017-0149-z.

4. Peckmezian T, Paxton SJ. A systematic review of outcomes following residential treatment for eating disorders. *European Eating Disorders Review*. 2020;28 (3):246–259. doi: https://doi.org/10.1002/ erv.2733.

5. Chang P, Delgadillo J, Waller G. Early response to psychological treatment for eating disorders: a systematic review and meta-analysis. *Clinical Psychology Review*. 2021;86:102032. doi: 10.1016/j.cpr.2021 .102032.

6. Eddy KT, Tabri N, Thomas JJ, Murray HB, Keshaviah A, Hastings E, et al. Recovery from anorexia nervosa and bulimia nervosa at 22-year follow-up. *Journal of Clinical Psychiatry*. 2017;78 (2):184–189. doi: 10.4088/JCP.15m10393.

7. Glasofer DR, Muratore AF, Attia E, Wu P, Wang Y, Minkoff H, et al. Predictors of illness course and health maintenance following inpatient treatment among patients with anorexia nervosa. *Journal of Eating Disorders*. 2020;8(1):69. doi: 10 .1186/s40337-020-00348-7.

8. American Psychological Association. *Diagnostic and Statistical Manual of Mental Disorders*. 5th ed. American Psychological Association Publishing; 2013.

9. Makino M, Tsuboi K, Dennerstein L. Prevalence of eating disorders: a comparison of Western and non-Western countries. *MedGenMed*. 2004;6(3):49.

10. Marques L, Alegria M, Becker AE, Chen CN, Fang A, Chosak A, et al. Comparative prevalence, correlates of impairment, and service utilization for eating disorders across US ethnic groups: implications for reducing ethnic disparities in health care access for eating disorders. *International Journal of Eating Disorders*. 2011;44(5):412–420. doi: 10 .1002/eat.20787.

11. Dinkler L, Yasumitsu-Lovell K, Eitoku M, Fujieda M, Suganuma N, Hatakenaka Y, et al. Development of a parent-reported screening tool for avoidant/restrictive food intake disorder (ARFID): initial validation and prevalence in 4-7-year-old Japanese children. *Appetite*. 2022;168:105735. doi: 10.1016/j.appet .2021.105735.

12. Feillet F, Bocquet A, Briend A, Chouraqui JP, Darmaun D, Frelut ML, et al. Nutritional risks of ARFID (avoidant restrictive food intake disorders) and related behavior. *Archives of Pediatrics*. 2019;26(7):437–441. doi: 10.1016/j.arcped .2019.08.005.

13. Yilmaz Z, Hardaway JA, Bulik CM. Genetics and epigenetics of eating disorders. *Advances in Genomics and Genetics*. 2015;5:131–150. doi: 10.2147/AGG.S55776.

14. Watson HJ, Yilmaz Z, Thornton LM, Hubel C, Coleman JRI, Gaspar HA, et al. Genome-wide association study identifies eight risk loci and implicates metabo-psychiatric origins for anorexia nervosa. *Natural Genetics*. 2019;51(8):1207–1214. doi: 10.1038/s41588-019-0439-2.

15. Dinkler L, Wronski ML, Lichtenstein P, Lundstrom S, Larsson H, Micali N, et al. Etiology of the broad avoidant restrictive food intake disorder phenotype in Swedish Twins Aged 6 to 12 Years. *JAMA Psychiatry*. 2023;80(3):260–269. doi: 10.1001/jamapsychiatry.2022.4612.

16. Walton E, Bernardoni F, Batury VL, Bahnsen K, Lariviere S, Abbate-Daga G, et al. Brain structure in acutely underweight and partially weight-restored individuals with anorexia nervosa: a coordinated analysis by the ENIGMA Eating Disorders Working Group. *Biological Psychiatry*. 2022;92(9):730–738. doi: 10.1016/j.biopsych.2022.04.022.

17. Bailer UF, Frank GK, Price JC, Meltzer CC, Becker C, Mathis CA, et al. Interaction between serotonin transporter and dopamine D2/D3 receptor radioligand measures is associated with harm avoidant symptoms in anorexia and bulimia nervosa. *Psychiatry Research*. 2013;211(2):160–168. doi: 10.1016/j.pscychresns.2012.06.010.

18. Cryan JF, O'Riordan KJ, Cowan CSM, Sandhu KV, Bastiaanssen TFS, Boehme M, et al. The microbiota-gut-brain axis. *Physiological reviews*. 2019;99(4):1877–2013. doi: 10.1152/physrev.00018.2018.

19. Becker AE, Burwell RA, Gilman SE, Herzog DB, Hamburg P. Eating behaviours and attitudes following prolonged exposure to television among ethnic Fijian adolescent girls. *British Journal of Psychiatry: Journal of Mental Science*. 2002;180:509–514. doi: 10.1192/bjp.180.6.509.

20. Stice E, Rohde P, Shaw H, Gau JM. Clinician-led, peer-led, and internet-delivered dissonance-based eating disorder prevention programs: effectiveness of these delivery modalities through 4-year follow-up. *Journal of Consulting and Clinical Psychology*. 2020;88(5):481–494. doi: 10.1037/ccp0000493.

21. Forney KJ, Brown TA, Holland-Carter LA, Kennedy GA, Keel PK. Defining "significant weight loss" in atypical anorexia nervosa. *International Journal of Eating Disorders*. 2017;50(8):952–962. doi: 10.1002/eat.22717.

22. Katzman DK, Guimond T, Spettigue W, Agostino H, Couturier J, Norris ML. Classification of children and adolescents with avoidant/restrictive food intake disorder. *Pediatrics*. 2022;150(3). doi: 10.1542/peds.2022-057494.

23. Nitsch A, Watters A, Manwaring J, Bauschka M, Hebert M, Mehler PS. Clinical features of adult patients with avoidant/restrictive food intake disorder presenting for medical stabilization: a descriptive study. *International Journal of Eating Disorders* 2023;56(5):978–990. doi: 10.1002/eat.23897.

24. Grilo CM. Why no cognitive body image feature such as overvaluation of shape/weight in the binge eating disorder diagnosis? *International Journal of Eating Disorders*. 2013;46(3):208–211. doi. https://doi.org/10.1002/eat.22082.

25. Gale C, Holliday J, Troop NA, Serpell L, Treasure J. The pros and cons of change in individuals with eating disorders: a broader perspective. International Journal of Eating Disorders. 2006;39(5):394–403. doi: 10.1002/eat.20250.

26. Levinson CA, Williams BM. Eating disorder fear networks: identification of central eating disorder fears. *International Journal of Eating Disorders*. 2020;53(12):1960–1973. doi: https://doi.org/10.1002/eat.23382.

27. Keys A. The residues of malnutrition and starvation. *Science*. 1950;112(2909):371–373.

28. Wyatt P, Berry SE, Finlayson G, O'Driscoll R, Hadjigeorgiou G, Drew DA, et al. Postprandial glycaemic dips predict appetite and energy intake in healthy individuals. *Natural Metabolism.* 2021;3 (4):523–529. doi: 10.1038/s42255-021-00383-x.

29. Kaye WH, Bulik CM, Thornton L, Barbarich N, Masters K. Comorbidity of anxiety disorders with anorexia and bulimia nervosa. *American Journal of Psychology.* 2004;161(12):2215–2221. doi: 161/12/2215 [pii] 10.1176/appi.ajp.161.12 .2215.

30. Miniati M, Benvenuti A, Bologna E, Maglio A, Cotugno B, Massimetti G, et al. Mood spectrum comorbidity in patients with anorexia and bulimia nervosa. *Eating and Weight Disorders.* 2018;23 (3):305–311. doi: 10.1007/s40519-016-0333-1.

31. Swinbourne JM, Touyz SW. The co-morbidity of eating disorders and anxiety disorders: a review. *European Eating Disorders Review.* 2007;15(4):253–274. doi: 10.1002/erv.784.

32. Kerr-Gaffney J, Harrison A, Tchanturia K. Social anxiety in the eating disorders: a systematic review and meta-analysis. *Psychological Medicine.* 2018;48 (15):2477–2491. doi: 10.1017/ S0033291718000752.

33. Svedlund NE, Norring C, Ginsberg Y, von Hausswolff-Juhlin Y. Symptoms of attention deficit hyperactivity disorder (ADHD) among adult eating disorder patients. *BMC Psychiatry.* 2017;17(1):19. doi: 10.1186/s12888-016-1093-1.

34. Fouladi F, Mitchell JE, Crosby RD, Engel SG, Crow S, Hill L, et al. Prevalence of alcohol and other substance use in patients with eating disorders. *European Eating Disorders Review.* 2015;23 (6):531–536. doi: 10.1002/erv.2410.

35. Hill LS, Reid F, Morgan JF, Lacey JH. SCOFF, the development of an eating disorder screening questionnaire. *International Journal of Eating Disorders.* 2010;43(4):344–351. doi: 10.1002/eat .20679.

36. Maguen S, Hebenstreit C, Li Y, Dinh JV, Donalson R, Dalton S, et al. Screen for Disordered Eating: improving the accuracy of eating disorder screening in primary care. *General Hospital Psychiatry.* 2018;50:20–25. doi: 10.1016/j .genhosppsych.2017.09.004.

37. Mehler PS. *Eating Disorders: A Guide to Medical Care and Complications.* 3rd ed. JHU Press; 2017.

38. Crone C, Fochtmann LJ, Attia E, Boland R, Escobar J, Fornari V, et al. The American Psychiatric Association practice guideline for the treatment of patients with eating disorders. *American Journal of Psychiatry.* 2023;180 (2):167–171. doi: 10.1176/appi.ajp .23180001.

39. Yahalom M, Spitz M, Sandler L, Heno N, Roguin N, Turgeman Y. The significance of bradycardia in anorexia nervosa. *Int J Angiol.* 2013;22(2):83–94. doi: 10.1055/ s-0033-1334138.

40. Ralph AF, Brennan L, Byrne S, Caldwell B, Farmer J, Hart LM, et al. Management of eating disorders for people with higher weight: clinical practice guideline. *Journal of Eating Disorders.* 2022;10(1):121. doi: 10.1186/s40337-022-00622-w.

41. Puckett L, Grayeb D, Khatri V, Cass K, Mehler P. A comprehensive review of complications and new findings associated with anorexia nervosa. *Journal of Clinical Medicine.* 2021;10(12). doi: 10 .3390/jcm10122555.

42. Gibson D, Watters A, Cost J, Mascolo M, Mehler PS. Extreme anorexia nervosa: medical findings, outcomes, and inferences from a retrospective cohort. *Journal of Eating Disorders.* 2020;8:25. doi: 10.1186/s40337-020-00303-6.

43. da Silva JSV, Seres DS, Sabino K, Adams SC, Berdahl GJ, Citty SW, et al. ASPEN consensus recommendations for refeeding syndrome. *Nutrition in Clinical Practice.* 2020;35(2):178–195. doi: https:// doi.org/10.1002/ncp.10474.

44. Consedine NS, Krivoshekova YS, Harris CR. Bodily embarrassment and judgment concern as separable factors in the

measurement of medical embarrassment: psychometric development and links to treatment-seeking outcomes. *British Journal of Health Psychology.* 2007;12(Pt 3):439–462. doi: 10.1348/135910706X118747.

45. Cachelin FM, Rebeck R, Veisel C, Striegel-Moore RH. Barriers to treatment for eating disorders among ethnically diverse women. *International Journal of Eating Disorders.* 2001;30(3):269–278. doi: 10.1002/eat.1084.

46. Foran AM, O'Donnell AT, Muldoon OT. Stigma of eating disorders and recovery-related outcomes: a systematic review. *European Eating Disorders Review.* 2020;28(4):385–397. doi: 10.1002/erv.2735.

47. Nechita DM, Bud S, David D. Shame and eating disorders symptoms: a meta-analysis. *International Journal of Eating Disorders.* 2021;54(11):1899–1945. doi: 10.1002/eat.23583.

48. Dahlenburg SC, Gleaves DH, Hutchinson AD. Anorexia nervosa and perfectionism: a meta-analysis. *International Journal of Eating Disorders.* 2019;52(3):219–229. doi: 10.1002/eat.23009.

49. Woolrich RA, Cooper MJ, Turner HM. A preliminary study of negative self-beliefs in anorexia nervosa: a detailed exploration of their content, origins and functional links to "not eating enough" and other characteristic behaviors. *Cognitive Therapy and Research.* 2006;30 (6):735–748. doi: 10.1007/s10608-006-9024-y.

50. Klein EM, Benecke C, Kasinger C, Brahler E, Ehrenthal JC, Strauss B, et al. Eating disorder psychopathology: the role of attachment anxiety, attachment avoidance, and personality functioning. *Journal of Psychosomatic Research.* 2022;160:110975. doi: 10.1016/j.jpsychores.2022.110975.

51. McAdams CJ, Efseroff B, McCoy J, Ford L, Timko CA. Social processing in eating disorders: neuroimaging paradigms and research domain organizational constructs. *Current Psychiatry Reports.*

2022;24(12):777–788. doi: 10.1007/s11920-022-01395-4.

52. Clinton D, Björck C, Sohlberg S, Norring C. Patient satisfaction with treatment in eating disorders: cause for complacency or concern? *European Eating Disorders Review.* 2004;12(4):240–246. doi: https://doi.org/10.1002/erv.582.

53. Heruc G, Hurst K, Casey A, Fleming K, Freeman J, Fursland A, et al. ANZAED eating disorder treatment principles and general clinical practice and training standards. *Journal of Eating Disorders.* 2020;8(1):63. doi: 10.1186/s40337-020-00341-0.

54. Haynos AF, Snipes C, Guarda A, Mayer LE, Attia E. Comparison of standardized versus individualized caloric prescriptions in the nutritional rehabilitation of inpatients with anorexia nervosa. *International Journal of Eating Disorders.* 2016;49(1):50–58. doi: 10.1002/eat.22469.

55. McNamara N, Parsons H. "Everyone here wants everyone else to get better": the role of social identity in eating disorder recovery. *British Journal of Social Psychology.* 2016;55(4):662–680. doi: 10.1111/bjso.12161.

56. de Vos JA, LaMarre A, Radstaak M, Bijkerk CA, Bohlmeijer ET, Westerhof GJ. Identifying fundamental criteria for eating disorder recovery: a systematic review and qualitative meta-analysis. *Journal of Eating Disorders.* 2017;5:34. doi: 10.1186/s40337-017-0164-0.

57. Atti AR, Mastellari T, Valente S, Speciani M, Panariello F, De Ronchi D. Compulsory treatments in eating disorders: a systematic review and meta-analysis. *Eating and Weight Disorders.* 2021;26(4):1037–1048. doi: 10.1007/s40519-020-01031-1.

58. Davis L, Walsh BT, Schebendach J, Glasofer DR, Steinglass JE. Habits are stronger with longer duration of illness and greater severity in anorexia nervosa. *International Journal of Eating Disorders.* 2020;53 (5):413–419. doi: 10.1002/eat.23265.

59. Lam RW, Levitt AJ, Levitan RD, Michalak EE, Cheung AH, Morehouse R, et al.

Efficacy of bright light treatment, fluoxetine, and the combination in patients with nonseasonal major depressive disorder: a randomized clinical trial. *JAMA Psychiatry.* 2016;73(1):56–63. doi: 10.1001/jamapsychiatry.2015.2235.

60. Levitan RD, Levitt AJ, Michalak EE, Morehouse R, Ramasubbu R, Yatham LN, et al. Appetitive symptoms differentially predict treatment response to fluoxetine, light, and placebo in nonseasonal major depression. *Journal of Clinical Psychiatry.* 2018;79(4). doi: 10.4088/JCP.17m11856.

61. Beauchamp MT, Lundgren JD. A systematic review of bright light therapy for eating disorders. *Primary Care Companion for CNS Disorders.* 2016;18(5). doi: 10.4088/PCC.16r02008.

62. Romo-Nava F, Guerdjikova AI, Mori NN, Scheer F, Burgess HJ, McNamara RK, et al. A matter of time: a systematic scoping review on a potential role of the circadian system in binge eating behavior. *Frontiers of Nutrition.* 2022;9:978412. doi: 10.3389/fnut.2022.978412.

63. Datta N, Matheson BE, Citron K, Van Wye EM, Lock JD. Evidence based update on psychosocial treatments for eating disorders in children and adolescents. *Journal of Clinical Child and Adolescent Psychology.* 2023;52(2):159–170. doi: 10.1080/15374416.2022.2109650.

64. Jewell T, Blessitt E, Stewart C, Simic M, Eisler I. Family therapy for child and adolescent eating disorders: a critical review. *Family Process.* 2016;55 (3):577–594. doi: 10.1111/famp.12242.

65. Van Wye E, Matheson B, Citron K, Yang HJ, Datta N, Bohon C, et al. Protocol for a randomized clinical trial for avoidant restrictive food intake disorder (ARFID) in low-weight youth. Contemporary Clinical Trials. 2023;124:107036. doi: 10.1016/j.cct.2022.107036.

66. Lock J, Robinson A, Sadeh-Sharvit S, Rosania K, Osipov L, Kirz N, et al. Applying family-based treatment (FBT) to three clinical presentations of avoidant/restrictive food intake disorder: Similarities and differences from FBT for anorexia nervosa. *International Journal of*

Eating Disorders. 2019;52(4):439–446. doi: https://doi.org/10.1002/eat.22994.

67. Spettigue W, Norris ML, Santos A, Obeid N. Treatment of children and adolescents with avoidant/restrictive food intake disorder: a case series examining the feasibility of family therapy and adjunctive treatments. *Journal of Eating Disorders.* 2018;6:20. doi: 10.1186/s40337-018-0205-3.

68. Atwood ME, Friedman A. A systematic review of enhanced cognitive behavioral therapy (CBT-E) for eating disorders. *International Journal of Eating Disorders.* 2020;53(3):311–330. doi: 10.1002/eat.23206.

69. Kaidesoja M, Cooper Z, Fordham B. Cognitive behavioral therapy for eating disorders: a map of the systematic review evidence base. *International Journal of Eating Disorders.* 2023;56(2):295–313. doi: 10.1002/eat.23831.

70. Bell C, Waller G, Shafran R, Delgadillo J. Is there an optimal length of psychological treatment for eating disorder pathology? *International Journal of Eating Disorders.* 2017;50(6):687–692. doi: 10.1002/eat.22660.

71. Brigham KS, Manzo LD, Eddy KT, Thomas JJ. Evaluation and treatment of avoidant/restrictive food intake disorder (ARFID) in adolescents. *Current Pediatric Reports.* 2018;6(2):107–113. doi: 10.1007/s40124-018-0162-y.

72. Hay P. A systematic review of evidence for psychological treatments in eating disorders: 2005-2012. *International Journal of Eating Disorders.* 2013;46 (5):462–469. doi: 10.1002/eat.22103.

73. Zeeck A, Herpertz-Dahlmann B, Friederich HC, Brockmeyer T, Resmark G, Hagenah U, et al. Psychotherapeutic treatment for anorexia nervosa: a systematic review and network meta-analysis. *Frontiers in Psychiatry.* 2018;9:158. doi: 10.3389/fpsyt.2018.00158.

74. Svaldi J, Schmitz F, Baur J, Hartmann AS, Legenbauer T, Thaler C, et al. Efficacy of psychotherapies and pharmacotherapies

for bulimia nervosa. *Psychological Medicine.* 2019;49(6):898–910. doi: 10 .1017/S0033291718003525.

75. Hilbert A, Petroff D, Herpertz S, Pietrowsky R, Tuschen-Caffier B, Vocks S, et al. Meta-analysis of the efficacy of psychological and medical treatments for binge-eating disorder. *Journal of Consulting and Clinical Psychology.* 2019;87(1):91–105. doi: 10.1037/ ccp0000358.

76. Steinberg D, Perry T, Freestone D, Bohon C, Baker JH, Parks E. Effectiveness of delivering evidence-based eating disorder treatment via telemedicine for children, adolescents, and youth. *Eating Disorders.* 2023;31(1):85–101. doi: 10.1080/ 10640266.2022.2076334.

77. Kaye WH, Wagner A, Fudge JL, Paulus M. Neurocircuity of eating disorders. *Current Topics in Behavioral Neurosciences.* 2011;6:37–57. doi: 10 .1007/7854_2010_85.

78. Attia E, Kaplan AS, Walsh BT, Gershkovich M, Yilmaz Z, Musante D, et al. Olanzapine versus placebo for out-patients with anorexia nervosa. *Psychological Medicine.* 2011;41 (10):2177–2182. doi: S0033291711000390 [pii] 10.1017/S0033291711000390.

79. Brambilla F, Garcia CS, Fassino S, Daga GA, Favaro A, Santonastaso P, et al. Olanzapine therapy in anorexia nervosa: psychobiological effects *International Clinical Psychopharmacology.* 2007;22 (4):197–204. doi: 10.1097/YIC .0b013e328080ca31.

80. Brambilla F, Monteleone P, Maj M. Olanzapine-induced weight gain in anorexia nervosa: involvement of leptin and ghrelin secretion? *Psychoneuroendocrinology.* 2007;32 (4):402–406. doi: 10.1016/j.psyneuen .2007.02.005.

81. Kafantaris V, Leigh E, Hertz S, Berest A, Schebendach J, Sterling WM, et al. A placebo-controlled pilot study of adjunctive olanzapine for adolescents with anorexia nervosa. *Journal of Child Adolescent Psychopharmacology.* 2011;21 (3):207–212. doi: 10.1089/cap.2010.0139.

82. Frank GK, Shott ME, Hagman JO, Schiel MA, DeGuzman MC, Rossi B. The partial dopamine D2 receptor agonist aripiprazole is associated with weight gain in adolescent anorexia nervosa. *International Journal of Eating Disorders.* 2017;50(4):447–450. doi: 10.1002/eat .22704.

83. Shapiro JR, Berkman ND, Brownley KA, Sedway JA, Lohr KN, Bulik CM. Bulimia nervosa treatment: a systematic review of randomized controlled trials. *International Journal of Eating Disorders.* 2007;40 (4):321–336. doi: 10.1002/eat.20372.

84. McElroy SL, Hudson J, Ferreira-Cornwell MC, Radewonuk J, Whitaker T, Gasior M. Lisdexamfetamine dimesylate for adults with moderate to severe binge eating disorder: results of two pivotal phase 3 randomized controlled trials. *Neuropsychopharmacology.* 2016;41 (5):1251–1260. doi: 10.1038/npp.2015.275.

85. Peat CM, Berkman ND, Lohr KN, Brownley KA, Bann CM, Cullen K, et al. Comparative effectiveness of treatments for binge-eating disorder: systematic review and network meta-analysis. *European Eating Disorders Review.* 2017;25(5):317–328. doi: 10.1002/erv .2517.

86. Stancil SL, Adelman W, Dietz A, Abdel-Rahman S. Naltrexone reduces binge eating and purging in adolescents in an eating disorder program. *Journal of Child and Adolescent Psychopharmacology.* 2019;29(9):721–724. doi: 10.1089/cap .2019.0056.

87. Guerdjikova AI, Walsh B, Shan K, Halseth AE, Dunayevich E, McElroy SL. Concurrent improvement in both binge eating and depressive symptoms with naltrexone/bupropion therapy in overweight or obese subjects with major depressive disorder in an open-label, uncontrolled study. *Advances in Therapy.* 2017;34(10):2307–2315. doi: 10.1007/ s12325-017-0613-9.

Chapter 26

Alcohol Use Disorder

Michael Weaver and Heather Webber

26.1 Introduction

Alcohol use disorder (AUD) is a prevalent medical condition characterized by the continuation of alcohol use despite negative consequences. AUD affects almost 15 million people over the age of 12 per year in the United States. Some of the major long-term negative health consequences of drinking alcohol include digestive problems, heart disease, stroke, liver disease, and cancer. Drinking alcohol can also result in emergency department visits for injuries or alcohol poisoning/overdose. In addition to these physical health consequences, AUD can have a negative impact on occupational performance, social relationships, and mental health. The good news is, there are guidelines to help health care providers identify who may be at risk to develop and who may be suffering from an AUD, and there are many evidence-based treatment options. In this chapter, we will outline the best practices for diagnosis, withdrawal management, long-term pharmacotherapy options, and resources for patients.

26.2 Diagnosis

Asking about alcohol use is important because alcohol use is related to health issues. Screening for alcohol use can help reduce alcohol intake, identify those at risk, and aid in preventing serious drinking problems. Drinking alcohol is incredibly common, so it is important to determine when someone's drinking is or may become problematic. During the screening, make the patient feel comfortable with discussing their alcohol use. You can start by stating that you screen everyone or that screening is a part of your standard procedures. Often, if someone's drinking is problematic, they may feel guilty or annoyed when asked about it. You can start with something like, "It is common for people to drink a 6-pack per day." This may make the patient more comfortable to disclose the real quantity and frequency of their own drinking.

Before screening for AUD, it is important to understand the criteria in the Diagnostic and Statistical Manual of Mental Disorders, 5th edition (DSM-5) and common definitions of problematic alcohol use. The DSM-5 criteria focus mostly on consequences related to drinking, inability to control drinking, craving, and withdrawal symptoms. Patients are diagnosed with a mild AUD if they report two to three symptoms, moderate if they report four to five symptoms, and severe if they report six or more. The Centers for Disease Control and Prevention (CDC) defines heavy drinking as 15 or more drinks per week for men and 8 or more drinks per week for women. Heavy drinking is a risk factor for experiencing alcohol-related problems.

You should also know the definition of a standard drink and be able to convert your patient's answers into standard drink form. For example, a 12-oz container of beer is considered to be one standard drink, but only up to 7% alcohol by volume. Also, bars tend to sell beer in pints, which are 16 oz rather than 12. Because of these nuances, people tend to misreport how much they are actually drinking. For more information on standard drink examples, see the National Institute on Alcohol Abuse and Alcoholism (NIAAA) standard drink guide: https://pubs.niaaa.nih.gov/publications/practitioner/PocketGuide/pocket_guide2.htm.

Understandably, many physicians will not have time to conduct a full clinical interview with their patients. The NIAAA has proposed a workflow for screening, brief intervention, and referral to treatment (SBIRT). The contents of the workflow have been reproduced in Figure 26.1.

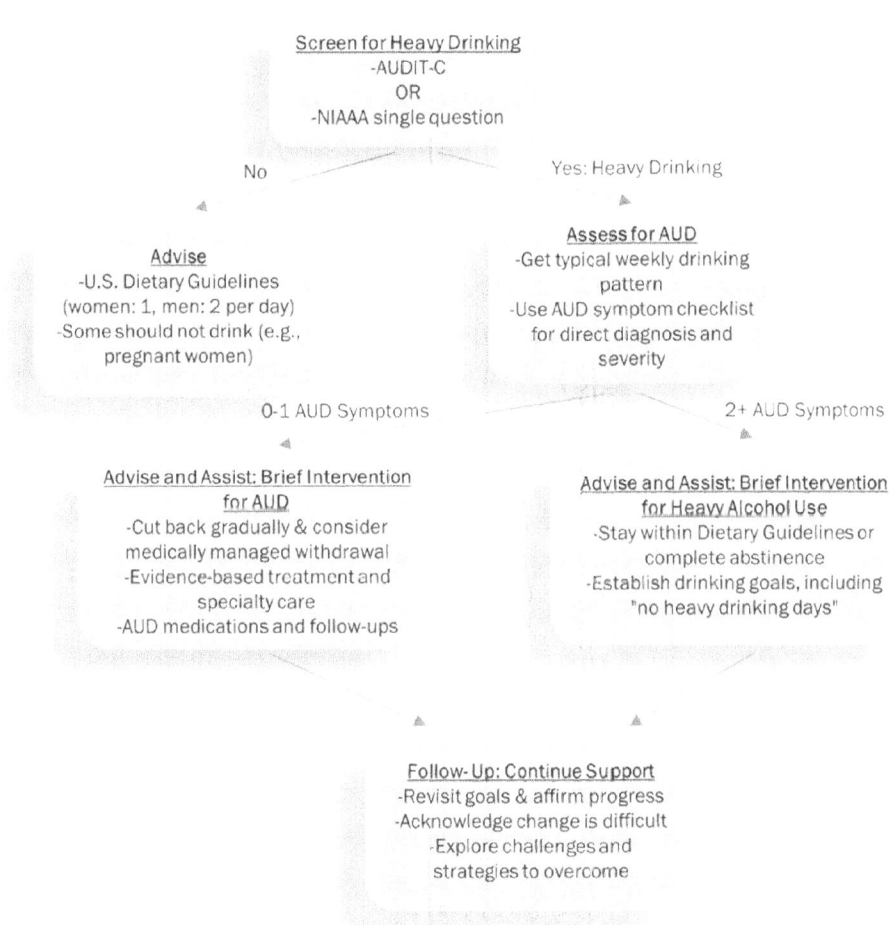

Figure 26.1 Screening, brief intervention, and referral to treatment workflow from NIAAA.

First, screen for heavy alcohol use using the AUDIT-C [1] or the NIAAA single screening question – "How many times in the past year have you had X or more drinks in a day?," where X = 4+ for women and 5+ for men. If the patient answers with 1+ days, then it is a positive test for heavy alcohol use and should be followed up with more questions regarding quantity and frequency in a typical week. In order to diagnose AUD or identify the severity of the patient's drinking problems, use the Alcohol Symptom Checklist [2] or a similar instrument. Note that other screening tools may be more useful for certain populations (adolescents or pregnant women), and resources for these can be found on the NIAAA website.

If the patient screens negative for heavy alcohol use, then provide information that can help prevent an escalation in drinking. The US Dietary Guidelines state that women should not have more than one drink per day and that men should not have more than two drinks per day. If the patient screens positive for heavy drinking or AUD, help them recognize the issue and recommend reducing their drinking gradually or consider medically managed withdrawal treatment. Not everyone will be ready to commit to making a change. This is a common response. In this case, inform the patient of alcohol's health risks, encourage thought and conversation concerning the pros and cons of drinking, and reiterate your willingness to help if they want it [3].

You may also have patients who are ready to consider getting help with reducing their alcohol use. Evidence shows that history taking alone can be therapeutic, so your interview has already started their recovery processes. Brief interventions (5- to 15-minute sessions during routine visits) can be used to help the patient start working on reducing their drinking or to motivate the patient to engage with more treatment. During brief interventions, you will work with the patient to help identify reasons for reducing their alcohol use. You can do this by linking their drinking with health problems or with other consequences they've experienced from drinking (e.g., not spending as much time with family). With the patient, you can help identify pros and cons of drinking. For example, some people may perceive that alcohol reduces their stress, and in response to this you can suggest that reducing alcohol use could actually make them feel and function better, thus reducing stress. Continue to offer your support and help identify a plan for change. Always follow up with the patient at the next visit to determine if any changes have been made and if any new strategies can be useful. See Table 26.1 for solutions for common pitfalls that can occur with AUD diagnosis and management.

26.3 Withdrawal Management

Patients may develop an acute alcohol withdrawal syndrome when chronic alcohol use is interrupted. Acute withdrawal is most safely managed in an inpatient setting if the patient has been drinking heavily, has a history of seizures or delirium tremens, or has unstable comorbid medical or psychiatric problems. Up to 20% of patients develop delirium tremens if left untreated. Recognition and effective treatment of alcohol withdrawal are important to prevent excess mortality due to complications.

Even when patients acknowledge heavy drinking, they often underestimate the amount, which may be due to minimization or because alcohol is an amnestic agent and drinkers quickly lose count of how much they have had to drink. There is significant individual variability in the threshold at which a patient may develop withdrawal, and

Table 26.1 AUD management pitfalls to avoid

Common Mistake	How to Avoid
"The patient didn't look like an alcoholic."	Screen for alcohol use.
"The patient said he was just a social drinker."	Obtain adequate history of alcohol consumption or previous alcohol withdrawal syndrome (AWS).
"He was still drunk when he came in."	Patients can develop AWS before or after their blood alcohol concentration is zero.
"I was too busy to check on that alcoholic patient."	Use standardized protocols with nurse autonomy to save time to initiate treatment with cross-tolerant medication for AWS.
"I didn't know her liver was that bad."	Avoid giving benzodiazepines with multiple metabolites to patients with hepatic impairment.
"I didn't think the patient would need to go to the ICU."	Know when to escalate level of care to a step-down or intensive care unit (ICU) for worsening AWS.
"I gave him phenytoin, but he had another seizure."	Use benzodiazepines or phenobarbital for AWS-related seizures, not other anticonvulsants.
"Her alcohol withdrawal is better, but she is still confused."	Give thiamine for Wernicke's encephalopathy.
"She doesn't drink much, but she takes a lot of sleeping pills."	Take use of sedatives into account (prescribed/illicit benzodiazepines, z-drugs), which can also cause withdrawal.
"This is the fourth time we've treated him for alcohol withdrawal."	Link to community resources for treatment of AUD to help prevent recidivism.

those who drink a majority of days out of a week are more likely to develop withdrawal due to tolerance. Not all daily drinkers will develop withdrawal, but it is difficult to predict who will and who will not. The best predictor of whether a patient will develop acute withdrawal is a past history of alcohol withdrawal.

The alcohol withdrawal syndrome has two phases, early and late. The signs and symptoms of early withdrawal usually develop within 48 hours of the last drink. The initial indication is elevation of vital signs (heart rate, blood pressure, temperature). Tremors develop next, first a fine tremor of the hands and fasciculation of the tongue, sometimes followed by gross tremors of the extremities. Disorientation and mild hallucinations (often auditory, occasionally visual) may develop as the syndrome progresses, accompanied by diaphoresis. Seizures are an early sign of alcohol withdrawal and may be the presenting symptom. Late alcohol withdrawal is also known as delirium tremens ("the DTs") and consists of worsening autonomic dysregulation that is responsible for much of the morbidity and mortality attributed to alcohol withdrawal. It begins after early withdrawal, usually 72 hours or more after the last drink, and peaks around 5 days. Some patients do not progress from early to late withdrawal, and the symptoms simply subside after a few days with or without treatment, but it is impossible to predict which patients will progress. The signs of late withdrawal consist of worsening diaphoresis, nausea and vomiting (which may result in aspiration pneumonia), delirium with frank hallucinations, and rapid, severe fluctuation in vital signs. Sudden changes in blood pressure and heart rate may result in complications such as myocardial infarction or a cerebrovascular event, and increased QT variability elevates the risk for serious cardiac arrhythmias. Hyperthermia is also associated with higher mortality. Progression to late withdrawal results in significant morbidity and even death, but adequate treatment of early withdrawal helps prevent progression to late withdrawal.

The revised Clinical Institute Withdrawal Assessment for Alcohol (CIWA-Ar) is commonly used to assess severity of withdrawal [4]. Regular assessment should continue until the withdrawal syndrome has come under control (CIWA-Ar score <6) for at least 24 hours. If no withdrawal signs have manifested after 48 hours, then it is usually safe to discontinue monitoring for withdrawal. Standardized algorithms with frequent assessment for signs of withdrawal also facilitate efficient treatment of patients at risk for withdrawal [5].

Pharmacotherapy is indicated for management of moderate to severe withdrawal, and any cross-tolerant medication may be used. It is inappropriate to give beverage alcohol to prevent or treat alcohol withdrawal. Both benzodiazepines and barbiturates effectively treat alcohol withdrawal.

Severe withdrawal (delirium tremens), manifested by abnormal and fluctuating vital signs with delirium, should be treated aggressively in an intensive care environment with sufficiently large doses of medication to suppress the withdrawal [6]. Medications with a rapid onset of action should be used intravenously for immediate effect. Lorazepam and diazepam have a rapid onset of action when given intravenously, although the duration of action is shorter than when given orally. For example, give lorazepam 1–4 mg every 10–30 minutes until the patient is calm but awake and the heart rate is <120 bpm. A continuous intravenous infusion may be warranted to control withdrawal symptoms, and the infusion rate can be titrated to the desired level of consciousness. After stabilization, the patient can be changed to an equivalent dose of a long-acting sedative-hypnotic and tapered.

No specific benzodiazepine is superior to any other for alcohol withdrawal treatment, although longer-acting benzodiazepines may allow for a smoother withdrawal course. Severe alcohol withdrawal refractory to high-dose benzodiazepines has been treated successfully with the addition of phenobarbital or propofol.

26.4 Long-Term Pharmacotherapy

There are several options for pharmacologic treatment of AUD. While inherently effective, medications for AUD are typically part of a larger treatment plan. When prescribing medications, it is best to instruct patients to consider taking them in combination with some other type of treatment (e.g., psychotherapy or Alcoholics Anonymous). Unfortunately, despite great promise, medications for treating AUD are underprescribed. Significant treatment barriers include compliance concerns, pricing, and apprehensions from providers concerning the efficacy of medications [3]. See Table 26.2 for a summary of pharmacotherapy options.

26.4.1 Naltrexone (Oral – ReVia, Injectable – Vivitrol)

The US Food and Drug Administration (FDA) approved oral naltrexone to treat AUD in 1994. Naltrexone works by blocking opioid receptors, which are responsible for the

Table 26.2 Pharmacotherapy options for AUD

Medication	Route of Administration	FDA-approved Dose	Common Side Effects
Naltrexone	Oral	50 mg daily	Somnolence, nausea, vomiting, decreased appetite, abdominal pain, insomnia, dizziness
Extended-Release Naltrexone	Intramuscular	380 mg monthly	Same as oral Naltrexone plus injection site reactions
Acamprosate	Oral	666 mg three times daily	Diarrhea
Disulfiram	Oral	250–500 mg daily	Drowsiness

Information partially taken from Kranzler and Soyka 2018 [10].

pleasurable effects of alcohol. Naltrexone does not cause a bad reaction to alcohol – it just makes drinking less "fun." It also reduces cravings and thoughts about drinking. Naltrexone is taken orally as one 50-mg dose per day. The side effect profile is favorable, with the only common side effect being nausea. Pairing the dose with meals can help. Naltrexone has the potential to worsen liver damage and cannot be taken if prescription opioids are needed for acute or chronic pain.

In 2006, the FDA approved an extended-release, intramuscular (IM) version of naltrexone for the treatment of AUD (Vivitrol). This is given monthly in the clinic as a 380-mg dose injected into the upper outer quadrant of the buttock. While there can be injection site problems, it is generally well tolerated by patients. It may help increase compliance, helps maintain a good serum level over time, and has an overall lower dose than the oral version, which can be helpful for preventing liver damage. It does not come in generic form, so one major setback of IM naltrexone is the pricing. While it is covered by insurance, each dose is about $1,200. Both forms of naltrexone should be taken for at least 6 months, which can be extended for another 3–6 months. Meta-analyses have shown that both routes of administration for naltrexone are effective at reducing the number of heavy drinking days [7]; however, a direct comparison between the two medications is still needed.

26.4.2 Acamprosate (Campral)

Acamprosate was approved by the FDA in 2004. The mechanism underlying acamprosate's effects are not well understood, but it is hypothesized that it might act as a partial co-agonist on NMDA (glutamate) receptors. Acamprosate primarily works by reducing cravings and other symptoms associated with protracted abstinence (e.g., sleep, anxiety). There are minimal side effects to acamprosate, including the potential for loose stool. Interestingly, the effects of acamprosate appear to be sustained at least for a whole additional year if prescribed for 12 months and then stopped. Acamprosate has some drawbacks – it does not treat withdrawal symptoms and has a larger dosing burden. It is prescribed as two large 333-mg pills three times a day. Meta-analyses have shown that acamprosate is best at helping maintain abstinence, an effect that is larger after a longer detoxification time [8].

26.4.3 Disulfiram (Antabuse)

The first medication approved by the FDA was disulfiram (Antabuse) in 1951. When taken in combination with alcohol, disulfiram leads to increased concentration of acetaldehyde. This interaction causes a very unpleasant reaction to alcohol, including flushing, heart palpitations, chest tightness, nausea, headache, and anxiety – a reaction that has been described as feeling similar to a heart attack. Importantly, even very small amounts of alcohol can cause the reaction, so patients should be warned to look out for over-the-counter medications and other preparations that might contain alcohol (e.g., cough syrup or mouthwash). Disulfiram can be helpful with avoiding slips or relapse by conditioning patients to avoid the unpleasant reaction, but it does not help with reducing cravings or initiation of abstinence. Disulfiram can affect the liver, can worsen psychotic symptoms, and is contraindicated for people with heart disease. For these reasons, disulfiram is not prescribed commonly and is not considered a primary medication for AUD. However, disulfiram can be helpful for those who have not had success with other medications and in situations where dosing can be monitored. It is taken orally once daily (500 mg, or 250 mg for those with liver disease) and will wear off within a few days.

26.4.4 Anticonvulsants (Off-Label Options)

Anticonvulsants are also promising options for the treatment of AUD. Anticonvulsants are generally well tolerated, lack abuse potential, and are already prescribed for multiple other indications (e.g., seizures, pain, anxiety). They are also useful for mild-to-moderate alcohol withdrawal syndrome, unlike the FDA-approved options described earlier. Two examples of anticonvulsants that show promise for treating AUD include gabapentin and topiramate. Gabapentin potentiates gamma amino butyric acid (GABA) through its interaction with voltage-sensitive calcium channels and potassium channels. It is taken two to three times a day with a wide dosing range that can be started low and worked up to a maximum dose of 3,600 mg in 24 hours. The main side effect with gabapentin is sedation. Topiramate enhances GABA by binding to the $GABA_A$ receptor. While the side effects are relatively mild, transient cognitive impairment, including word-finding, can occur. Both have been shown to decrease the percentage of heavy drinking days [9].

26.5 Resources for Patients

Alcoholics Anonymous (AA) is a fellowship of men and women who share their experiences, strength, and hope with each other to solve their common problem and help others recover from AUD. The only requirement for membership is a desire to stop drinking; the primary purpose is to stay sober and help others achieve sobriety. There are no dues or fees for membership, and AA is not affiliated with any religion, politics, or organization. There are 12 consecutive activities, or steps, to achieve during the recovery process. Alcoholics Anonymous produces positive outcomes in many members, and patients can become involved with AA before, during, after, or instead of professional treatment. The approach of AA often results in development of coping skills similar to those taught in structured psychosocial treatment settings, which leads to reductions in alcohol consumption [11]. Physicians who identify patients with alcohol problems can recommend that patients attend AA meetings and provide local contact information to patients. Attending one meeting per week, on average, appears to be the minimum threshold to realize benefit, and higher meeting frequency is associated with progressively greater rates of abstinence.

Research has tried to pinpoint the means by which AA works. The key ingredients appear to be helping people make positive changes in their social networks (e.g., disassociating themselves from heavy drinkers and increasing ties with abstainers/low-risk drinkers) and enhancing coping skills and self-efficacy for abstinence when encountering high-risk social situations [12].

Some people will not go to AA meetings, perhaps because of the religious-sounding ideology or some other aspect of the culture that rubs them the wrong way. There are several alternative mutual support groups that may appeal to those who are not interested in AA. Self-Management and Recovery Training (SMART Recovery) is a four-point program that emphasizes cognitive behavioral techniques. See their website at www.smartrecovery.org.

Secular Organization for Sobriety (SOS) is a mutual-help organization without the religious overtones of AA. Instead of 12 steps there are 9 principles, although there is some overlap with the Twelve Steps and Twelve Traditions of AA. More information can be found at www.sossobriety.org.

Al-Anon is a meeting to support family members (or anyone who cares about a person with an alcohol problem) of someone with AUD. Like AA, these meetings are free and open to the public, and are often held in the same building as AA meetings. Family members will learn how to be helpful for loved ones with AUD without enabling their behavior. Research has shown sustained attendance at Al-Anon benefits families through improved quality of life, increased self-esteem, and decreased depression [13]. Ask families if they are familiar with Al-Anon and encourage attendance. Even if the patient with AUD is not interested in recovery, these meetings are helpful.

References

1. D. A. Dawson, B. F. Grant, F. S. Stinson, Y. Zhou. Effectiveness of the derived Alcohol Use Disorders Identification Test (AUDIT-C) in screening for alcohol use disorders and risk drinking in the US general population. *Alcohol: Clin Exp Res* 2005; **29**: 844–854.

2. K. A. Hallgren, T. E. Matson, M. Oliver, K. Witkiewitz, J. F. Bobb, A. K. Lee, R. M. Caldeiro, D. Kivlahan, K. A. Bradley. Practical assessment of alcohol use disorder in routine primary care: performance of an alcohol symptom checklist. *J Gen Intern Med* 2022; **37**: 1885–1893.

3. J. Knox, D. S. Hasin, F. R. Larson, H. R. Kranzler. Prevention, screening, and treatment for heavy drinking and alcohol use disorder. *Lancet Psychiat* 2019; **6**: 1054–1067.

4. J. T. Sullivan, K. Sykora, J. Schneiderman, et al. Assessment of alcohol withdrawal: the revised clinical institute withdrawal assessment for alcohol scale (CIWA-Ar). *Br J Addict* 1989; **84**: 1353–1357.

5. C. D. Lansford, C. H. Guerriero, M. J. Kocan, et al. Improved outcomes in patients with head and neck cancer using a standardized care protocol for postoperative alcohol withdrawal. *Arch Otolaryngol Head Neck Surg* 2008; **134**: 865–872.

6. M. F. Weaver. Dealing with the DTs: managing alcohol withdrawal in

hospitalized patients. *The Hospitalist* 2007; **11**: 22–25.

7. C. E. Murphy, R. C. Wang, J. C. Montoy, E. Whittaker, M. Raven. Effect of extended-release naltrexone on alcohol consumption: a systematic review and meta-analysis. *Addiction* 2022; **117**: 271–281.

8. N. C. Maisel, J. C. Blodgett, P. L. Wilbourne, K. Humphreys, J. W. Finney. Meta-analysis of naltrexone and acamprosate for treating alcohol use disorders: when are these medications most helpful?. *Addiction* 2013; **108**: 275–293.

9. C. J. Hammond, M. J. Niciu, S. Drew, A. J. Arias. Anticonvulsants for the treatment of alcohol withdrawal syndrome and alcohol use disorders. *CNS Drugs* 2015; **29**: 293–311.

10. H. R. Kranzler, M. Soyka. Diagnosis and pharmacotherapy of alcohol use disorder: a review. *JAMA* 2018; **320**: 815–824.

11. J. Morgenstern, E. Labouvie, B. S. McCrady, et al. Affiliation with Alcoholics Anonymous after treatment: a study of its therapeutic effects and mechanisms of action. *J Consult Clin Psychol* 1997; **65**: 768–777.

12. J. F. Kelly, R. L. Stout, M. Magill, et al. The role of Alcoholics Anonymous in mobilizing adaptive social network changes: a prospective lagged mediational analysis. *Drug Alcohol Depen* 2011; **114**: 119–126.

13. C. Timko, M. Halvorson, C. Kong, et al. Social processes explaining the benefits of Al-Anon participation. *Psychol Addict Behav* 2015; **29**: 856–863.

Other Substance Use Disorders

Thanh Thuy Truong

27.1 Introduction

Substance use disorders (SUD) present significant public health challenges. In 2021, the National Survey on Drug Use and Health (NSDUH) estimated that among people aged 12 and older, 57.8% used tobacco, alcohol, or an illicit drug in the past month – a marker of current use. Among these, 19.5% used a tobacco product and 14.3% used an illicit drug. The most-used illicit drug was marijuana, with 18.7% (52.5 million people) using it in the past year, highest among young adults aged 18–25, followed by adults >26 years old, then adolescents. The percentage of people aged 12 or older meeting criteria for SUD was 25.6% of people ages 18–25, 16.1% of people age 26 or older, and 8.5% of adolescents ages 12–17 [1]. Overdose death rates remain high with the rise of illicit synthetic opioids such as fentanyl [2].

27.2 Screening

A medical evaluation should always include a screening for substance use. Substance intoxication and withdrawal often induce physiologic and psychiatric symptoms that can make it challenging to establish a diagnosis. In the clinic, using the single question, "How many times in the past year have you used an illegal drug or used a prescription medication for nonmedical reasons?" is a sensitive screen for drug use. A response of at least one time is positive for unhealthy drug use [3]. A positive screen prompts a more comprehensive assessment to determine current impact of use on the person's life and the presence of a SUD.

27.3 Diagnosis of a Substance Use Disorder

Substance use alone is not sufficient for a diagnosis of SUD. Rather, SUD is diagnosed based on 11 criteria in the DSM-5 [4]. The person must demonstrate a pattern of substance use that causes significant impairment or distress, meeting at least two criteria within a 12-month period. The criteria can be grouped into three main categories:

Loss of Control

1. Substance is often taken in larger amounts or over a longer period than was intended
2. Persistent desire or unsuccessful efforts to cut down or control use
3. Craving or strong desire or urge to use
4. Recurrent use in physically hazardous situations
5. Continued use despite knowledge of persistent psychological or physical problems caused or exacerbated by the substance

Adverse Consequences

6. A great deal of time is spent to obtain, use, or recover from the substance's effects
7. Continued use despite recurrent social or interpersonal problems
8. Use resulting in a failure to fulfill major role obligations at work, school, or home
9. Important social, occupational, or recreational activities are reduced or given up

Physiological Dependence

(Note that tolerance and withdrawal to a prescribed medicine do not count toward diagnosis of SUD.)

10. Tolerance
11. Withdrawal

SUD severity is based on the number of criteria met: 2–3 = mild, 4–5 = moderate, 6 or more = severe. Early remission is not meeting any criteria (except for craving) for at least 3 months, and sustained remission is not meeting criteria for 12 months.

27.3.1 Drug Testing

Toxicology screening is an important component of the diagnostic evaluation but not sufficient to diagnose a SUD. Drug testing can be performed through various means, including urine, blood, hair, and saliva tests, as described in Table 27.1. The most used test is urine immunoassay for common substances. The clinician should be aware of potential false positives and limitation in detecting common synthetic substances. Table 27.2 summarizes information on urine toxicology screens. Toxicology screens are helpful tools to determine the pattern of use and potential risk of overdose, especially if the individual is combining multiple substances. They can also be used to monitor treatment progress and assess if the patient is taking a medication as prescribed. Many controlled medications have street value, thus clinicians prescribing controlled medications should routinely test for the presence of the drug in the patient's system. An example of a medication frequently diverted is buprenorphine, thus a qualitative test is preferred to assess appropriate use [5–7]. This example applies to commonly diverted controlled substances such as stimulants.

27.4 Neurobiology of Addiction

Many models have been proposed to identify brain structures involved in addictive processes (Table 27.3). Volkow identified four brain circuits involved in the development of addiction:

1. *Reward circuit* in the nucleus accumbens (NAc) and the ventral pallidum
2. *Motivation/drive circuit* in the orbitofrontal cortex (OFC) and the subcallosal area
3. *Memory and learning circuit* in the amygdala and the hippocampus
4. *Control circuit* in the prefrontal cortex (PFC) and the anterior cingulate gyrus (ACG)

Dopaminergic neurons directly innervate these circuits and connect directly and indirectly to other sites via glutamatergic projections. It is thought that in individuals with SUD, the rewarding experience of the drug is enhanced in the motivation/drive circuits. This enhancement is due to the higher reward of the drug, which increases DA in the NAc many times greater compared to natural reinforcers such as food and sex [8]. Recurrent

Table 27.1 Toxicology screens [23]

Test Type	Advantages	Disadvantages
Immunoassay, urine	• Rapid and widely accessible • Noninvasive	• Higher likelihood of false positives and negatives, urine tampering. • Shorter detection window compared to hair
GC-MS/LC-MS, urine	• High accuracy, often used for confirmation testing	• Often takes longer for results • Higher cost
Dipstick (POC)	• Rapid, cost effective	• Lower accuracy than other tests
Saliva	• Noninvasive • Can get observed testing • Quick results • Parent drug is usually present in higher concentrations compared to urine.	• Smoking, mouthwash, food may interfere with results • More expensive than urine analysis • Smaller detection windows compared to urine, hair, and sweat.
Hair	• Detects drug use in the past 3 month • May be considered in forensic settings, CPS cases	• Expensive • Cannot evaluate recent drug exposures • Results may be affected by certain hair treatments
Blood	• Harder to tamper/adulterate results • Helpful to test for biomarkers of alcohol use disorder such as: MCV, LFT, GGT, CDT20	• Shorter duration of detection

substance use leads to progressive structural and functional disruption in these brain regions. SUD development can be conceptualized as involving three stages [9]:

1. Binge/intoxication: positive reinforcement

   • *Neurocircuit*: NAc, ventral pallidum

2. Withdrawal/negative affect: loss of reward (negative reinforcement)

   • *Neurocircuit*: amygdala, habenula, and hypothalamus

3. Preoccupation/anticipation ("craving")

   • *Neurocircuit*: PFC, OFC, ACG

Drugs create short- and long-term changes in these systems to reinforce drug-seeking behavior. Table 27.4 summarizes common substances and their mechanism of action.

Table 27.2 Substances on the urine toxicology screen [23, 24]

Substance Class	Duration of Detection	False Positives	Notes
Amphetamines	1–3 days	Amantadine, Bupropion, Chlorpromazine, Despiramine, Trazodone, Labetalol, Promethazine, Pseudoephedrine	
Cannabis	Single use: 2–3 days Chronic heavy use: >30 days	PPIs, NSAID, efavirenz, hemp-containing foods	
Cocaine	2–5 days	Coca leaf tea	Detects benzoylecgonine
Barbiturates	Short-acting: 1–4 days Long acting: 3 weeks	NSAIDs, Phenytoin	Long acting (i.e., phenobarbital), may be used in some withdrawal regimens, and may be detected for up to weeks
Opioids	1–4 days	Diphenhydramine, poppy seeds, quinine, quinolones, rifampin, Dextromethorphan	Tests for morphine metabolites; does not detect synthetic opioids such as hydrocodone, oxycodone, buprenorphine, methadone, fentanyl
PCP	7–14 days	Dextromethorphan, diphenhydramine, ibuprofen, tramadol, venlafaxine	
Benzodiazepines	Short-acting: 3 days Long-acting: 30 days	Sertraline, Efavirenz, Oxaprozin	Tests for diazepam metabolites, thus may not detect clonazepam, lorazepam, and alprazolam

27.5 Management of Intoxication/Withdrawal

All clinicians will encounter patients going through intoxication and withdrawal of various substances, many times a combination of substances. These states increase the risk of danger to themselves and/or others and the likelihood of ongoing substance use or relapse. Patients who are experiencing severe psychiatric symptoms such as psychosis, mania, or

Table 27.3 Neurobiology of addictive processes

Circuit	Brain Regions	Description	Stage of SUD
Reward	Nucleus accumbens (NAc) Ventral pallidum/Ventral tegmental area	Reward and motivation Neurotransmitter: Dopamine	Binge/intoxication; Involves large surges of DA in NAc
Memory and learning	Amygdala	Processing emotions Neurotransmitter: serotonin, Dopamine, glutamate, GABA	Withdrawal/negative affect stage Involves recruitment of
	Hippocampus	Memory consolidation and recall Neurotransmitter: serotonin, dopamine, glutamate, GABA	brain stress systems when the substance is removed
	Thalamus	Relays information/ serotonin, dopamine, glutamate, GABA	
	Hypothalamus	Homeostasis Neurotransmitter: serotonin, dopamine, glutamate GABA	
Control	Prefrontal cortex (PFC) and the anterior cingulate cortex (ACG)	Executive function Neurotransmitter: dopamine, serotonin, norepinephrine	Preoccupation-anticipation stage Involves impulsivity and loss of executive control over substance use
Motivation/ drive	Orbitofrontal cortex (OFC) Subcallosal area	Regulates impulses Neurotransmitter: dopamine, serotonin	Preoccupation-anticipation stage Involved in compulsivity and impulsivity

suicidal ideation often need to be hospitalized if symptoms do not resolve in the emergency room. Even when the clinician strongly suspects substance intoxication or withdrawal to be the cause, patients at imminent danger to themselves or others should be offered hospitalization. If the patient lacks decision-making capacity and is at imminent risk, involuntary hospitalization should be considered. Table 27.5 summarizes presentations of common substances and management. Patients entering treatment during an intoxication or withdrawal should be assessed for the presence of SUD and referred to the appropriate SUD treatment. The American Society of Addiction Medicine (ASAM) Patient Placement Criteria can assist in determining level of care (i.e., inpatient, residential, or outpatient) [10]. In general, patients needing 24/7 medical management should be referred to an inpatient facility. A residential treatment program is best for patients needing a controlled environment due to a high risk of relapse or living in an unstable/unsafe environment. Outpatient is appropriate for patients who have insight into their condition, not at high risk of a complicated withdrawal, psychiatrically stable, and have good social support.

Table 27.4 Mechanism of action of common substances

Substance	Mechanism of Action
Nicotine	Agonist at nicotinic acetylcholine receptors, leading to the release of dopamine in the mesolimbic area, the corpus striatum, and the frontal cortex. Nicotine also modulates the activity of norepinephrine, acetylcholine, serotonin, GABA, glutamate, and endorphins
Cannabis (delta-9-tetrahydrocannabinol)	Acts on CB1 and CB2 receptors; CB1 is the main receptor found in the CNS, highest in the cerebellum, basal ganglia, hippocampus, and cerebral cortex. THC stimulates the DA release in the NAc and prefrontal cortex. CB2 receptors are mostly found in immune cells, where may regulate immune function and inflammation.
Cocaine	Blocks the reuptake of dopamine, serotonin, and norepinephrine
Amphetamines	Increases the release of dopamine and norepinephrine by inhibiting vesicular monoamine transport (VMAT) and blocks reuptake of these neurotransmitters
Opioids	Agonist at mu, delta, and kappa opioid receptors in the brain and periphery
PCP	Acts as a noncompetitive antagonist at the N-methyl-D-aspartate (NMDA) receptor
Benzodiazepines	Facilitates the binding of gamma-aminobutyric acid (GABA) to GABA receptors

27.6 Treatment

SUD recovery involves a complex matrix of psychotherapy, motivational interviewing, medications, psychosocial interventions, and peer recovery. Most patients with SUD do not believe they need treatment, and most do not seek treatment [1]. All clinicians will encounter the patient who is entering treatment mainly due to external pressures such as from family or work. The transtheoretical model outlines five main stages of change:

1. *Precontemplation* – The individual may have limited awareness of how the substance is negatively affecting their lives. They are not yet ready to change.
2. *Contemplation* – The individual is considering making a change but may feel ambivalent about taking action.
3. *Preparation* – The individual is preparing to take action. They may set goals, gather information, and make plans for change.
4. *Action* – The individual is actively making changes to their behavior.
5. *Maintenance* – The individual has successfully changed their behavior and is working to maintain their new habits.

Motivational interviewing is a collaborative process that elicits the person's own motivation for change [11]. Different techniques are used depending on the stage. For example, someone in the precontemplation stage may benefit from developing

Table 27.5 Management of substance intoxication and withdrawal

Substance	Intoxication	Withdrawal	Management
Tobacco/Nicotine	Euphoria, increased alertness, decreased appetite, weight loss, nausea, vomiting, dizziness, tremors, sweating, tachycardia, hypertension	Irritability, restlessness, and agitation, anxiety, depressed mood, difficulty concentrating, increased appetite, weight gain, insomnia, headaches, fatigue	**Intoxication:** most patients will only need supportive care. For nicotine poisoning, activated charcoal can be used. **Withdrawal:** Long-acting nicotine replacement products
Carnnabinoids	Altered mental status, conjunctival injection, nystagmus, tachycardia, slurred speech, ataxia, and appetite stimulation, delusions, hallucinations, paranoia	Irritability, restlessness, nervousness, insomnia, nightmares or vivid dreams, loss of appetite, depressed mood, tremor (mild), body temperature elevation (mild),	**Intoxication:** reassurance, rest in a quiet environment, supportive care. Benzodiazepines and antispychotics may be used for severe anxiety and psychosis, respectively. **Withdrawal:** supportive care, symptomatic treatment for insomnia, gabapentin 1,200 mg/day in divided doses has evidence for withdrawal and craving [25]
CNS depressants alcohol, barbiturates, benzodiazepines	Sedation, confusion, disorientation, slurred speech, ataxia, disinhibition, dizziness, impaired psychomotor performance, poor memory, emotional lability, irritability, depression, and suicidal gestures or attempts; at high doses, can cause respiratory depression/arrest, coma, and death	Insomnia, anxiety, panic attacks, tremor, nausea, vomiting, elevated blood pressure and pulse rate, irritability, agitation, sweating, hyperactive reflexes, pleading for drugs, grand mal seizures, confusion, delirium, psychosis	**Intoxication:** supportive care, intubation if needed. Flumazenil has a limited role because it can precipitate seizures. Consider using in patients who are known not to be chronic users or a child who had an accidental ingestion. **Withdrawal:** Sedatives/alcohol: transition to long-acting benzodiazepines for alcohol/sedative withdrawal, monitor withdrawal using Clinical Institute Withdrawal Assessment Alcohol Scale Revised (CIWA-AR)
CNS stimulants ecstasy (MDMA), cocaine,	Euphoria with acute use and dysphoria with chronic use,	Depression, anxiety, irritability, suicidal ideation, impaired	**Intoxication:** Supportive care for dehydration and hyperthermia, phentolamine

Table 27.5 (cont.)

Substance	Intoxication	Withdrawal	Management
methamphetamines, amphetamines (speed)	increased energy with acute use and fatigue with chronic use, hypersexuality, decreased appetite, delusions, suspiciousness, paranoid psychosis, insomnia, weight loss Sympathetic nervous system activation: pupillary dilation, hypertension, tachycardia, hyperthermia, cardiac arrest, stroke, seizures	concentration, sleep disturbances, increased appetite, aches and pains, tremors, sweating, and headaches	for hypertensive crisis, benzodiazepines for agitation and seizures. Antipsychotics may be used if benzodiazepines are insufficient or there is severe psychosis, but it increases risk of neuroleptic malignant syndrome. **Withdrawal:** supportive care, provide environmental safety.
Hallucinogens (LSD, Psilocybin, Ayahuasca, etc...)	Visual hallucinations, flushed face, pupillary dilation, fine tremor, increased blood pressure and pulse rate, increased body temperature, hyperreflexia, muscle weakness, tremor, dizziness, weakness, nausea, vomiting, paresthesia, labile mood, anxiety, panic attacks, depression, flashbacks	None known, but some patients may experience flashbacks to the intoxication long after use	**Intoxication:** Reassurance, rest in a quiet environment, supportive care. Benzodiazepines for severe agitation.
Opioids	Analgesia, drowsiness, euphoria, nausea, vomiting, pupillary constriction or pinpoint pupils	Lacrimation, rhinorrhea, yawning, irritability, sweating, restlessness, tremor, insomnia,	**Intoxication:** Supportive care, naloxone (multiple doses may be needed for fentanyl overdose) **Withdrawal:** Use Clinical Opiate Withdrawal Scale

Table 27.5 (cont.)

Substance	Intoxication	Withdrawal	Management
	(may be dilated with meperidine), constipation, suppression of cough reflex, grand mal seizures (particularly with tramadol), hypotension, respiratory depression, pulmonary edema, respiratory arrest, coma, death	piloerection, abdominal cramps, nausea, vomiting, diarrhea, muscle and bone pain, tachycardia and hypertension	(COWS) to assess severity and guide management. Buprenorphine and methadone are first-line and may be initiated then tapered over several days; symptomatic treatment may include clonidine for anxiety/hypertension, NSAIDs for muscle aches, sedating medications for sleep (i.e., trazodone, benzodiazepine, hypnotics, mirtazapine)
Phencyclidines	Agitation, tachycardia, hypertension, ataxia, slurred speech, vertical and horizontal nystagmus, delusions, hallucinations, aggression, hyperthermia, rigidity, rhabdomyolysis and acute renal failure, grand mal seizures, death	Depression, anxiety	**Intoxication:** Supportive care for dehydration and hyperthermia, phentolamine for hypertensive crisis, benzodiazepines for agitation and seizures. Antipsychotics may be used if benzodiazepines are insufficient or there is severe psychosis

ambivalence or discrepancy. Questions that may be helpful at this stage include "How does use of X align with your values and how does it not?" and "What benefits might you get if you were to stop using?" Evidence-based therapies for various SUD include cognitive-behavioral therapy, dialectical behavior therapy, and contingency management [12–14].

27.6.1 Harm Reduction

Harm reduction is a person-centered approach that aims to minimize the negative consequences of drug use without requiring abstinence. The goal is then to improve quality of life and engage the patient in health care. Examples of harm reduction interventions include providing clean needles, distributing naloxone for opioid overdose prevention, and providing education and resources to reduce the risk of overdose and other negative health outcomes. Initiatives may address barriers to care such as poverty, transportation, and housing [15].

27.6.2 Medications

Among the SUDs, alcohol, opioid, and tobacco use disorders have FDA-approved medications that should be offered to every patient (see Chapter 26 for more detail on alcohol use disorder). For tobacco use disorder, varenicline, bupropion, and nicotine replacement are effective to reduce craving and recurrence. Varenicline has the highest efficacy in comparison studies [16]. The duration of therapy may vary with each patient; a longer duration of treatment with varenicline (24 weeks) may increase cessation rates [17]. Varenicline has demonstrated safety and efficacy in individuals with co-occurring psychiatric disorders, prompting the removal of the FDA black box warning in 2016 [18].

For opioid use disorder (OUD), medications include the opioid agonists buprenorphine and methadone, and the opioid antagonist naltrexone [19]. Oral naltrexone has a limited role in OUD, but the long-acting injectable naltrexone has demonstrated noninferiority to buprenorphine [20]. For other SUDs, we encourage use of evidence-based pharmacotherapy to reduce craving and risky behaviors or to improve overall functioning. The extensive literature in pharmacological management of stimulants SUD is beyond the scope of this chapter.

27.6.3 Managing Co-occurring Conditions

Many patients with SUD also have co-occurring psychiatric conditions such as bipolar disorder, depression, anxiety, and psychotic disorders. Similarly, SUDs are common among psychiatric patients and lead to worse medical and psychiatric outcomes. Most patients with schizophrenia die from cardiovascular diseases that are exacerbated by high rates of tobacco use [21, 22]. Therefore, patients need a comprehensive treatment that addresses co-occurring medical illnesses, psychiatric disorders, and SUD.

27.7 Ongoing Challenges

Common substances are now more potent, such as methamphetamine and cannabis, and the emergence of new psychoactive substances has presented growing challenges. The latter often elude standard toxicology screenings. Multi-substance use is also common and can make it challenging to determine the cause of a toxidrome. The optimal approach for managing SUD involves a collaborative effort from an interdisciplinary team.

References

1. Substance Abuse and Mental Health Services Administration (SAMHSA). Key substance use and mental health indicators in the United States: results from the 2021 National Survey on Drug Use and Health. 2021. Available at: www .samhsa.gov/data/sites/default/files/ reports/rpt39443/ 2021NSDUHFFRRev010323.pdf (accessed June 24, 2024).

2. National Institute for Drug Abuse. Overdose death rates. 2021. www .drugabuse.gov/drug-topics/trends-statistics/overdose-death-rates (accessed June 28, 2021).

3. Smith PC, Schmidt SM, Allensworth-Davies D, Saitz R. A single-question screening test for drug use in primary care. *Arch Intern Med* 2010; **170**: 1155–1160.

4. American Psychiatric Association, ed. *Diagnostic and Statistical Manual of Mental Disorders: DSM-5*. 5th ed. American Psychiatric Association; 2013.

5. Donroe JH, Holt SR, O'Connor PG, Sukumar N, Tetrault JM. Interpreting quantitative urine buprenorphine and norbuprenorphine levels in office-based clinical practice. *Drug Alcohol Depend* 2017; **180**: 46–51.

6. Accurso AJ, Lee JD, McNeely J. High prevalence of urine tampering in an office-based opioid treatment practice detected by evaluating the norbuprenorphine to buprenorphine ratio. *J Subst Abuse Treat* 2017; **83**: 62–67.

7. Holt SR, Donroe JH, Cavallo DA, Tetrault JM. Addressing discordant quantitative urine buprenorphine and norbuprenorphine levels: case examples in opioid use disorder. *Drug Alcohol Depend* 2018; **186**: 171–174.

8. Volkow ND, Fowler JS, Wang G-J. The addicted human brain: insights from imaging studies. *J Clin Invest* 2003; **111**: 1444–1451.

9. Miller SC, Fiellin DA, Rosenthal RN, Saitz R, American Society of Addiction Medicine, eds. *The ASAM Principles of Addiction Medicine*. 6th edition. Wolters Kluwer; 2019.

10. ASAM Criteria Intake Assessment Guide. Default. www.asam.org/asam-criteria/criteria-intake-assessment-form (accessed December 4, 2022).

11. Miller WR, Rollnick S. *Motivational Interviewing: Helping People Change*. 3rd ed. Guilford Press; 2013.

12. Buckner JD, Ecker AH, Beighley JS, Zvolensky MJ, Schmidt NB, Shah SM et al. Integrated cognitive behavioral therapy for comorbid cannabis use and anxiety disorders. *Clin Case Stud* 2016; **15**: 68–83.

13. Barry DT, Beitel M, Cutter CJ, Fiellin DA, Kerns RD, Moore BA et al. An evaluation of the feasibility, acceptability, and preliminary efficacy of cognitive-behavioral therapy for opioid use disorder and chronic pain. *Drug Alcohol Depend* 2019; **194**: 460–467.

14. Hand DJ, Ellis JD, Carr MM, Abatemarco DJ, Ledgerwood DM. Contingency management interventions for tobacco and other substance use disorders in pregnancy. *Psychol Addict Behav J Soc Psychol Addict Behav* 2017; **31**: 907–921.

15. Stancliff S, Phillips BW, Maghsoudi N, Joseph H. Harm reduction: front line public health. *J Addict Dis* 2015; **34**: 206–219.

16. Gonzales D, Rennard SI, Nides M, Oncken C, Azoulay S, Billing CB et al. Varenicline, an α4β2 nicotinic acetylcholine receptor partial agonist, vs sustained-release bupropion and placebo for smoking cessation: a randomized controlled trial. *JAMA* 2006; **296**: 47–55.

17. Schnoll R, Leone F, Veluz-Wilkins A, Miele A, Hole A, Jao NC et al. A randomized controlled trial of 24-weeks of varenicline for tobacco use among cancer patients: efficacy, safety, and adherence. *Psychooncology* 2019; **28**: 561–569.

18. Anthenelli RM, Benowitz NL, West R, Aubin LS, McRae T, Lawrence D et al. Neuropsychiatric safety and efficacy of varenicline, bupropion, and nicotine patch in smokers with and without psychiatric disorders (EAGLES): a double-blind, randomised, placebo-controlled clinical trial. *The Lancet* 2016; **387**: 2507–2520.

19. Abuse NI on D. How effective are medications to treat opioid use disorder? Natl. Inst. Drug Abuse. www.drugabuse.gov/publications/research-reports/medications-to-treat-opioid-addiction/efficacy-medications-opioid-use-disorder (accessed June 30, 2021).

20. Tanum L, Solli KK, Latif Z-H, Benth JŠ, Opheim A, Sharma-Haase K et al. Effectiveness of injectable extended-release naltrexone vs daily

buprenorphine-naloxone for opioid dependence: a randomized clinical noninferiority trial. *JAMA Psychiatry* 2017; **74**: 1197–1205.

21. Bizzarri JV, Sbrana A, Rucci P, Ravani L, Massei GJ, Gonnelli C et al. The spectrum of substance abuse in bipolar disorder: reasons for use, sensation seeking and substance sensitivity. *Bipolar Disord* 2007; **9**: 213–220.

22. Callaghan RC, Veldhuizen S, Jeysingh T, Orlan C, Graham C, Kakouris G et al. Patterns of tobacco-related mortality among individuals diagnosed with schizophrenia, bipolar disorder, or depression. *J Psychiatr Res* 2014; **48**: 102–110.

23. Moeller KE, Kissack JC, Atayee RS, Lee KC. Clinical interpretation of urine drug tests: what clinicians need to know about urine drug screens. *Mayo Clin Proc* 2017; **92**: 774–796.

24. Levy S, Weitzman ER, Marin AC, Magane KM, Wisk LE, Shrier LA. Sensitivity and specificity of S2BI for identifying alcohol and cannabis use disorders among adolescents presenting for primary care. *Subst Abuse* 2021; **42**: 388–395.

25. Nielsen S, Gowing L, Sabioni P, Le Foll B. Pharmacotherapies for cannabis dependence. *Cochrane Database Syst Rev* 2019; **2019**: CD008940.

Autistic Spectrum Disorders

Taiwo T. Babatope, Antonio F. Pagán, Caroline W. McCool, Natalie R. Parks, Nermin Koch, Laura M. Welch, and Parnaz Daghighi

28.1 Clinical Description

Autism spectrum disorder (ASD) is defined by the American Psychiatric Association as a neurodevelopmental disorder involving (a) persistent deficits in social communication and interactions and (b) restricted, repetitive patterns of behavior, interests, or activities [1]. The first Diagnostic Statistical Manual (DSM) by the APA categorized ASD as a childhood subtype of schizophrenia–though ASD was eventually separated from schizophrenia, becoming its own diagnosis [2]. ASD evolved into a diagnostic spectrum with the publication of the DSM-5 and DSM-5-TR (see Table 28.1 for full criteria), which consolidated unreliably diagnosed subtypes such as Asperger's disorder, pervasive developmental disorder not otherwise specified, and childhood disintegrative disorder under the ASD diagnosis [3, 4]. As a result of the conceptualization of autism as a spectrum disorder, significant variations in patients' social, communicative, and intellectual abilities have been observed [1]. Diagnosis of ASD is made based on behavioral presentation and reporting of symptoms from the "early developmental period" as defined by the DSM-5-TR [1]. Although substantial heterogeneity exists between and within individuals across development, a set of core diagnostic features of ASD can be reliably identified by trained clinicians, namely social interactions, communication, and restricted, repetitive, or sensory behaviors [5, 6]. ASD is associated with significant impairment in multiple domains of adaptive functioning and has several theoretical causes [5, 7, 8]. Individuals who meet criteria for ASD need varying levels of psychosocial support to achieve relative independence, with some needing continuous care into adulthood [9].

28.1.1 Diagnostic Criteria

ASD is defined and diagnosed based on behavioral observations and reporting of symptoms. The DSM-5-TR criteria for ASD define the disorder in terms of (a) persistent impairment in areas of social communication and interaction and (b) restricted, repetitive patterns of behaviors, interests, or activities [1]. An ASD diagnosis also includes one of three severity levels to indicate the level of support currently needed. In the DSM-5-TR, diagnostic criteria under *persistent deficits in social communication and social interaction* was updated to clarify that "all of" the deficits are required for diagnosis. Further, the DSM-5-TR includes specifiers that can accompany an ASD diagnosis, such as whether the person has another neurodevelopmental, mental, or behavioral disorder. However, the DSM-5-TR updates the wording from "disorder" to "problem," broadening the criteria to also include problems that do not fully meet criteria as separate diagnosable conditions. ASD should be differentiated from other disorders, including but not limited to attention-deficit/hyperactivity disorder (ADHD), intellectual developmental disorder, language

Table 28.1 DSM 5 TR diagnostic criteria for autism [1]

A. Persistent deficits in social communication and social interaction across multiple contexts, as manifested by all of the following, currently or by history:

 1. Deficits in social-emotional reciprocity, ranging, for example, from abnormal social approach and failure of normal back-and-forth conversation; to reduced sharing of interests, emotions, or affect; to failure to initiate or respond to social interactions.

 2. Deficits in nonverbal communicative behaviors used for social interaction, ranging, for example, from poorly integrated verbal and nonverbal communication; to abnormalities in eye contact and body language or deficits in understanding and use of gestures; to a total lack of facial expressions and nonverbal communication.

 3. Deficits in developing, maintaining, and understanding relationships, ranging, for example, from difficulties adjusting behavior to suit various social contexts; to difficulties in sharing imaginative play or in making friends; to absence of interest in peers.

B. Restricted, repetitive patterns of behavior, interests, or activities, as manifested by at least two of the following, currently or by history:

 1. Stereotyped or repetitive motor movements, use of objects, or speech (e.g., simple motor stereotypies, lining up toys or flipping objects, echolalia, idiosyncratic phrases).

 2. Insistence on sameness, inflexible adherence to routines, or ritualized patterns of verbal or nonverbal behavior (e.g., extreme distress at small changes, difficulties with transitions, rigid thinking patterns, greeting rituals, need to take same route or eat same food every day).

 3. Highly restricted, fixated interests that are abnormal in intensity or focus (e.g., strong attachment to or preoccupation with unusual objects, excessively circumscribed or perseverative interests).

 4. Hyper- or hyporeactivity to sensory input or unusual interest in sensory aspects of the environment (e.g., apparent indifference to pain/temperature, adverse response to specific sounds or textures, excessive smelling or touching of objects, visual fascination with lights or movement).

C. Symptoms must be present in the early developmental period (but may not become fully manifest until social demands exceed limited capacities, or may be masked by learned strategies in later life).

D. Symptoms cause clinically significant impairment in social, occupational, or other important areas of current functioning.

E. These disturbances are not better explained by intellectual developmental disorder (intellectual disability) or global developmental delay. Intellectual developmental disorder and autism spectrum disorder frequently co-occur; to make comorbid diagnoses of autism spectrum disorder and intellectual developmental disorder, social communication should be below that expected for general developmental level.

disorders, selective mutism, stereotypic movement disorder, and obsessive-compulsive disorder (OCD). See Table 28.1 for full diagnostic criteria for ASD.

ASD can be diagnosed across the life span; however, symptoms may differ across developmental periods with some symptoms not manifesting until social demands exceed limited capacities [1]. Early signs of ASD often include delayed verbal and nonverbal communication including deficits in articulation, expression, and reception. Additional early signs include reduced social engagement, joint attention, smiling, and eye contact, decreased response to their own name beginning at 12 months of age, higher rates of atypical behaviors with objects (e.g., spinning and unusual visual regard), repetitive motor mannerisms (e.g., hand flapping), and sensory hyperresponsiveness [10].

ASD is a lifelong neurodevelopmental disorder that can also be diagnosed as an adult if symptoms are present in the "early developmental period," which is generally considered to be around 2 years old [11]. Autistic adults often have symptoms related to social and communication difficulties, repetitive behaviors, sensory processing difficulties, and issues with executive function and theory of mind [12]. One reason for a missed diagnosis in childhood is that individuals who have a higher Intelligence Quotient (IQ) require less educational support, thus achieving optimal functional outcomes in adulthood (e.g., full-time employment) [13]. Another reason for delayed diagnosis is that symptoms can be "masked" by other disorders such as ADHD or OCD [14]. A third reason for a missed diagnosis is that adults, females in particular, may learn behavioral coping strategies that help "camouflage" or mask symptoms (e.g., mimicking small talk, feigning eye contact, and practicing conversations ahead of social situations) [15].

28.2 Epidemiology/Etiology

28.2.1 Prevalence

In the 1960s and 1970s, the prevalence of ASD was low (from 0.4 to 2/1,000) likely due to poor survey methods (i.e., head counts of children in smaller communities who were diagnosed with a severe phenotype of ASD). Heterogeneous methods of diagnosis and surveying design cause prevalence differences between studies, which cannot be attributed with certainty to survey methods or true population differences. However, recent years have seen a general trend toward increased prevalence of ASD in the United States [16]. Per the Centers for Disease Control and Prevention Autism and Developmental Disabilities Monitoring Network program, the combined prevalence per 1,000 children was 23.0 in 2018 compared to 6.7 in 2000 [17]. ASD is known to occur in all socioeconomic, racial, and ethnic groups, although some studies have shown an increased prevalence in white and Hispanic children. However, social determinants of health, such as access to care and testing, cannot be ruled out as confounders to prevalence rates. Finally, ASD is more than four times as common in males compared to age-matched females [17].

28.2.2 Etiology

Autism spectrum disorders are heterogeneous, complex, multifactorial disorders with a largely unknown etiology. Despite advances in understanding ASD, the majority of cases do not have an identified underlying cause. In the early 20th century, the predominant theories on the etiology of ASD came from a psychogenic approach, which stated that ASD was caused by emotional or psychological factors rather than biological or physical factors [7]. Today it is understood that no single factor is causally associated with ASD. Instead, many risk factors for ASD have been identified [8].

Genetics

Advancements in research on ASD have uncovered a complex and significant genetic component in the etiology of ASD. For example, more than 40% of patients diagnosed with ASD are concurrently diagnosed with genetic or chromosomal abnormalities. Although there is a 70–90% heritability estimates for ASD, the molecular diagnostic yield is quite low. This is likely related to a multifactorial etiology, complex interplay of environmental factors, and the recognition of nearly 800 causative genes and their variations. Thus, there is not a clinically cohesive or shared model for genetic or biomarker causation for ASD. Common co-occurring genetic syndromes include tuberous sclerosis, fragile X, Rett syndrome, and mitochondrial dysfunction, and these syndromes collectively are reported in 10–20% of ASD cases. In families in which a second child is diagnosed with ASD, recurrence rates can be as high as 30% [18].

Promising biomarkers include genetic clusters, certain chromosomes, markers for mitochondrial function, oxidative stress, DNA methylation, and immune function [19]. In many cases, ASD seems to be caused by a combination of several abnormal genes acting in concert. Most chromosomes have been implicated in the presence of ASDs throughout literature on chromosomal aberrations. However, specifically aberrations on the long arm of chromosome 15 and structural abnormalities of the sex chromosomes have been reported most frequently [20]. Through extensive study using chromosomal microarray, several additional chromosomal sites have been proven to be associated with increased risk of ASD. In addition to chromosome 15 and the sex chromosomes, specifically X, disorders involving chromosomes 2, 3, 7, 16, 17, and 22 have also been identified to be linked to increased occurrence of ASD [20].

Environmental Factors

Additional risk factors for an ASD diagnosis include increased parental age at birth and premature birth, which are theorized to be due to older gametes having an increased probability of carrying mutations, resulting in prematurity and other obstetrical complications [21]. A variety of pre- and postnatal factors have been identified. Maternal diseases such as pregestational/gestational diabetes mellitus and peripartum infections with pathogens like rubella and cytomegalovirus are associated with ASD. Additionally, prolonged fever and maternal inflammation have been associated with ASD through mechanisms involving inflammatory cytokines. Perinatal drug associations have also been found, including valproic acid, thalidomide, and potentially misoprostol and serotonin reuptake inhibitors. Exposure to substances such as ethanol, cocaine, and heavy metals, along with folic acid deficiency, has also been associated with ASD diagnosis.

28.3 Evaluations

28.3.1 Clinical Assessments

The American Academy of Pediatrics recommends screening for ASD at 18 and 24 months to ensure systematic monitoring for early signs of ASD [22]. General developmental screening tools at early well-child doctor visits identify language, cognitive, and motor delays but may not be sensitive to social symptoms associated with identification of ASD [22, 23]. Table 28.2 shows a summary of selected assessment tools for autism spectrum disorders [24]. Thus, parental identification of social communication deficits at home and around peers is vital.

While screening tools can be helpful for early identification, "expert clinical opinion" is necessary for diagnosis [25–27]. Primary care providers should refer positive screen results

Table 28.2 Summary of selected assessment instruments of ASD [24]

Scale (see legend)	Uses	Age Range	Method of Administration
Autism Behavior Checklist	Screening	children	parent rated
Childhood Autism Rating Scale	Screening	children	clinician rated
Checklist for Autism in Toddlers	Screening	toddlers	parent rated
Communication and Symbolic Behavior Scales Developmental Profile Infant-Toddler Checklist	Screening	toddlers	parent rated
Autism Screening Questionnaire	Screening	child/adult	parent rated
Autism Quotient	Screening	child/adult	self or parent rated
Childhood Autism Screening Test	Screening	4–11 years	parent rated
Asperger Syndrome Diagnostic Scale	Screening	5–18 years	parent or teacher rated
Gilliam Asperger's Disorder Scale	Screening	3–22 years	parent or teacher rated
Asperger Syndrome Diagnostic Interview	Screening	child/adult	interview + clinician rated
Social Responsiveness Scales	Screening	4–18 years	parent or teacher rated
Autism Diagnostic Interview–Revised	diagnostic	child/adult	interview + clinician rated
Diagnostic Interview for Social and Communication Disorders	diagnostic	child/adult	interview + clinician rated
Autism Diagnostic Observation Schedule	diagnostic	child/adult	semistructured interactive session

to appropriate specialists (i.e., developmental neuropsychologists) for a comprehensive ASD evaluation, an audiology evaluation, and early intervention services simultaneously [28]. The three essential objectives of comprehensive evaluations should be to provide a definitive diagnosis, explore differential diagnoses and comorbidities, and ultimately determine the child's overall level of adaptive functioning for intervention planning [29].

A complete psychiatric assessment must be conducted with careful consideration of DSM-5-TR diagnostic criteria [24]. Historical information should be obtained (e.g., pregnancy, neonatal, and developmental history). Reports from previous evaluations should be reviewed and the child's response to previous evaluations should be determined [30]. Medical assessments should include a physical examination, analyses of medical history including immunizations, allergies or unusual medication responses, and routine laboratory testing [30]. Audiological and visual examinations should be conducted.

Diagnostic genetic testing is recommended to identify molecular diagnosis for individuals with suspected developmental delay of undetermined etiology. In cases of confirmed clinical diagnosis of ASD, intellectual disorder, and/or global developmental delay, chromosomal microarray (CMA) and the fragile X gene testing are tier 1 standard of care. Other factors noted during the history or physical examination might suggest specific genetic diagnosis and require different tests including the phosphatase and tensin homolog, methyl CpG binding protein 2, or the karyotype analysis [31]. Alternatively, if tier 1 genetic studies return with no clinically relevant findings and the patient has evidence of unresolved medical findings, further testing such as whole exome sequencing could be performed [31]. Involvement of genetics specialists is often recommended to help with this investigative process.

Metabolic workup is recommended at the same time or soon after CMA and fragile X DNA testing [32]. Table 28.3 summarizes first-tier laboratory investigations that should be ordered for all patients who present with global developmental delay and/or intellectual disability without a recognizable constellation of symptoms [33].

Neurologic consultation should be prioritized if epilepsy is suspected. In cases of comorbid intellectual or global developmental delay, or a decline in functioning, neuroimaging and an electroencephalogram (EEG) should be obtained. Certain developmental disorders, most notably Landau-Kleffner syndrome, also should be ruled out. In this condition, a highly distinctive EEG abnormality is present and associated with development of marked aphasia [34].

28.3.2 Comorbidities

Common comorbid and differential neurodevelopmental disorders with autism include ADHD, global developmental delay or intellectual disability, language or learning disorder, social communication disorder, stereotypic movement disorder, or Tourette's disorder [35–43]. Intellectual disability is a critical area of assessment, as ASD has been linked to intellectual impairment, with nearly 70% of individuals with ASD scoring below-average IQ [35, 36]. Typically, a clinical psychologist may administer the Wechsler Intelligence Scale for Children-IV (WISC-IV) or similar tests, including achievement tests [37–39]. In addition, the Behavior Assessment System for Children and the Vineland Adaptive Behavior Scales (Vineland) for ASD diagnosis and classification can be used [40–42]. Care collaboration between the patient's primary care provider and other organizations (e.g., school) is vital for treatment planning. Evaluation of multiple streams of development, including cognitive, communication, motor, and adaptive skills, may be best accomplished by multidisciplinary team evaluations, including psychology, speech and language, occupational therapy, physical therapy, and special education [43].

Mental and behavioral disorders are also common comorbid and differential disorders with ASD [44–66]. Several studies have documented high rates of psychiatric comorbidities in individuals with ASD, including mood disorders, such as depression and bipolar disorders [44–48]. Internalizing symptoms may be misinterpreted as core features of autism. Regarding bipolar disorders, the flight of ideas or elevated energy could strongly suggest that individuals with ASD are manic or hypomanic [49–51]. Reported prevalence of **anxiety** in ASD varies widely, with estimates ranging from 13.6% to 84.1% [52–56]. A recent systematic review has identified clinically significant levels of

Table 28.3 First-tier laboratory investigations [33]

Blood laboratory Investigations*

Complete Blood Count (CBC)	
Comprehensive Metabolic panel (CMP)	Electrolytes to calculate anion gap (sodium, potassium, carbon dioxide, chloride), glucose, calcium, blood urea nitrogen (BUN), creatinine, BUN/creatinine ratio, estimated glomerular filtration rate (eGFR), total protein, albumin, globulin, albumin/globulin ratio, bilirubin, alkaline phosphatase (ALP), aspartate amino transferase (AST), alanine amino transferase (ALT)
Lead level	When risk factors for exposure are present
Thyroid stimulating hormone (TSH)	
Amino acids	
Acylcarnitine profile, carnitine	Free and total
Homocysteine	
Ammonia	
Lactate	
Ferritin, vitamin B12	When dietary restriction or pica are present
Copper and ceruloplasmin	Consider as first line investigation when hepatomegaly, dystonia, abnormal liver function tests are present
Biotinidase	Consider when severe hypotonia and seizures are present.

Urine laboratory Investigations*

Urine	Organic acids, creatine metabolites, purines, pyrimidines, glycosaminoglycans
Perform testing after 4h to 8h of fasting *	

anxiety with up to 39.6% for various disorders (e.g., generalized anxiety disorder, OCD) [56–63]. Individuals with ASD also present with comorbid ADHD 50% to 70% of the time [64, 65]. There have been reports that schizophrenia disorders and ASD do not co-occur at elevated rates [66]. The prevalence of OCD in the general population of children and adolescents is between 2% and 4%, whereas in children with ASD it is between 2.6% and 37.2% [56, 63].

Neurological and medical conditions can also be comorbid or differential diagnosis with ASD, including cerebral palsy, epilepsy, Landau Kleffner syndrome, mitochondrial disorders, or neonatal encephalopathy [22, 46]. Children with autism are also more prone to a variety of neurological disorders, sleep disorders (80% occurrence rate), and gastrointestinal (GI) disorders (46% to 84% occurrence rate). Some genetic disorders are also more common in children with ASD [55]. For individuals with known syndromic conditions, the services of orthopedists and respiratory therapists may be required [30].

28.4 Clinical Presentation

Parents of autistic children most often report concerns related to abnormal childhood developmental trajectory and a history of unusual behaviors, with variability in ages where features suggestive of ASD are most noticeable [67, 68]. Infants diagnosed with ASD appear to have relatively intact eye contact and social smile at 6 months of age [69–73]. However, the frequency and quality of these social behaviors decline between 6 and 12 months old [71]. Symptoms of impaired social interactions often become more apparent around 12 months of age [74]. Such symptoms include a lack of responsiveness to name, atypical object exploration, repetitive behaviors, and nonverbal communication deficits [75–81]. The ASD diagnosis can be reliably made in the second year of life, and these early diagnoses are relatively stable over time [74, 82].

28.4.1 Clinical Course

Changes in core deficits in communication, social, and restricted and repetitive behaviors associated with autism differ among individuals. The trajectory of core symptoms in diagnosed children are variable, with improvement only in some behaviors and with different timing across behaviors [83]. Autism spectrum disorder is considered a stable diagnosis, and the majority of children given this diagnosis still meet criteria at follow-up appointments [84]. Even among individuals with significant improvements, substantial gains are usually not enough to move them into the normal range of functioning. Individuals who no longer meet criteria for an ASD diagnosis are usually those who would have previously been diagnosed as having pervasive developmental disorder-not otherwise specified (PDD-NOS) using DSM-IV criteria [85].

Long-term follow-up studies indicate that there is considerable heterogeneity in social role attainment outcomes for persons with autism [86]. The majority of autistic individuals remain dependent on their families or professional service providers for assistance with tasks of daily living. However, some adults live independently, marry, attend college, work in competitive jobs, and develop a large network of friends. Even among the employed, most jobs are poorly paid and do not provide a living wage. There is a subgroup of between 15% and 25% of adults with autism who show more favorable outcomes [87].

Individual prognostic factors have not been consistently replicated, and outcomes for individual children cannot be reliably predicted. Some difficulties in establishing prognostic factors include sampling bias in previous longitudinal studies as well as expansion of the diagnosis in DSM-5, leading to higher-functioning individuals meeting criteria for ASD [88]. However, some factors that have been studied to contribute to better outcomes include higher IQ, lower levels of social impairment, and early language abilities [89–91]. It is possible that adequate functioning in adulthood for individuals with autism is dependent as much or more on the degree of support offered by families, friends, and service providers as on basic intelligence and language skills. All-cause mortality risk is increased twofold in people with ASD [92]. Mortality risk in people has been found to be at its height in childhood and lower in young and middle adulthood [93].

28.4.2 Functional Impairment

Individuals with ASD struggle to develop social relationships. It remains unclear whether the lower rate of social relationships of adults with autism implies a lack of desire or motivation for friendships or a lack of skills needed to form and maintain desired social relationships [94–95]. Substantially fewer studies have examined the extent of impairment in the domain of restricted and repetitive behaviors compared to the communication and social deficits of autism. Limited available evidence suggests that most persons with autism remain impaired in the social communication domain across the life course. There is, however, some evidence that the qualitative nature of repetitive behaviors and stereotyped interests changes over time [96]. Further, less is known regarding the causes of various physical and mental comorbidities [97–103].

28.4.3 Financial Burden

The financial burden on families of children with ASD is correlated with the existing societal financial safety net. Poorer outcomes are expected when the family carries a substantial share of the cost to support the development of children with ASD, especially in lower-income households where access to resources remains limited [104].

28.5 Treatment

28.5.1 Behavioral Interventions

The goal of ASD treatment is to minimize the effects of developmental delays and maximize the child's ability in areas of speech and language abilities, motor skills, social/emotional skills, and cognitive skills. Several different behavioral interventions have been developed and used in different settings such as clinics, schools, and at home. Children with ASD, especially those with higher IQ and better language and motor skills, can make immense progress with early diagnosis and interventions [105, 106].

Patients with developmental delays should be evaluated by speech, occupational, and physical therapists to identify needed interventions. Many states provide free Early Child Intervention services for qualifying individuals from birth until 3 years old. The services designate an Individualized Family Service Plan (IFSP) for every eligible child to assess needs, provide services, and assess progress. When children start school, they can also benefit from specialized Individualized Education Plans (IEP) from age 3 years through high school or until age 21. Some states also provide services beyond age 21 [107]. Funding for both IFSPs and IEPs are provided through the Individuals with Disabilities Education Act, which was developed to provide government services for individuals with disabilities. Services provided by IFSPs and IEPs can differ from state to state; however, they all aim to improve symptoms in areas of communication, behavior, socializing, and self-care depending on the specific needs of the child.

Several different behavioral interventions have been developed to improve communication and social skills beyond the toddler years and into adulthood for individuals with ASD. Applied behavior analysis (ABA) techniques are widely studied and commonly implemented. ABA is an evidenced-based treatment where desired behaviors are reinforced and undesired behaviors are discouraged by measuring antecedents and consequences to certain behaviors [108, 109]. The ABA treatment plan includes seven dimensions, generality, effective, technological, applied, conceptually systematic, analytic, and behavioral [108, 109]. The most commonly used techniques are discrete trial training (DTT) and pivotal response training (PRT) [110–113]. PRT is based on play and initiated by the child who requires motivation. DTT involves teaching skills, after breaking them into smaller components, by instruction and reinforcement [113, 114]. There are several other behavioral therapy approaches to improve communication and social skills for children with autism, including picture exchange communication system and other alternative approaches based on writing, drawing, or pointing [115, 116].

Sensory sensitivity is one of the hallmark symptoms of ASD, and sensory integration therapy can be used to improve overwhelming sensory stimuli such as loud noises, tactile sensitivities, and bright lights for the child [117]. However, parent support and education are integral in treatment, since the learned behaviors need to be reinforced at home as well. Autism support groups can also help parents connect with others, find support, and share information for different treatment options and resources available nationally and within the community.

28.5.2 Pharmacological Treatments

There are no curative treatments for the core features of ASD. However, medications are often used to target comorbid conditions or problematic behaviors that interfere with progress or pose safety concerns. Importantly, pharmacological treatments should be used second line and in conjunction with behavioral interventions described in the preceding sections [118–120].

Common targets of medications for ASD include irritability, cognitive rigidity, anxiety, obsessions, and sleep [121]. Antipsychotics have the most evidence for reducing aggressive behavior, although they should be used with caution due to potential significant side effects of weight gain, sedation, and extrapyramidal movements. Risperidone and Aripiprazole are the only antipsychotics FDA-approved for irritability associated with ASD, although others are often used [92, 122]. Antipsychotic medications can also be used for repetitive behaviors and severe cognitive rigidity [123, 124].

Stimulants, α-2 agonists (Clonidine, Guanfacine), and Atomoxetine are prescribed for comorbid ADHD symptoms [125]. Although evidence is mixed for their efficacy and tolerability in autistic populations, selective serotonin reuptake inhibitors (SSRIs) can be used for comorbid anxiety, OCD, or depressive disorders [121]. There are no FDA-approved medications for sleep disturbances in ASD, but melatonin is considered first line should behavioral interventions alone fail. Referral to a sleep specialist should also be considered if behavioral interventions and melatonin are ineffective [121].

Extra caution should be used when prescribing medications to patients with ASD given increased sensitivity to side effects and observed paradoxical reactions to certain medication types, namely benzodiazepines and diphenhydramine. Thus, any medication prescribed should be started at low doses and increased slowly [118]. Psychoeducation should be provided to families with potential side effects to monitor for, particularly with patients who have low verbal skills and may have difficulty communicating their needs.

28.5.3 Alternative Treatment Options

Given the limitations of pharmacotherapy in treating ASD individuals, families often search for alternative treatments in hopes of enhancing their child's quality of life. These treatments can range from having poor evidence but minimal risks (such as yoga, music therapy, or vitamin C supplementation) to being potentially harmful, time intensive, and expensive (intravenous immunoglobulin, chelation, or hyperbaric oxygen therapy) [120, 126, 127]. While a physician should approach these conversations with empathy and humility, it is very important to always ask families about additional supplements, over-the-counter medications, alternative treatments, or special diets being given to patients and to consider their safety and possible interactions with other treatments [127].

References

1. American Psychiatric Association. *Diagnostic and Statistical Manual of Mental Disorders: DSM-5-TR*. American Psychiatric Association; 2022.

2. American Psychiatric Association. *Diagnostic and Statistical Manual of Mental Disorders: DSM*. American Psychiatric Association; 1952.

3. American Psychiatric Association. *Diagnostic and Statistical Manual of Mental Disorders: DSM-5*. American Psychiatric Association; 2013.

4. Lord C, Elsabbagh M, Baird G, Veenstra-Vanderweele J. Autism spectrum disorder. *Lancet*. 2018;392 (10146):508–520.

5. Lord C, Rutter M, Goode S, Heemsbergen J, Jordan H, Mawhood L, Schopler E. Autism diagnostic observation schedule: a standardized observation of communicative and social behavior. *J Autism Dev Disord*. 1989;19(2):185–212.

6. Regier DA, Narrow WE, Clarke DE, Kraemer HC, Kuramoto SJ, Kuhl EA, Kupfer DJ. DSM-5 field trials in the United States and Canada, part II: test-retest reliability of selected categorical diagnoses. *Am J Psychiatry*. 2013;170 (1):59–70.

7. Kanner L. Autistic disturbances of affective contact. *Nervous Child*. 1943;2 (3):217–250.

8. Mandy W, Lai MC. Towards sex-and gender-informed autism research. *Autism*. 2017;21(6):643–645.

9. Campisi L, Imran N, Nazeer A, Skokauskas N, Azeem MW. Autism spectrum disorder. *Br Med Bull*. 2018;127 (1):91–100.

10. Ozonoff S, Iosif AM, Baguio F, Cook IC, Hill MM, Hutman T, Rogers SJ, Rozga A, Sangha S, Sigman M, Steinfeld MB. A prospective study of the emergence of early behavioral signs of autism. *J Am Acad Child Adolesc Psychiatry*. 2010;49 (3):256–266.

11. Huang Y, Arnold SR, Foley KR, Trollor JN. Diagnosis of autism in adulthood: a scoping review. *Autism*. 2020;24 (6):1311–1327.

12. Howlin P, Magiati I. Autism spectrum disorder: outcomes in adulthood. *Curr Opin Psychiatry*. 2017;30(2):69–76.

13. Lehnhardt FG, Gawronski A, Volpert K, Schilbach L, Tepest R, Vogeley K. Psychosocial functioning of adults with late diagnosed autism spectrum disorders: a retrospective study. *Fortschritte der Neurologie-Psychiatrie*. 2011;80(2):88–97.

14. Pehlivanidis A, Papanikolaou K, Mantas V, Kalantzi E, Korobili K, Xenaki LA, Vassiliou G, Papageorgiou C. Lifetime co-occurring psychiatric disorders in newly diagnosed adults with attention deficit hyperactivity disorder (ADHD) or/and autism spectrum disorder (ASD). *BMC Psychiatry*. 2020;20(1):1–2.

15. McQuaid GA, Lee NR, Wallace GL. Camouflaging in autism spectrum disorder: examining the roles of sex, gender identity, and diagnostic timing. *Autism*. 2022;26(2):552–559.

16. Fombonne, E. Editorial: the rising prevalence of autism. *J Child Psychol Psychiatr*. 2018;59:717–720.

17. Centers for Disease Control and Prevention [Internet]. U.S. Department of Health and Human Services. Facts about CDC's autism and developmental disabilities monitoring (ADDM) network.

cdc.gov. Updated January 14, 2022; cited January 12, 2023. Available from www .cdc.gov/ncbddd/autism/materials/addm-factsheet.html.

18. Genovese A, Butler MG. Clinical assessment, genetics, and treatment approaches in autism spectrum disorder (ASD). *Int J Mol Sci.* 2020;21(13):4726.

19. Goldani AA, Downs SR, Widjaja F, Lawton B, Hendren RL. Biomarkers in autism. *Front Psychiatry.* 2014;12(5):100.

20. Gillberg C. Chromosomal disorders and autism. *J Autism Dev Disord.* 1998;28 (5):415–425.

21. Hodges H, Fealko C, Soares N. Autism spectrum disorder: definition, epidemiology, causes, and clinical evaluation. *Transl Pediatr.* 2020;9(Suppl 1):S55–S65.

22. Zwaigenbaum L, Bauman ML, Fein D, Pierce K, Buie T, Davis PA, Newschaffer C, Robins DL, Wetherby A, Choueiri R, Kasari C. Early screening of autism spectrum disorder: recommendations for practice and research. *Pediatrics.* 2015;136 (Supplement_1):S41–S59.

23. Pinto-Martin JA, Young LM, Mandell DS, Poghosyan L, Giarelli E, Levy SE. Screening strategies for autism spectrum disorders in pediatric primary care. *J Dev Behav Pediatr.* 2008;29(5):345–350.

24. Volkmar F, Siegel M, Woodbury-Smith M, King B, McCracken J, State M. Practice parameter for the assessment and treatment of children and adolescents with autism spectrum disorder. *J Am Acad Child Adolesc Psychiatry.* 2014;53 (2):237–257.

25. Chawarska K, Klin A, Paul R, Volkmar F. Autism spectrum disorder in the second year: stability and change in syndrome expression. *J Child Psychol Psychiatr.* 2007;48(2):128–138.

26. Bishop SL, Luyster R, Richler J, Lord CA. *Diagnostic Assessment: Autism Spectrum Disorders in Infants and Toddlers.* Guilford Press; 2008.

27. Volkmar FR, Klin A, Siegel B, Szatmari P, Lord C, Campbell M, Freeman BJ, Cicchetti DV, Rutter M, Kline W,

Buitelaar J. Field trial for autistic disorder in DSM-IV. *Am J Psychiatry.* 1994;151 (9):1361–1367.

28. Monteiro SA, Dempsey J, Berry LN, Voigt RG, Goin-Kochel RP. Screening and referral practices for autism spectrum disorder in primary pediatric care. *Pediatrics.* 2019;144(4):e20183326.

29. Brian JA, Zwaigenbaum L, Ip A. Standards of diagnostic assessment for autism spectrum disorder. *Paediatr Child Health.* 2019;24(7):444–451.

30. Volkmar F, Cook Jr E, Pomeroy J, Realmuto G, Tanguay P. Summary of the practice parameters for the assessment and treatment of children, adolescents, and adults with autism and other pervasive developmental disorders: American Academy of Child and Adolescent Psychiatry. *J Am Acad Child Adolesc Psychiatry.* 1999;38 (12):1611–1616.

31. Muhle RA, Reed HE, Vo LC, Mehta S, McGuire K, Veenstra-VanderWeele J, Pedapati E. Clinical diagnostic genetic testing for individuals with developmental disorders. *J Am Acad Child Adolesc Psychiatry.* 2017;56(11):910.

32. Moeschler JB, Shevell M, Committee on Genetics, Moeschler JB, Shevell M, Saul RA, Chen E, Freedenberg DL, Hamid R, Jones MC, Stoler JM. Comprehensive evaluation of the child with intellectual disability or global developmental delays. *Pediatrics.* 2014;134(3):903–918.

33. Bélanger SA, Caron J. Evaluation of the child with global developmental delay and intellectual disability. *Paediatr Child Health.* 2018;23(6):403–410.

34. Camfield P, Camfield C. Epileptic syndromes in childhood: clinical features, outcomes, and treatment. *Epilepsia.* 2002;43:27–32.

35. Joseph RM, Tager-Flusberg H, Lord C. Cognitive profiles and social-communicative functioning in children with autism spectrum disorder. *J Child Psychol Psychiatry.* 2002;43(6):807–821.

36. Hao G, Layton TL, Zou XB, Li DY. Evaluating autism in a Chinese

population: the clinical autism diagnostic scale. *World J Pediatr.* 2014;10:160–163.

37. Wechsler D, Kodama H. *Wechsler Intelligence Scale for Children.* Psychological Corporation; 1949.

38. Wechsler D. *Wechsler Preschool and Primary Scale of Intelligence – Fourth Edition.* The Psychological Corporation; 2012.

39. Burns TG. Wechsler Individual Achievement Test-III: what is the 'gold standard' for measuring academic achievement? *Appl Neuropsychol.* 2010;17 (3):234–236.

40. Reynolds CR, Kamphaus RW. *The Clinician's Guide to the Behavior Assessment System for Children (BASC)* Guilford Press; 2002.

41. Sparrow SS, Cicchetti DV. *The Vineland Adaptive Behavior Scales.* Allyn & Bacon; 1989.

42. Layton T. Early assessment in autism spectrum disorders. *J Psychol Abnorm Child.* 2014;3(4):130.

43. Steiner AM, Goldsmith TR, Snow AV, Chawarska K. Practitioner's guide to assessment of autism spectrum disorders in infants and toddlers. *J Autism Dev Disord.* 2012;42(6):1183–1196.

44. Volkmar FR, Klin A. Issues in the Classification of Autism and Related Conditions. In Volkmar FR, Paul R, Klin A, Cohen D, eds. *Handbook of Autism and Pervasive Developmental Disorders.* John Wiley & Sons; 2005.

45. Hedley D, Young R. Social comparison processes and depressive symptoms in children and adolescents with Asperger syndrome. *Autism.* 2006;10:139–153.

46. Munesue T, Ono Y, Mutoh K, Shimoda K, Nakatani H, Kikuchi M. High prevalence of bipolar disorder comorbidity in adolescents and young adults with high-functioning autism spectrum disorder: a preliminary study of 44 outpatients. *J Affect Disord.* 2008;111 (2–3):170–175.

47. Simonoff E, Pickles A, Charman T, Chandler S, Loucas T, Baird G. Psychiatric

disorders in children with autism spectrum disorders: prevalence, comorbidity, and associated factors in a population-derived sample. *J Am Acad Child Adolesc Psychiatry.* 2008;47(8):921–929.

48. Simonoff E, Jones CR, Pickles A, Happé F, Baird G, Charman T. Severe mood problems in adolescents with autism spectrum disorder. *J Child Psychol Psychiatry.* 2012;53(11):1157–1166.

49. Lainhart JE, Folstein SE. Affective disorders in people with autism: a review of published cases. *J Autism Dev Disord.* 1994;24(5):587–601.

50. Joshi G, Biederman J, Petty C, Goldin RL, Furtak SL, Wozniak J. Examining the comorbidity of bipolar disorder and autism spectrum disorders: a large controlled analysis of phenotypic and familial correlates in a referred population of youth with bipolar I disorder with and without autism spectrum disorders. *J Clin Psychiatry.* 2013;74(6):6865.

51. Skeppar P, Thoor R, Agren S, Isakson AC, Skeppar I, Persson BA, Fitzgerald M. Neurodevelopmental disorders with comorbid affective disorders sometimes produce psychiatric conditions traditionally diagnosed as schizophrenia. *Clin Neuropsychiatry.* 2013;10 (3–4):123–134.

52. Bellini S. Social skill deficits and anxiety in high-functioning adolescents with autism spectrum disorders. *Focus Autism Other Dev Disabl.* 2004;19(2):78–86.

53. Bradley EA, Summers JA, Wood HL, Bryson SE. Comparing rates of psychiatric and behavior disorders in adolescents and young adults with severe intellectual disability with and without autism. *J Autism Dev Disord.* 2004;34:151–161.

54. Kim JA, Szatmari P, Bryson SE, Streiner DL, Wilson FJ. The prevalence of anxiety and mood problems among children with autism and Asperger syndrome. *Autism.* 2000;4(2):117–132.

55. Lidstone J, Uljarević M, Sullivan J, Rodgers J, McConachie H, Freeston M, Le

Couteur A, Prior M, Leekam S. Relations among restricted and repetitive behaviors, anxiety and sensory features in children with autism spectrum disorders. *Res Autism Spectr Disord.* 2014;8(2):82–92.

56. Van Steensel FJ, Bögels SM, Perrin S. Anxiety disorders in children and adolescents with autistic spectrum disorders: a meta-analysis. *Clin Child Fam Psychol Rev.* 2011;14:302–317.

57. Evans DW, Canavera K, Kleinpeter FL, Maccubbin E, Taga K. The fears, phobias and anxieties of children with autism spectrum disorders and down syndrome: comparisons with developmentally and chronologically age matched children. *Child Psychiatry Hum Dev.* 2005;36:3–26.

58. Gadow KD, Devincent CJ, Pomeroy J, Azizian A. Comparison of DSM-IV symptoms in elementary school-age children with PDD versus clinic and community samples. *Autism.* 2005;9(4):392–415.

59. Weisbrot DM, Gadow KD, DeVincent CJ, Pomeroy J. The presentation of anxiety in children with pervasive developmental disorders. *J Child Adolesc Psychopharmacol.* 2005;15(3):477–496.

60. de Bruin EI, Ferdinand RF, Meester S, de Nijs PF, Verheij F. High rates of psychiatric co-morbidity in PDD-NOS. *J Autism Dev Disord.* 2007;37:877–886.

61. Gillott A, Standen PJ. Levels of anxiety and sources of stress in adults with autism. *J Intellect Disabil.* 2007;11(4):359–370.

62. Sukhodolsky DG, Scahill L, Gadow KD, Arnold LE, Aman MG, McDougle CJ, Tierney E, Williams White S, Lecavalier L, Vitiello B (2008) Parent-rated anxiety symptoms in children with pervasive developmental disorders: frequency and association with core autism symptoms and cognitive functioning. *J Abnorm Child Psychol.* 36(1):117–128.

63. Geller DA. Obsessive-compulsive and spectrum disorders in children and adolescents. *Psychiatr Clin.* 2006;29(2):353–370.

64. Hours C, Recasens C, Baleyte JM. ASD and ADHD comorbidity: what are we talking about? *Front Psychiatry.* 2022;13:154.

65. Al-Beltagi M. Autism medical comorbidities. *World J Clin Pediatr.* 2021;10(3):15.

66. Volkmar FR, Cohen DJ. Comorbid association of autism and schizophrenia. *Am J Psychiatry.* 1991;148(12):1705–1707.

67. Whitehouse AJ, Evans K, Eapen V, Wray J. *A National Guideline for the assessment and Diagnosis of Autism Spectrum Disorders in Australia.* Autism Cooperative Research Centre (CRC); 2018.

68. La Roche MJ, Bush HH, D'Angelo E. The assessment and treatment of autism spectrum disorder: a cultural examination. *Practice Innovations.* 2018;3(2):107.

69. Bryson SE, Zwaigenbaum L, Brian J, Roberts W, Szatmari P, Rombough V, McDermott C. A prospective case series of high-risk infants who developed autism. *J Autism Dev Disord.* 2007;37:12–24.

70. Landa RJ, Holman KC, Garrett-Mayer E. Social and communication development in toddlers with early and later diagnosis of autism spectrum disorders. *Arch Gen Psychiatry.* 2007;64(7):853–864.

71. Ozonoff S, Iosif AM, Baguio F, Cook IC, Hill MM, Hutman T, Rogers SJ, Rozga A, Sangha S, Sigman M, Steinfeld MB. A prospective study of the emergence of early behavioral signs of autism. *J Am Acad Child Adolesc Psychiatry.* 2010;49(3):256–266.

72. Young GS, Merin N, Rogers SJ, Ozonoff S. Gaze behavior and affect at 6 months: predicting clinical outcomes and language development in typically developing infants and infants at risk for autism. *Dev Sci.* 2009;12(5):798–814.

73. Zwaigenbaum L, Bryson S, Lord C, Rogers S, Carter A, Carver L, Chawarska K, Constantino J, Dawson G, Dobkins K, Fein D. Clinical assessment and management of toddlers with suspected

autism spectrum disorder: insights from studies of high-risk infants. *Pediatrics.* 2009;123(5):1383–1391.

74. Rogers SJ. What are infant siblings teaching us about autism in infancy? *Autism Res.* 2009;2(3):125–137.

75. Nadig AS, Ozonoff S, Young GS, Rozga A, Sigman M, Rogers SJ. A prospective study of response to name in infants at risk for autism. *Arch Pediatr Adolesc Med.* 2007;161(4):378–383.

76. Kim SH, Lord C. Restricted and repetitive behaviors in toddlers and preschoolers with autism spectrum disorders based on the Autism Diagnostic Observation Schedule (ADOS). *Autism Res.* 2010;3 (4):162–173.

77. Ozonoff S, Macari S, Young GS, Goldring S, Thompson M, Rogers SJ. Atypical object exploration at 12 months of age is associated with autism in a prospective sample. *Autism.* 2008;12(5):457–472.

78. Landa R, Garrett-Mayer E. Development in infants with autism spectrum disorders: a prospective study. *J Child Psychol Psychiatry.* 2006;47(6):629–638.

79. Paul R, Fuerst Y, Ramsay G, Chawarska K, Klin A. Out of the mouths of babes: vocal production in infant siblings of children with ASD. *J Child Psychol Psychiatry.* 2011;52(5):588–598.

80. Presmanes AG, Walden TA, Stone WL, Yoder PJ. Effects of different attentional cues on responding to joint attention in younger siblings of children with autism spectrum disorders. *J Autism Dev Disord.* 2007;37:133–144.

81. Yoder P, Stone WL, Walden T, Malesa E. Predicting social impairment and ASD diagnosis in younger siblings of children with autism spectrum disorder. *J Autism Dev Disord.* 2009;39:1381–1391.

82. Chawarska K, Klin A, Paul R, Macari S, Volkmar F. A prospective study of toddlers with ASD: short-term diagnostic and cognitive outcomes. *J Child Psychol Psychiatry.* 2009;50(10):1235–1245.

83. Pickles A, McCauley JB, Pepa LA, Huerta M, Lord C. The adult outcome of children referred for autism: typology and prediction from childhood. *J Child Psychol Psychiatry.* 2020;61(7):760–767.

84. Brignell A, Harwood RC, May T, Woolfenden S, Montgomery A, Iorio A, Williams K. Overall prognosis of preschool autism spectrum disorder diagnoses. *Cochrane Database Syst Rev.* 2022;9(9):CD012749.

85. Woolfenden S, Sarkozy V, Ridley G, Williams K. A systematic review of the diagnostic stability of autism spectrum disorder. *Res Autism Spectr Disord.* 2012;6(1):345–354.

86. Roux AM, Shattuck PT, Cooper BP, Anderson KA, Wagner M, Narendorf SC. Postsecondary employment experiences among young adults with an autism spectrum disorder. *J Am Acad Child Adolesc Psychiatry.* 2013;52 (9):931–939.

87. Shattuck PT, Narendorf SC, Cooper B, Sterzing PR, Wagner M, Taylor JL. Postsecondary education and employment among youth with an autism spectrum disorder. *Pediatrics.* 2012;129 (6):1042–1049.

88. Henninger, N. A., & Taylor, J. L. (2013). Outcomes in adults with autism spectrum disorders: a historical perspective. *Autism*;17(1):103–116.

89. Mason D, Capp SJ, Stewart GR, Kempton MJ, Glaser K, Howlin P, Happé F. A Meta-analysis of outcome studies of autistic adults: quantifying effect size, quality, and meta-regression. *J Autism Dev Disord.* 2021;51(9):3165–3179.

90. Howlin P, Moss P, Savage S, Rutter M. Social outcomes in mid- to later adulthood among individuals diagnosed with autism and average nonverbal IQ as children. *J Am Acad Child Adolesc Psychiatry.* 2013;52(6):572–581.e1.

91. Kirby AV, Baranek GT, Fox L. Longitudinal predictors of outcomes for adults with autism spectrum disorder: systematic review. *OTJR Occup Particip Health.* 2016;36(2):55–64.

92. Hirota T, King BH. Autism spectrum disorder: a review. *JAMA.* 2023;329 (2):157–168.

93. Rutter M. Pathways from childhood to adult life. *J Child Psychol Psychiatry.* 1989;30(1):23–51.

94. Mesibov GB, Schopler E, Caison W. The adolescent and adult psychoeducational profile: assessment of adolescents and adults with severe developmental handicaps. *J Autism Dev Disord.* 1989;19:33–40.

95. Orsmond GI, Krauss MW, Seltzer MM. Peer relationships and social and recreational activities among adolescents and adults with autism. *J Autism Dev Disord.* 2004;34:245–256.

96. Seltzer MM, Shattuck P, Abbeduto L, Greenberg JS. Trajectory of development in adolescents and adults with autism. *Ment Retard Dev Disabil Res Rev.* 2004;10(4):234–247.

97. Ghaziuddin M, Weidmer-Mikhail E, Ghaziuddin N. Comorbidity of Asperger syndrome: a preliminary report. *J Intellect Disabil Res.* 1998;42(4):279–283.

98. Bradley E, Bolton P. Episodic psychiatric disorders in teenagers with learning disabilities with and without autism. *Br J Psychiatry.* 2006;189(4):361–366.

99. Leyfer OT, Folstein SE, Bacalman S, Davis NO, Dinh E, Morgan J, Tager-Flusberg H, Lainhart JE. Comorbid psychiatric disorders in children with autism: Interview development and rates of disorders. *J Autism Dev Disord.* 2006;36:849–861.

100. Simonoff E, Pickles A, Charman T, Chandler S, Loucas T, Baird G. Psychiatric disorders in children with autism spectrum disorders: prevalence, comorbidity, and associated factors in a population-derived sample. *J Am Acad Child Adolesc Psychiatry.* 2008;47(8):921–929.

101. Joshi G, Wozniak J, Petty C, Martelon MK, Fried R, Bolfek A, Kotte A, Stevens J, Furtak SL, Bourgeois M, Caruso J. Psychiatric comorbidity and functioning in a clinically referred population of adults with autism spectrum disorders: a comparative study. *J Autism Dev Disord.* 2013;43:1314–1325.

102. Schieve LA, Gonzalez V, Boulet SL, Visser SN, Rice CE, Braun KV, Boyle CA. Concurrent medical conditions and health care use and needs among children with learning and behavioral developmental disabilities: National Health Interview Survey, 2006–2010. *Res Dev Disabil.* 2012;33(2):467–476.

103. Kohane IS, McMurry A, Weber G, MacFadden D, Rappaport L, Kunkel L, Bickel J, Wattanasin N, Spence S, Murphy S, Churchill S. The co-morbidity burden of children and young adults with autism spectrum disorders. *PLoS ONE.* 2012;7(4):e33224.

104. McCall BP, Starr EM. Effects of autism spectrum disorder on parental employment in the United States: evidence from the National Health Interview Survey. *Community, Work & Family.* 2018;21(4):367–392.

105. Helt M, Kelley E, Kinsbourne M, Pandey J, Boorstein H, Herbert M, et al. Can children with autism recover? If so, how? *Neuropsychol Rev.* 2008;18(4):339–366

106. Dawson G. Early behavioral intervention, brain plasticity, and the prevention of autism spectrum disorder. *Dev Psychopathol.* 2008;20(3):775–803

107. Early Childhood Technical Assistance Center. The Individuals with Disabilities Education Act IIDEA [Internet]. North Carolina: UNC; 2023 (cited February 1, 2023). Available from: https://ectacenter.org/idea.asp.

108. Foxx RM. Applied behavior analysis treatment of autism: the state of the art. *Child Adolesc Psychiatr Clin N Am.* 2008;17(4):821–834

109. Virués-Ortega J. Applied behavior analytic intervention for autism in early childhood: meta-analysis, meta-regression and dose-response meta-analysis of multiple outcomes. *Clin Psychol Rev.* 2010;30(4):387–399

110. Erba HW. Early intervention programs for children with autism: conceptual frameworks for implementation. *Am J Orthopsychiatry.* 2000;70(1):82–94.

111. Stahmer AC, Ingersoll B, Carter C. Behavioral approaches to promoting play. *Autism.* 2003;7(4):401–413.

112. Verschuur R, Didden R, Lang R, Sigafoos J, Huskens B. Pivotal response treatment for children with autism spectrum disorders: a systematic review. *Rev J Autism Dev Disord.* 2013;1(1):34–61.

113. Lei J, Ventola P. Pivotal response treatment for autism spectrum disorder: current perspectives. *Neuropsychiatr Dis Treat.* 2017;13:1613–1626.

114. Jobin A. Varied treatment response in young children with autism: a relative comparison of structured and naturalistic behavioral approaches. Autism. 2020;24(2):338–351.

115. Bondy AS, Frost LA. The picture exchange communication system. *Semin Speech Lang.* 1998;19(4):373–388.

116. Bernier A, Ratcliff K, Hilton C, Fingerhut P, Li CY. Art interventions for children with autism spectrum disorder: a scoping review. *Am J Occup Ther.* 2022;76(5):7605205030.

117. Bodison SC, Parham LD. Specific sensory techniques and sensory environmental modifications for children and youth with sensory integration difficulties: a systematic review. *Am J Occup Ther.* 2018;72(1):7201190040p1–7201190040p11.

118. Aishworiya R, Valica T, Hagerman R, Restrepo B. An update on psychopharmacological treatment of autism spectrum disorder. *Neurotherapeutics.* 2022;19(1):248–262.

119. Masi A, DeMayo MM, Glozier N, Guastella AJ. An overview of autism spectrum disorder: heterogeneity and treatment options. *Neurosci Bull.* 2017;33(2):183–193.

120. Kevelson SD, Rahman J, Veenstra-VanderWeele J. Autism Spectrum Disorders. In Dulcan MK, ed., *Dulcan's Textbook of Child and Adolescent Psychiatry.* 3rd ed. American Psychiatric Association Publishing; 2022:146–151.

121. Dulcan MK, Ballard RR, Jha P, Sadhu JM, eds. *Concise Guide to Child and Adolescent Psychiatry.* 5th ed. American Psychiatric Association Publishing; 2018:41–50.

122. Deb S, Roy M, Limbu B, Akrout Brizard B, Murugan M, Roy A, Santambrogio J. Randomised controlled trials of antipsychotics for people with autism spectrum disorder: a systematic review and meta-analysis. *Psychol Med.* 2023;53(16):7964–7972.

123. Zhou MS, Nasir M, Farhat LC, et al: Meta-analysis: pharmacologic treatment of restricted and repetitive behaviors in autism spectrum disorders. *J Am Acad Child Adolesc Psychiatry.* 2021;60:35–45.

124. Fieiras C, Chen MH, Escobar Liquitay CM, Meza N, Rojas V, Franco JVA, Madrid E. Risperidone and aripiprazole for autism spectrum disorder in children: an overview of systematic reviews. *BMJ Evidence-Based Med.* 2023;28(1):7–14.

125. Accordino RE, Kidd C, Politte LC, Henry CA, McDougle CJ. Pharmacological interventions in autism spectrum disorder. *Expert Opin Pharmacother.* 2016;17(7):937–952.

126. Sadock BJ, Sadock VA, Ruiz P, Kaplan HI. *Kaplan and Sadock's Synopsis of Psychiatry.* 11th ed. Wolters Kluwer; 2015.

127. Höfer J, Hoffmann F, Bachmann C. Use of complementary and alternative medicine in children and adolescents with autism spectrum disorder: a systematic review. *Autism.* 2017;21(4):387–402.

Attention Deficit/Hyperactivity Disorder

Cesar A. Soutullo

29.1 Introduction

Attention deficit/hyperactivity disorder (ADHD) is a neurodevelopmental disorder that appears in childhood and has a high prevalence (5.9%) [1]. It is about 2:1 in male:female frequency, but the rate in clinical settings can be as high as 9:1, as females may have just inattention and thus may escape clinical detection until they fail in academics at a later age [2].

ADHD was first described by European authors: Weikgard in Germany (1775), Crichton in United Kingdon (1798), Hoffmann in Germany (1845), Bourneville, Boulanger and Paul-Boncour in France (1887–1901), Still in United Kingdom (1902), Rodriguez-Lafora in Spain (1917), and Kramer and Pillnow in Germany (1932) [2]. These researchers and clinicians gradually defined a behavioral syndrome in young children, initially attributed to a "lack of moral control," then thought to be brain-based and genetic in origin. It was found in some children who suffered post–viral lethargic encephalitis associated with the 1918–1920 N1H1 influenza pandemic that started in Kansas (US), known as the Spanish Flu. Initially the disease was called hyperkinetic disorder (the term used until ICD-10) or minimal brain damage/dysfunction, renamed ADD in DSM-III (1980), and eventually changed ADHD, with three presentations: predominantly inattentive, hyperactive/impulsive, or combined [3].

29.2 Definition, Clinical Characteristics, and Diagnosis

The current DSM-5-TR [3] definition requires a clinical diagnosis, with the presence of the following:

1. Developmentally inappropriate levels of hyperactive-impulsive and/or inattentive symptoms for at least 6 months
2. Symptoms must be present in at least two settings (e.g., home, school)
3. Symptoms must cause impairment
4. Some of the symptoms and impairments first occurred prior to age 12
5. No other disorder (medical, psychiatric or medication, substance or toxic exposure, or environmental) can better explain the symptoms.

Unlike prior editions, ICD-11 [4] now has criteria similar to DSM and defines ADHD as a "persistent pattern (at least 6 months) of inattention and/or hyperactivity-impulsivity that has a direct negative impact on academic, occupational or social functioning."

There is significant developmental and contextual variability: Younger children are more likely to present with hyperactivity/impulsivity, school-age children are more likely

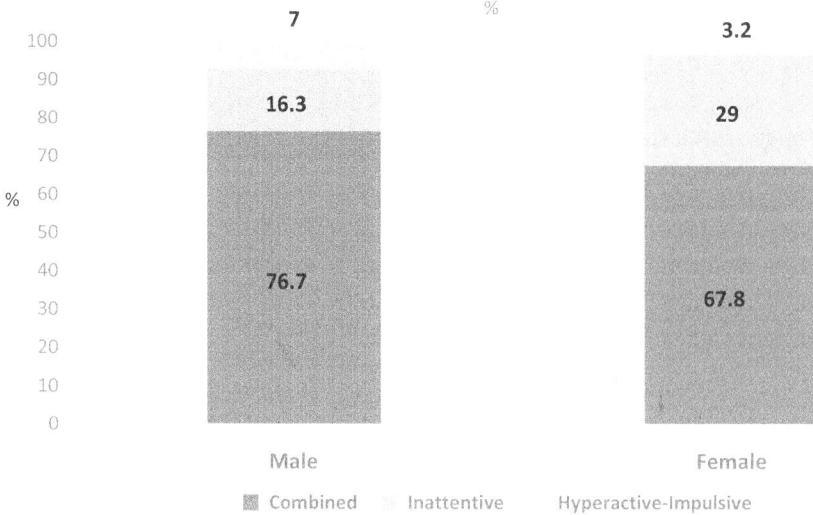

Figure 29.1 ADHD presentation (%) by sex.

to show the three key symptoms (hyperactivity/impulsivity and inattention), and adolescents, females, and adults may lose most, or all, their hyperactivity and retain inattention and impulsivity. Due to the lack of longitudinal stability, DSM and ICD dropped the prior subdivision in "subtypes" and coined the term "presentations": predominantly inattentive (more frequent in females: 29% vs 16.3% in males), predominantly hyperactive impulsive (the least frequent), and combined (the more frequent both in boys: 76.7% and girls: 67.8%) [2, 3] (Figure 29.1).

Younger boys present clinically with behavioral problems secondary to their hyperactivity/impulsivity as well as academic underachievement. These children present a bit before or immediately after first grade, when the rules and routines at school become more rigorous, and worsen as the academic expectations increase. Depending on the type of preschool education (less or more structured), symptoms may have more or less impact. For example, if the child is expected to sit down and work on reading and writing, their symptoms may impact more and differ from neurotypically developing children. If the level of academic and behavioral expectation is lower, or there is a lot of one-on-one supervision, symptoms may be present but not impact until later grades of primary school. Girls or children with a more inattentive presentation may remain undetected until later ages, closer to 10–12 years, when they start having academic difficulties. This is related to the gradual reduction in parent support and the increasing academic demands/expectations that require more independent and efficacious work, complex schedules, assignments, and self-regulation.

ADHD is associated with significant, often severe longitudinal morbidity including academic impairment (lower rates of high school and college graduation, that leads to low self-esteem), behavioral problems (oppositional defiant [ODD] and conduct disorders [CD] linked to peer rejection and risky behaviors), and medical problems (increased risk of accidents, accidental poisoning, encounters with the law and substance use, higher rates of teen pregnancy and sexually transmitted diseases, obesity, and early death, accidents, violence [impulsivity], and lower rates of access to preventive medicine and healthy lifestyle habits). It is also associated with lower duration of relationships and employment, causing important personal and societal loss and economic burden (US$19.4 billion/year in the United States) [2–7].

Contrary to popular belief, ADHD is neither a predominantly academic problem nor a benign/cosmetic issue. However, some of these negative outcomes are preventable and respond to treatment [6], but adherence to medication and other forms of treatment tends to be suboptimal [8, 9].

A recent review of clinical guidelines found they all emphasize the need to screen for ADHD and for a complete clinical history, including standardized rating scales to diagnose ADHD. Guidelines point out that there is no laboratory or psychological test for ADHD [10]. The most used rating scale to determine the presence and severity of ADHD symptoms is the ADHD-RS [11], with versions that are parent- and teacher-rated. There are validated versions for preschoolers [12], also available in Spanish [13] and other languages. This rating scale is frequently used in research as a clinician-scored scale that collects information from the parents as well as observational information from the child. In adults, the Adult ADHD Self-report Scale is the standard of care [14]. These are very useful tools to identify the presence and severity of symptoms as well as to track improvement of symptoms over time in an evidence-based, measurement-based care model. However, these instruments are not diagnostic, as they can be (falsely) positive in other medical or psychiatric conditions. The diagnosis in ADHD remains totally clinical, based on parents interview, child examination, collateral information from teachers, coaches, and others, and ruling out other medical, developmental, learning, psychiatric, or substance use problems [2, 3].

Along these lines, these is no neuropsychological test that can diagnose ADHD [15], but a good neuropsychological evaluation can assess some of the most widely accepted theories about neuropsychological deficits in ADHD. These may include working memory, processing speed (that can be tested along with intellectual function with IQ testing), sustained attention and inhibitory control (tested with Stroop test and CPT), motor control, divided attention/task switching (Trail Making), cognitive flexibility (WCST), planning (Tower of London), and affect regulation. This is a rapidly developing area, but there is no single test that can make a diagnosis.

29.3 Epidemiology

ADHD, like most neurodevelopmental disorders, is more frequent in males, with an estimated international prevalence of 5.9% [1]. There are no significant international differences between North America and Europe, Asia, Africa, South America, and Oceania [1]. There is also no evidence of an increasing epidemiological prevalence over time in the last three decades [1]. Studies in the United States and Sweden found more likelihood of diagnosis over the last years (increasing administrative prevalence). However, both the rates of diagnosis and treatment in most countries are still way below 2%, showing that more than half of the children (and most adults) with ADHD still remain undiagnosed [16]. Rates of ADHD in adults are about 2.2%, and 1.5% in persons over age 50 [2].

29.4 Etiology

ADHD is a highly heritable polygenic brain-based disorder (77% heritability), with some environmental causes, mostly problems during pregnancy and delivery (low birth weight, exposure to nicotine or alcohol in utero, birth hypoxia, severe neglect, and brain injury) [2]. Many genetic and environmental risk factors accumulate to cause the disorder, with evidence of gene–environment (GxE) interactions. ADHD in not produced by negative parenting, but severe psychosocial deprivation, abuse, or neglect can produce clinical pictures similar to ADHD. This was well documented by Dr. Rutter in United Kingdom, who studied chronically neglected institutionalized orphans in the Socialist Republic of Romania under Ceauşescu, who eventually were adopted by British families.

There is no single gene that has been identified as cause of ADHD, but there are several genes that may explain low percentage of the variance. Among the candidate genes, some have been identified, such as ANKK1, DAT1, LRP5, LRP6, SNAP25, ADGRL3, DRD4, and BAIAP2 [2]. Most of these genes are expressed in the brain and are involved in the formation of proteins that play key roles in dopamine or other amines' reuptake or transport, as well as receptors and some synaptic connectivity proteins [2]. GxE interactions make some children more sensitive to environmental stressors depending on their genetic characteristics. For example, studies found an association between COMT Met/Met polymorphism and executive function deficits (higher impulsivity) and higher number of sexual partners [17]. There is also preliminary data on DRD3 haplotypes, prenatal maternal smoking, and higher rates of resistance to medications (stimulants) and having both genetic and exposure to nicotine in utero has a multiplying effect on treatment resistance [18].

There are also genes involved in the expression of the disorder (type of symptoms, association with executive function deficits or other neuropsychological testing alterations, comorbidity with autism spectrum, tics/Tourette, mood, and anxiety disorders), response to treatment, sensitivity to adverse events, and persistence of the disorder into adulthood.

Four decades of neuroimaging and neuropsychological research have helped to develop a model to understand ADHD, and its key neuropsychological findings include alteration in structure, function, and connectivity of frontoparietal attentional, reward, executive control, and motor network circuits [2].

1. Alteration in frontal and anterior cingulate circuits involved in the modulation of "executive function" (sustained and divided attention, resistance to distraction, ability to shift tasks and still finish the task, and working memory).
2. Alteration in basal ganglia circuits involved in reward processing (nucleus accumbens), impulse control, and delayed aversion.
3. Difficulty in modulating emotional responses coming from limbic circuits and the amygdala.
4. Alterations in functional connectivity and inability to turn off circuits or switch activity from circuits such as the default mode network and activate frontal "task-relevant" circuits when there is a demand to perform a task, or ventral attentional networks (involved in self-instructions) [19]. These findings are based on functional neuroimaging studies in children with ADHD versus controls that found hypoactivation mostly in systems involved in executive function (frontoparietal network) and attention (ventral attentional network), and hyperactivation predominantly in the default, ventral attention, and somatomotor networks. In adults with ADHD they found hypoactivation in the frontoparietal system and hyperactivation in the visual, dorsal attention, and default networks [19].

5. There is also evidence of persistent volumetric and functional connectivity abnormalities in patients who continue to show symptoms of ADHD in adulthood (persistent ADHD), and at least partial resolution of some of these deficits both with medication treatment and in patients who no longer have symptoms in adulthood [20].

29.5 Treatment of ADHD

The treatment of ADHD is multimodal in nature and involves a series of strategies in three domains that generally should be combined for a better result. They also need to evolve and adapt to the needs of the child, adolescent, emerging adult, and fully independent adults, family, school/academic or work demands, and clinical characteristics including strengths and difficulties in specific areas: verbal, nonverbal abilities, and others. These three interventions have demonstrated efficacy when combined and include [2, 21–24]:

1. Psychoeducation and parent training in behavioral modification (behavioral therapy).
2. School/academic intervention, after a detailed evaluation, to compensate for difficulties and use strengths as leverage.
3. Safe and effective medication management [21–24] with stimulants or nonstimulants:

   a. Stimulants: Dopamine transporter inhibitors (methylphenidate or dextroamphetamine)
   b. Nonstimulants: mostly norepinephrine (NE) agents: alfa 2 agonists (guanfacine, clonidine) or NE reuptake inhibitors (atomoxetine, viloxazine).

The treatment plan must be agreed with parents and patient, based on a set of target symptoms and prioritized realistic treatment goals (Figure 29.2). These goals and target symptoms may respond to different components of the multimodal treatment and should be reevaluated periodically once they are achieved, or new problems arise, in a

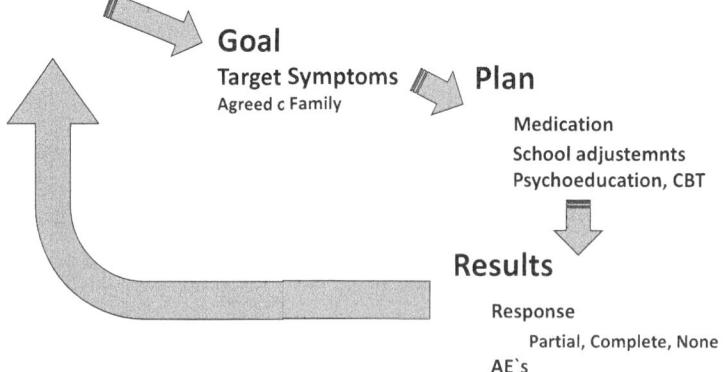

PDCA. Plan, Do, Check, Adjust

Evaluation: ADHD. Biological Brain Disorder that produces behaviors

Goal
Target Symptoms
Agreed c Family

Plan
Medication
School adjustemnts
Psychoeducation, CBT

Results
Response
Partial, Complete, None
AE`s

Figure 29.2 PDCA model for ADHD multimodal treatment planning, establishing target symptoms and goals with the family, and readjustment depending on results and new emerging problems.

model similar to that of continuous improvement and performance evaluation (quality improvement).

29.5.1 Medication Efficacy and Effectiveness

A detailed description of each medication available for ADHD in children, adolescents, and adults is beyond the scope of this manual and can be found elsewhere [21–24]. There are several medications available that have been approved for ADHD, but this widely varies among different countries (Figure 29.3).

29.5.1.1 Stimulants in ADHD

- **Methylphenidate (MPH) and Dex-MPH.** It has many different galenic forms (tablets, capsules, oral solutions and patches), with different delivery systems (immediate, extended release, osmotic delivery system, or modified release with biphasic pellets), the racemic form dexmethylphenidate (d-MPH), and its combination with the pro-drug ser-d-MPH.
- **Dextroamphetamine.** It also has several galenic formulations, delivery systems, immediate- and extended-release forms, mixed salts, and the pro-drug lisdexamphetamine. Pro-drugs are medications that are bound to an amino acid and are inactive outside the body and activated inside. This is a protective mechanism to minimize risk of substance abuse.

Stimulants are the most effective medications in ADHD with an effect size range from 0.8 to 1.1 [23]. An effect size (ES) (Cohen's D or Standardized Mean Difference) higher

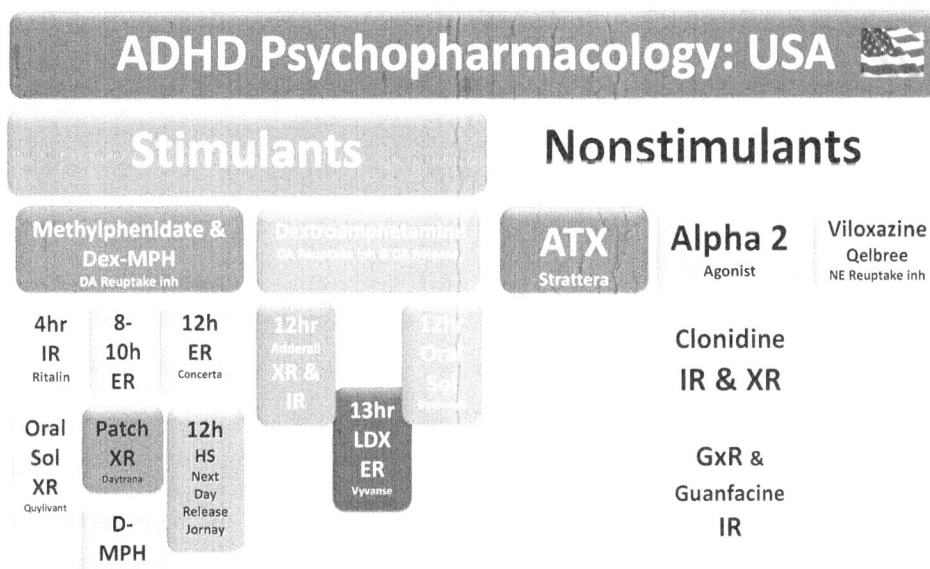

Figure 29.3 Medications approved in the USA for ADHD. A good resource that we recommend to our trainees is the downloadable table of current medications available at: www.adhdmedicationguide.com [26].

than 0.8 is considered high, and between 0.5–0.8 is considered medium. ES is calculated dividing the difference in means between the two groups (medication vs placebo in this case), divided by the standard deviation (SD). For a similar difference between groups, a low SD will yield a high ES.

The ES of d-amphetamine is higher than that of MPH, but tolerability to d-amphetamines tends to be a bit worse [23], so current guidelines tend to favor MPH as the first-line treatment [21–24]. If there is no response, the doctor should switch to d-amphetamine. However, the choice between MPH and d-amphetamine is a matter of parents and physician preference. Some guidelines value cost-effectiveness, not just efficacy and tolerability [24]. Lisdexamphetamine is the only extended-release d-amphetamine available in Europe. Due to its relatively recent release, and its cost, with similar or slightly better efficacy than MPH, it was approved by the European Medications Agency (EMA) as second line, after the patient fails or does not tolerate MPH. As medicine advances, and cost of testing drops, pharmacogenetic testing and other tools for precision medicine will be used to identify individual rates of preferential responders or nonresponders, as well as fast or slow metabolizers, for different medications [25].

Stimulants are very safe and work fast, but in order to be effective, the dose needs to be sufficient and individually titrated, as they have a dose–response curve [21–22]. The dose needs to be gradually increased, usually every week, to reach a full response, if tolerated (start low and increase slow, but don´t stay in a subtherapeutic dose). Once we reach a possible therapeutic dose that is reasonably tolerated, we wait there to see a full response, as some symptoms may take longer to improve. In general, MPH therapeutic range starts at around 1 mg/kg/day, but it can vary from child to child. It is important to know that d-MPH has double the potency of MPH, so the equivalent dose should be half of that of MPH. The approximate equivalence of MPH to d-amphetamine is also 2:1, but in general d-amphetamine may be a bit more effective, so lower doses may be sufficient. Sometimes, a nonresponder who has been previously treated may respond to simply a higher dose.

Preferential Response to MPH or d-Amphetamine

About 69% of patients will have a (partial or complete) response to d-amphetamine, and 57% will respond to methylphenidate. Twenty-eight percent will have a preferential response to d-amphetamine, 16% will have a preferential response to methylphenitate, and 41% percent will respond to either of the two molecules [27]. So, in theory, we can obtain a significant response in 85% of patients, but 15% will be nonresponders to stimulants (Figure 29.4).

29.5.1.2 Nonstimulants in ADHD

For patients that do not respond to stimulants, have a partial response, or do not tolerate them due to adverse events (AEs), or if parents do not want to use stimulants, the nonstimulants are good alternatives. The development of nonstimulants was seeking to avoid the reward DA pathway (nucleus accumbens), having no abuse potential, and avoiding the classification as Schedule II N medications (high potential for abuse). It also was trying to avoid the observed effect of stimulants as potentially worsening on tics, due to its effect on the cortico-striatal DA pathway. They are a bit less effective, with effect sizes ranging from 0.4 to 0.6 (medium range), and they also take longer to work [22, 23].

Meta-analysis
Differential Response to Stimulants

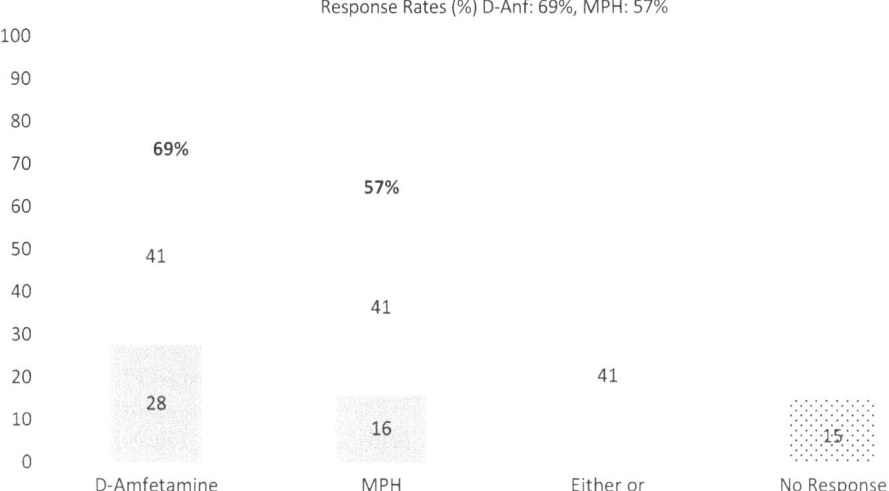

Response Rates (%) D-Anf: 69%, MPH: 57%

Figure 29.4 Differential response to stimulants.
Adapted from Arnold LE. Methylphenidate vs. amphetamine: comparative review. *J Att Disord*. 2000;3(4), 200–211.

Norepinephrine Reuptake Inhibitors

The benefits of NE reuptake inhibitors in ADHD were known since the 1980s with the off-label use of tricyclic antidepressants, but they never reach significance in the clinical trials to obtain the US Food and Drug Administration (FDA) approval. In the early 2000s Atomoxetine was approved for ADHD in the United States, Europe, and other countries as the first nonstimulant, a possible alternative to stimulants.

- **Atomoxetine.** This medication may take up to 12 weeks to achieve a full response, but you can see a partial response at 4 weeks of fully therapeutic dose [28]. Atomoxetine is started at 0.5 mg/kg/day for the first week or two and then increased to the full therapeutic dose of 1.2 mg/kg/day. There is no evidence that pushing the dose higher may have any more benefits than waiting a bit longer on 1.2 mg/kg/d, but some patients may respond to 1.4–1.6 mg/kg/day. Atomoxetine may have a bimodal response pattern to which patients either do or do not respond. In a meta-analysis of atomoxetine studies by Newcorn, almost half of the patients (47%) had a much improved clinical response, 40% had no response, and only 13% had a minimal response. No baseline predictors of the response were found, except having some response by week 4 of treatment, which predicted a response by 12 weeks (sensitivity 81%, specificity 72%, positive predictive value 75%, and negative predictive value 79%) [28]. There is preliminary functional neuroimaging evidence of the possible prediction of response to methylphenidate versus atomoxetine in patients who showed striatal activation [29].
- **Viloxazine-ER.** Viloxazine extended-release was approved in 2021 by the FDA for the treatment of ADHD in children and adolescents (ages 6–17 years). Viloxazine is a novel nonstimulant with norepinephrine reuptake inhibitor properties, and may also

have serotonergic signaling activity in the brain [30]. The recommended titration for children (ages 6–11) is to start at 100mg/day on week 1 and increase by 100 mg/day every week until reaching 400mg/day (required dose for 43% of the children in the studies). For adolescents (ages 12–17) you can start at 200 mg/day on week 1 (that was enough for 39% of the adolescents in the studies) and then increase to 300 or 400 mg/day (required for 39% of adolescents in the study). In the clinical trials it started to separate from placebo after week 1, but the effect was maximum at week 4. It can show some partial efficacy at 50% of these recommended doses.

Alpha-2 Agonists

The alpha-2 agonists guanfacine and clonidine also work through the NE system, by activating the alpha-2 postsynaptic receptor. They enhance NE signaling, thus improving the signal-to-noise ratio, as opposed to DA agents like stimulants that reduce the noise. Guanfacine is more selective than clonidine, and thus produces less cardiovascular/blood pressure effects and less sedation.

- **Guanfacine.** Guanfacine needs to be titrated slowly, starting at 1mg/day on week 1, then 2mg/d on week 2, and so on. If we use the immediate-release formulation, the dose should be divided in AM and PM (bid). The extended-release (XR) formulation can be given once a day in AM, or if not tolerated (sedation, fatigue, low blood pressure), it can be given at bedtime. The usual therapeutic dose is 0.1 mg/kg/day. So, for example, a 30-kg child may respond to 3 mg. It takes longer than stimulants to work, but not as much as atomoxetine, and you can see a partial response when you reach 50% of the target dose. Some children may need a slower titration or cannot reach the full recommended dose but may respond to lower doses.
- **Clonidine.** Clonidine dosing can be tricky due to the decimals, so caution must be in place to avoid mistakes. The range of therapeutic dose is 0.15–0.25 mg/kg/day. It should be titrated carefully, and the rule is not to increase the dose more than 0.05 mg every 3 days [31]. It also has an XR formulation.

29.5.1.3 Stimulant and Nonstimulant Combination

Stimulants and nonstimulants can be combined; if there is a partial response to stimulants and insufficient response to nonstimulant, one can try to use lower doses of both agents to target different receptors (DA and NA).

29.5.2 Safety and Tolerability

ADHD medications are very safe and relatively easy to use by a trained physician. The use of stimulants is limited in the case of very small children (preschoolers) or children who develop adverse events (AEs). The most frequent AEs are decreased appetite (which may result in weight loss), delayed sleep onset, and other, less frequent adverse events such as worsening or developing anxiety, mood changes, including worsening irritability, flattened affect/excessive sadness, or sensitivity to criticism.

Some of these AEs can be minimized by gradual titration of dose, increasing toward a therapeutic dose every 7–10 days, giving the medication as early as possible in AM (to avoid sleep disturbances at night), trying to stay on the same dose every day (not stopping medication on weekends), since there is some accommodation, and eventually decreasing the dose if AEs do not improve and are moderate or severe. Other, less frequent AEs are headaches, GI problems (heartburn), worsening or onset of motor or vocal tics, and even psychotic symptoms. In this last case, the medication should be discontinued, and a urine toxicity screen in indicated to rule out substance use.

Due to the mild chronotropic effect of stimulants, children with known history of cardiac arrythmias, known cardiac malformations, or family history of sudden death need pediatric cardiology clearance before starting a stimulant or other medication for ADHD (such as alfa-2 agonists). The same cardiac clearance is needed if the child develops paroxystic tachycardia, dizziness, or fainting on exertion or at rest.

The nonstimulants may have a different set of AEs, such as decreased blood pressure, bradycardia and dizziness/fainting spells, or sedation / decreased energy with alfa-agonists clonidine and guanfacine. Atomoxetine may induce sedation or difficulty in sleep onset, changes in appetite, but not as intense as stimulants, and poor gastrointestinal tolerability.

29.5.3 Non-Approved or Non-Effective Agents in ADHD

There are some agents that have been used in ADHD due to some beneficial effects but that are not approved in any country for children or adults with ADHD [2, 22, 23]. These include NE tricyclic antidepressants (mostly desipramine and nortriptyline), not recommended due to severe cardiac risks, poor tolerability, and narrow therapeutic range; bupropion, venlafaxine, and reboxetine. Risperidone has been used in small children with ADHD to control irritability and agitation or temper outbursts, but there is no evidence of its efficacy for ADHD core symptoms.

There is no evidence of the beneficial effect of elimination diets (except maybe elimination of artificial food coloring, with a very low effect size <0.2), omega 3 fatty acids, alternative medicine/herbal remedies, or cannabis products [2, 32].

29.5.4 Nonpharmacological Treatments in ADHD

Nonpharmacological treatments for ADHD are recommended as first-line treatment in preschoolers [24] and as adjunctive treatment to pharmacological management in all ages, mostly behavioral management training for parents and academic interventions [2, 21, 22, 24].

29.5.4.1 Psychotherapy

Psychotherapeutic interventions that have demonstrated moderate efficacy in ADHD include parent training for preschool children and cognitive-behavioral therapy, with strong emphasis on the behavioral aspects and organizational skills [2]. There is little evidence that cognitive training or social skills training improve ADHD symptoms or academic achievement [2], but computerized cognitive training may improve verbal working memory [32–34]. Cognitive-behavioral therapy may be more effective for the non-core ADHD symptoms that are frequently comorbid, such as oppositional defiant symptoms, anxiety, and problems in parent–child interaction [22].

29.5.4.2 Academic Intervention

After a careful evaluation and specific academic intervention, accommodations and modifications should be put in place for every child with ADHD [2]. These include remediation in areas where there is a delay (reading, writing, math), accommodations (when there is no change in the curricular content but the methodology is changed, for example oral exams in children with writing difficulties), and modifications (significant curricular changes described in an Individual Educational Plan [IEP]). In the United States, the accommodations are listed in a "504 Plan," described in Section 504 of the Rehabilitation Act of 1973, which prohibits discrimination on the basis of disability in schools. They remain under General Education, and the child stays in the least restrictive environment, as opposed to children in Special Education with an IEP, who may be placed in a self-contained classroom for part of or the entire day. Parents have the right to request an evaluation at school and adequate accommodations and remediation depending on the child's needs.

References

1. Polanczyk GV, Willcutt EG, Salum GA, Kieling C, Rohde LA. ADHD prevalence estimates across three decades: an updated systematic review and meta-regression analysis. *Int J Epidemiol.* 2014;43(2):434–442.

2. Faraone SV, Banaschewski T, Coghill D, et al. The World Federation of ADHD International Consensus Statement: 208 Evidence-based Conclusions about the Disorder, Neuroscience and Biobehavioral Reviews 2021, https://doi.org/10.1016/j.neubiorev.2021.01.022

3. American Psychiatric Association. (2022). *Diagnostic and Statistical Manual of Mental Disorders* (5th ed., text rev.). https://doi.org/10.1176/appi.books.9780890425787

4. International Classification of Diseases, Eleventh Revision (ICD-11), World Health Organization (WHO) 2019/2021.

5. Ruiz-Goikoetxea M, Cortese S, Aznárez-Sanado M, et al. Risk of unintentional injuries in children and adolescents with ADHD and the impact of ADHD medications: a systematic review and meta-analysis. *Neurosci Biobehav Rev.* 2017 Nov 18. [Epub ahead of print].

6. Boland H, DiSalvo M, Fried R, et al. A literature review and meta-analysis on the effects of ADHD medications on functional outcomes. *J Psychiatr Res.* 2020;123:21–30.

7. Pelham WE, Page TF, Altszuler AR, Gnagy EM, Molina BSG, Pelham WE. The long-term financial outcome of children diagnosed with ADHD. *J Consult Clin Psychol.* 2020;88(2):160–171.

8. Baweja R, Soutullo CA, Waxmonsky JC. Review of barriers and interventions to promote engagement for pediatric ADHD. *World J Psychiatry.* 2021; 11 (12):1206–1227.

9. Biederman J, Fried R, DiSalvo M, et al. Evidence of low adherence to stimulant medication among children and youths with ADHD: an electronic health records study. *Psychiatric Services.* 2019;70 (10):874–880.

10. Pliszka SR, Pereira-Sanchez V, Robles-Ramamurthy B. A review of clinical practice guidelines in the diagnosis and treatment of attention deficit/hyperactivity disorder. *Child Adolesc Psychiatric Clin N Am.* 2022; 31:569–581.

11. DuPaul GJ, Power TJ, Anastopoulos AD, Reid R. *ADHD Rating Scale – 5 for Children and Adolescents: Checklists, Norms, and Clinical Interpretation.* 2nd ed. Guilford Press; 2016.

12. McGoey KE, DuPaul GJ, Haley E, Shelton TL. Parent and teacher ratings of attention-deficit/hyperactivity disorder in preschool: the ADHD rating scale-IV preschool version. *J Psychopathol Behav Assess.* 2007;29(4):269–276.

13. Marín-Méndez JJ, Borra-Ruiz MC, Álvarez-Gómez MJ, McGoey KE, Soutullo C. Normative ADHD-RS-preschool data in a community sample in Spain. *Atten Disord.* 2019;23(6):615–623.

14. Adler L, Kessler RC, Spencer T, WHO. Adult ADHD Rating Scale. https://add .org/wp-content/uploads/2015/03/adhd-questionnaire-ASRS111.pdf.

15. De Freitas de Sousa A, Meneghetti Coimbra I, Marrone Castanho J, Polanczyk GV, Rhode LA. Attention Deficit Hyperactivity Disorder. In Rey JM, Martin A, eds., *JM Rey's IACAPAP e-Textbook of Child and Adolescent Mental Health*. International Association for Child and Adolescent Psychiatry and Allied Professions: 2020.

16. Cortese S. Pharmacologic treatment of attention deficit-hyperactivity disorder. *N Eng J Med.* 2020;383(11):1050–1056.

17. Bousman CA, Cherner M, Atkinson JH, Heaton RK, Grant I, Everall IP, the HNRC Group. COMT Val158Met polymorphism, executive dysfunction, and sexual risk behavior in the context of HIV infection and methamphetamine dependance. *Interdisciplinary Perspectives on Infectious Diseases.* 2010. https://doi .org/10.1155/2010/678648. www.hindawi .com/journals/ipid/2010/678648/.

18. Pagerols M, Richarte V, Sánchez-Mora C, Garcia-Martínez I, Corrales M, Corominas M, Cormand B, Casas M, Ribasés M, Ramos-Quiroga JA. Pharmacogenetics of methylphenidate response and tolerability in ADHD. *Pharmacogenomics J.* 2017;17(1):98–104.

19. Cortese S, Kelly C, Chabernaud C, Proal E, Di Martino A, Milham MP, Castellanos FX. Toward systems neuroscience of ADHD: a meta-analysis of 55 fMRI studies. *Am J Psychiatry.* 2012;169 (10):1038–1055.

20. Mattfeld AT, Gabrieli JD, Biederman J, Spencer T, Brown A, Kotte A, Kagan E, Whitfield-Gabrieli S. Brain differences between persistent and remitted attention deficit hyperactivity disorder. *Brain.* 2014;137(Pt 9):2423–2428.

21. Wolraich L, Hagan JF, Allan C, et al. Clinical practice guideline for the diagnosis, evaluation, and treatment of attention-deficit/hyperactivity disorder in children and adolescents. *Pediatrics.* 2019;144(4):e20192528.

22. Coghill D, Banaschewski T, Cortese S, Asherson P, Brandeis D, Buitelaar J, et al. The management of ADHD in children and adolescents: bringing evidence to the clinic: perspective from the European ADHD Guidelines Group (EAGG). *Eur Child Adolesc Psychiatry.* 2021. [cited January 11, 2022]. https://doi.org/10 .1007/s00787-021-01871-x.

23. Cortese S, Adamo N, Del Giovane C, Mohr-Jensen C, Hayes AJ, Carucci S, et al. Comparative efficacy and tolerability of medications for attention-deficit hyperactivity disorder in children, adolescents, and adults: a systematic review and network meta-analysis. *Lancet Psychiatry.* 2018;5(9):727–738.

24. National Institute for Health and Care Excellence [NICE]. Attention deficit hyperactivity disorder: diagnosis and management (NICE guideline [NG87]). *Progress in Neurology and Psychiatry.* 2018 [cited March 30, 2022]. Available from: www.nice.org.uk/guidance/ng87.

25. Buitelaar J, Bölte S5, Brandeis D, Caye A, Christmann N, Cortese S, Coghill D, Faraone SV, Franke B, Gleitz M, Greven CU, Kooij S, Teixeira Leffa D, Rommelse N, Newcorn JH, Polanczyk GV, Rohde LA, Simonoff E, Stein M, Vitiello B, Yazgan Y, Roesler M, Doepfner M, Banaschewski T. Toward precision medicine in ADHD. *Front Behav Neurosci.* 2022;16:900981.

26. Adeshman A. 2023. www.adhdmedicationguide.com.

27. Arnold LE. Methylphenidate vs. amphetamine: comparative review. *J Att Disord.* 2000;3(4), 200–211.

28. Newcorn JH, Sutton VK, Weiss MD, Sumner CR. Clinical responses to atomoxetine in attention-deficit/ hyperactivity disorder: the Integrated Data Exploratory Analysis (IDEA) study. *J Am Acad Child Adolesc Psychiatry.* 2009;48(5):511–518.

29. Schulz KP, Bédard AV, Fan J, Hildebrandt TB, Stein MA, Ivanov I, Halperin JM, Newcorn JH. Striatal activation predicts differential therapeutic responses to methylphenidate and

atomoxetine. *J Am Acad Child Adolesc Psychiatry*. 2017;56(7):602–609.e2.

30. Nasser A, Hull JT, Chaturvedi SA, Liranso T, Odebo O, Koshelef AR, Nicholas Fry N, Cutler AJ, Rubin J, Stefan Schwabe S, Childress A. A phase III, randomized, double-blind, placebo-controlled trial assessing the efficacy and safety of viloxazine extended-release capsules in adults with attention-deficit/hyperactivity disorder. *CNS Drugs*. 2022;36:897–915.

31. Martin A, Scahill L, Kratochvil CJ, eds. *Pediatric Psychopharmacology: Principles and Practice*. 2nd ed. Oxford University Press; 2010.

32. Sonuga-Barke E, Brandeis D, Cortese S, Daley D, Ferrin M, Holtmann M, Stevenson J, Danckaerts M, van der Oord S, Döpfner M, Dittmann RW, Simonoff E, Zuddas A, Banaschewski T, Buitelaar J, Coghill D, Hollis C, Konofal E, Lecendreux M, Wong ICK, Sergeant J, the European ADHD Guidelines Group. Nonpharmacological interventions for ADHD: systematic review and meta-analyses of randomized controlled trials of dietary and psychological treatments. *Am J Psychiatry*. 2013;170 (3):275–289.

33. Cortese S, Ferrin M, Brandeis D, et al. Cognitive training for attention-deficit/ hyperactivity disorder: meta-analysis of clinical and neuropsychological outcomes from randomized controlled trials. *J Am Acad Child Adolesc Psychiatry*. 2015;54 (3):164–174. Erratum in: *J Am Acad Child Adolesc Psychiatry*. 2015 May;54(5):433.

34. Westwood SJ, Parlatini V, Rubia K, Cortese S, Sonuga-Barke EJS, Banaschewski T, Baeyens D, Bölte S, Brandeis D, Buitelaar J, Carucci S, Coghill D, Daley D, Döpfner M, Ferrin M, Galera C, Hollis C, Holtmann M, Purper-Ouakil D, Nagy P, Santosh P, Simonoff E, Soutullo CA, Stringaris A, Thapar A, van der Oord S, van den Hoofdakker BJ, Zuddas A, European ADHD Guidelines Group (EAGG). Computerized cognitive training in ADHD: a meta-analysis of randomized controlled trials with blinded and objective outcomes. *Mol Psychiatry*. 2023. https://doi.org/10.1038/s41380-023-02000-7. Online ahead of print.

Delirium and Other Medical Conditions Presenting with Psychiatric Symptoms

Silvia Hafliger

30.1 Introduction

Delirium is the most common neuropsychiatric syndrome in the medical setting. The sudden onset of acute brain dysfunction has been recognized since ancient times. As early as 500 BC, terms like phrenitis (agitated state) and lethargus (somnolence) were used to describe mental status changes in the setting of head trauma, fever, or poisoning [1].

This chapter straddles medicine, neurology, and psychiatry, encouraging the clinician to think holistically, how to recognize and treat the condition, and describes medical illnesses that can present with psychiatric symptoms such as endocrinopathies, limbic encephalitis (paraneoplastic syndromes), and Wilson's disease.

When working as a consulting psychiatrist, six principles need to be kept in mind:

1. Is this a psychiatric presentation of a medical illness?

    a. Depression as a harbinger of pancreatic cancer
    b. Anxiety in setting of a pulmonary embolism or hemorrhage
    c. Cognitive loss in the setting of brain cancer

2. Is this a psychiatric complication of medical treatment?

    a. Prednisone inducing mania in a post-transplant patient
    b. Immunomodulating drugs like interferon exacerbating or causing depression

3. Is this a medical presentation of a psychiatric illness?

    a. Delirium tremens in alcohol use disorder
    b. Heart arrythmias in setting of an eating disorder
    c. Nonepileptic seizures or chronic pain in conversion/somatic illness disorder

4. Is this a medical complication of psychiatric treatment?

    a. Neuroleptic malignant syndrome in setting of anti-dopaminergic drug use or withdrawal
    b. Serotonin syndrome with use of selective serotonin reuptake inhibitor and other serotonergic drugs like Linezolid
    c. Obesity and metabolic syndrome from second-generation antipsychotic medication
    d. Toxic megacolon due to Clozaril

5. Is this a presentation of comorbid psychiatric and medical illness?

    a. A patient with schizophrenia presenting with CHF

6. Is this a psychological reaction to medical illness?

   a. A patient reacting with grief, anger, and despair in setting of being told of cancer or end organ failure [2].

30.2 Delirium

Delirium has many names (ICU psychosis, toxic metabolic encephalopathy, acute confusion, "sundowning"), but all the labels can be thought of as acute brain failure, which in turn is a harbinger of significant cognitive, medical, and psychosocial dysfunction often lasting far longer than the initial presentation [3]. This condition has been underrecognized, undertreated, and often accepted as a cost associated with severe illness or ICU stays. A delirium episode affects patients, family, and caregivers profoundly and is never easily forgotten. It impacts individuals' identity, sense of autonomy, and behaviors.

30.2.1 Case Vignette

Mrs. J. is a 72-year-old widow, living alone, former teacher with prior medical history of congestive heart failure (treated with digoxin, amiodarone, and diuretics), diabetes (receiving Metformin), and osteoporosis (on alendronate). She is admitted for left hip fracture in the setting of a fall. She undergoes hip replacement surgery. Three days after her surgery nursing staff notices a change in her personality. She is described as withdrawn, quiet, not participating with a physical therapist. The medical staff requests a psychiatric consult to address a possible "acute nosocomial depression."

On psychiatric examination she appears somnolent. She is unable to sustain attention to questions and keeps stating that she wants to go home. She is not able to state the reason for admission and feels that the staff is harming her. She has not been eating as believes that she is being poisoned. Her sleep is impaired. She describes a yellow hue when looking at the wall.

You conduct a chart review and find an elevated WBC at 11.2, urine analysis is leukosterase positive, and her digoxin level is 2.5. Speaking to her daughter, you establish that Mrs. J. has no prior history of depression and was functionally independent before admission.

You diagnose hypoactive delirium in the setting of urinary tract infection and digitalis toxicity.

After her digitalis toxicity is treated and her urinary tract infection is resolved, her mental status returns to normal.

30.2.2 Clinical Presentation

Delirium was introduced to DSM-3 in 1980. Currently the DSM- 5TR criteria for delirium are:

A. Disturbance in attention and awareness

B. The disturbance presents acutely and fluctuates.

C. There is a change in cognition, memory, language, visuospatial ability, and perception.

D. The disturbance is not due to preexisting mental illness such as schizophrenia or neurocognitive disorder.

E. The disturbance is a direct consequence of a physiologic disturbance / medical illness / substance intoxication or withdrawal.

From a psychopathological standpoint, there are five core domains affected in delirium:

1. Cognitive deficits: impaired memory, abstract thinking, decreased executive function, impaired language
2. Attentional deficits: inability to focus, sustain and shift attention
3. Circadian rhythm disturbance: Sleep fragmentation and night day reversal
4. Emotional dysregulation: Fear, perplexity, anxiety, irritability, and anger
5. Psychomotor dysregulation: Agitation, picking, restlessness [4].

Moreover, five phenotypes for delirium have been described:

1. Subsyndromal delirium: characterized by restlessness, irritability, anxiety, and nightmares, without clear impairment in level of consciousness
2. Hyperactive delirium: More commonly seen in younger patients (with hyperdopaminergic or withdrawal states), present in about 10% of patients with delirium
3. Hypoactive delirium: More common in elderly patients, frequently associated with end organ failure or underlying neurocognitive disorder; seen in about 67 % of patients
4. Mixed delirium with features of hyperactivity and somnolence
5. Protracted / persistent delirium. Despite improvement of underlying medical illness or recovery from surgery, the patient continues to show fluctuation in attention and cognitive dysfunction often described as "brain fog."

While cases of hyperactive delirium are more easily recognized and treated, hypoactive delirium is commonly more insidious, prolonged, and difficult to diagnose, resulting in poorer outcomes.

30.2.3 Prevalence and Prognosis

The prevalence of delirium in the community is between 1% and 2%, but general hospital delirium rates are higher, ranging from 18% to 35% of admissions. In other words, one out of five hospitalized patients develop delirium. The prevalence increases even more in the ICU setting, and between 80% and 90% of end-of-life patients experience delirium.

Moreover, delirium leads to longer and more costly hospital stays. There is increased morbidity due to falls, decubitus ulcers, and feeding difficulties. In addition, the presence of delirium foretells a higher mortality rate both during the index admission and post discharge. Cognitive and functional decline post discharge often lead to nursing home admissions. Lastly, patients are at increased risk for PTSD/depression and dementia [5].

30.2.4 Vulnerability and Precipitating Factors

Diminished brain reserve, as seen in the elderly or very young patients or patients with underlying neurocognitive disorders, increases the risk for delirium. Patients with alcohol use disorder, traumatic brain injury, seizures, intellectual disability, prior cerebral vascular accident (CVA), and sensory impairment are vulnerable to developing delirium. Precipitating risk factors include severity of medical illness, polypharmacy, dehydration, immobility, and pain [6].

30.2.5 Diagnosis

Delirium is a great "masquerader," and the psychiatrist must assume that an acute change in mental status is due to delirium until proven otherwise [7]. Psychiatrists are in a unique position to evaluate mental status, search and identify underlying causes of delirium, treat agitation, and offer education and support to patients and families.

When facing a case of delirium, three history questions are critical:

1. What is the patient's baseline cognitive function?
2. What is the time frame of the symptoms?
3. What medications have been administered?

Collateral history from family or nursing staff is essential.

Delirium and neurocognitive disorder often overlap but can be distinguished by history regarding cognitive and functional abilities. Neurocognitive disorders present slowly, with gradual decline in an awake and alert patient. Memory complaints predominate.

Delirium presents acutely with fluctuating awareness and attention in a setting of underlying medical illness. Screening tools such as the Confusion Assessment Method (CAM / CAM-ICU) or the 4AT (Rapid Clinical Test for Delirium) can assist with diagnosis. A careful physical exam looking for tremors, asterixis, clonus, and motor deficits also needs to be performed.

Careful chart review with focus on medications administered or recently discontinued, laboratory review including renal, hepatic, and thyroid functions, complete blood count, urine culture, and urine drug screen are essential. Reviewing prescription drug monitoring sites might provide clues regarding controlled substance use or misuse. In addition, checking vital sign records, looking for periods of hypo- or hypertension, tachycardia, or fever, is also important. An electroencephalogram is often helpful in distinguishing depression from hypoactive delirium or inconvulsive status epilepticus. In delirium, the normal dominant alpha rhythm is replaced with diffuse delta slowing. An electrocardiogram, looking for arrhythmias and QTC prolongation, is also recommended.

Moreover, a good collaboration and communication with neurology and the medical/surgical team are essential aiming at the identification and treatment of the underlying cause of delirium (see the next section). Last, whenever working up a patient for delirium, ensuring physical safety and making sure the patient and the family remain calm and reassured are essential, sometimes with the help of sitters/one-to-one monitoring. See Section 30.2.8 for further details.

30.2.6 Etiology

When searching for underlying causes of delirium, nine categories must be carefully evaluated.

1. **Toxins**: Drugs administered or withdrawn. Offenders are digoxin, amiodaron, lidocaine, mexiletine, meperidine, quinolone antibiotics, opioids and benzodiazepines. Drugs of abuse include, among others, alcohol, PCP/cocaine, synthetic THC, ketamine, bath salts, and inhalants.
2. **Metabolic**: Electrolyte abnormalities such has hypo- or hypernatremia, hypo- or hyperglycemia, hypo- or hypercalcemia, hypoxia or hypercapnia, uremia, liver failure, vitamin deficiencies such as B12, thiamine (Wernicke encephalopathy)

3. **Infections**: Urinary tract infections are common and often overlooked, cellulitis, sepsis, pneumonia, meningitis, encephalitis, COVID-19.
4. **Endocrine abnormalities**: Hypo- or hyperthyroid, adrenal insufficiency
5. **Primary CNS injury**: Global hypoperfusion, hypertensive encephalopathy (posterior reversible encephalopathy syndrome/PRES), CVA ischemic or hemorrhagic, neurocognitive disorders, especially Lewy body dementia
6. **Autoimmune**: CNS vasculitis, cerebral lupus, autoimmune encephalitis
7. **Seizures**: Nonconvulsive status epilepticus, prolonged ictal state
8. **Cancer**: Brain metastasis form lung, breast, melanoma, CNS lymphoma, glial tumors
9. **Terminal**: End-of-life delirium: multi-organ failure [8].

It is important to keep in mind that, often, there is no one unique etiology for delirium. In those cases, the brain is being affected by multiple overlapping insults, at variable levels of intensity.

30.2.7 Pathophysiology

Currently there is no clear unifying theory, but there seems to be a final common pathway leading to the behavioral presentation of acute brain failure. Several hypotheses have been proposed, such as neuroinflammatory reactions, neurotransmitter imbalance (elevated dopamine / suppressed acetylcholine, increased glutamate, serotonergic dysfunction), neuroendocrine changes with alteration in HPA axis, metabolic dysfunctions, oxidative stress, disruptions in the circadian rhythm, and network dysconnectivity [9].

30.2.8 Treatment

The experience of delirium is uniquely terrifying, and 50% of patients remember the episode. Often patients fear that they were "going insane" or that they have "lost their mind." Giving the condition a name is reassuring to patients and families.

Finding and treating the underlying cause of delirium are essential. Preventive measures such as identifying patients at risk, avoiding polypharmacy, early mobilization, avoidance of urinary and nasogastric catheters, maintaining a regular day and nighttime pattern, avoidance of dehydration, minimal use of opioid and benzodiazepines, use of hearing aid and glasses, and the involvement of family to provide reassurance and orientation are important.

Nonpharmacological Interventions for Delirium

In the ICU implementation of the so-called ABCDEF bundle has helped reduce delirium:

- A stands for assessing/managing and preventing pain.
- B stands for spontaneous breathing and awakening trials.
- C is for choosing sedation that is less likely to cause delirium (avoiding benzodiazepines and propofol).
- D stands for delirium detection.
- E is for early mobilization and exercise.
- F is a reminder to involve family members.

Once a patient is transferred to a regular floor or rehab unit, maintaining a regular sleep schedule and avoiding nighttime testing or unnecessary vital signs and blood work are important.

Making sure patients have hearing aids, eyeglasses, and a calendar will help with orientation. Removal of indwelling catheters and urinary catheters will decrease infection risks and aid in mobilization.

Pharmacological Management of Delirium

Alcohol withdrawal delirium (delirium tremens) is the only delirious state treated with benzodiazepines. The management of delirium tremens is discussed in Chapter 26.

There are no FDA-approved medications for delirium. A recently conducted randomized placebo-controlled trial concluded that haloperidol and ziprasidone did not reduce the duration of delirium [10]. However, clinicians have used and continue to use dopamine-blocking agents to control agitation in hyperactive delirium. Haloperidol, due to its ease of administration and relative safety, remains the drug of choice. The goal is to calm and not to obtund the patient. Depending on the degree of agitation, oral haloperidol is dosed from 2–5 mg bid to 10 mg bid. When administering haloperidol and other antipsychotics for delirium, especially in the case of intravenous haloperidol, it is important to monitor the QTc interval in order to prevent potentially lethal ventricular arrhythmias such as torsades de pointes. If the QTc interval is greater than 500 msec or there is a 25% increase from baseline, haloperidol should be avoided. Risk factors for torsades include female gender, hypokalemia, hypomagnesemia, and alcohol use disorder. Second-generation antipsychotic medications can be used as well. Olanzapine 5–10 mg at bedtime has shown to be beneficial. Aripiprazole 2–10 mg daily is a suitable alternative when there is concern for QTC prolongation. Quetiapine 12.5–50 mg at bedtime has been used in elderly or Parkinson's disease patients who exhibit nighttime agitation. If antipsychotics are used, it is important to treat patients with the lowest dose and for the shortest time. Patients should not remain indefinitely on antipsychotics upon discharge [11].

In addition, alpha 2 adrenergic agonists have been used for sedation and analgesia in the ICU setting. Dexmedetomidine is administered intravenously, as a continuous drip or at nighttime, to calm agitated patients. It causes less respiratory depression and is less deliriogenic than fentanyl or propofol. Clonidine, an oral or transdermal alpha 2 agonist, has been used in non-ICU patients to control agitation. Valproic acid, a glutamate antagonist, either oral or as an IV formulation, can be used as treatment or as adjunctive drug for agitation. Melatonin 3–5 mg at bedtime is used to normalize sleep patterns.

Since delirium PTSD and depression are common in the aftermath of delirium, patients need to be monitored after discharge from ICU or hospital. Cognitive decline is common, as delirium can be an accelerating/precipitating factor for dementia. In a study of ICU survivors with a history of delirium, cognitive scores like patients with moderate traumatic brain injury or mild Alzheimer dementia were observed at a 3-month follow-up [12].

Last, allowing patients and families to process the delirium experience is important. ICU diaries used by families have reduced caregiver stress. A history of delirium predisposes a patient to have new, recurrent episodes of delirium, and preventive measures should be implemented, particularly in the case of new hospitalizations or planned surgical interventions.

30.3 Medical Illnesses Presenting with Psychiatric Symptoms

Several medical conditions can present with psychiatric symptoms or syndromes other than delirium (Table 30.1), and different DSM-5TR sections include categories

Table 30.1 Medications and medical conditions commonly associated with delirium

Medications

Opioids

Benzodiazepines (intoxication and withdrawal)

Histamine (H2 receptor) antagonists: Famotidine

Agents with anticholinergic effect: Diphenhydramine, Benztropine, Oxybutynin, certain antidepressants

Muscle relaxants: Baclofen, Cyclobenzaprine

Steroids

Anti-malaria medications: Mefloquine

Antibiotics: Ciprofloxacin

Immunomodulators: Interferon alpha, Il 2

Chemotherapy agents: Cytarabine

Medical Conditions

Hepatic encephalopathy (liver cirrhosis)

Uremia (end-stage renal disease)

Lupus and other autoimmune conditions

Endocrine disorders: thyroid disorders, adrenal diseases

Cerebrovascular accidents

Seizures

Central nervous system infections: meningitis, herpetic encephalitis, syphilis

Aacquired immunodeficiency syndrome (AIDS)

Central nervous system tumors

secondary to a medical condition. As examples, some of these conditions are discussed below, but the list provided is far from exclusive:

A. Thyroid disorders frequently present with psychiatric symptoms.

    1. Hyperthyroidism: Graves' disease is the most common form of thyroid hormone over production. Thyroid receptor auto antibodies stimulate the thyroid follicular cells to produce excessive amounts of T4 and T3. Patients have low TSH and high T4 and T3. Patients frequently present with weight loss, heat intolerance, tachycardia, and exophthalmos. Neuropsychiatric symptoms are elevated levels of anxiety, emotional lability, panic attacks, mania, psychosis, and delirium.

    2. Thyroid storm is a life-threatening complication of hyperthyroidism and can be triggered by surgery or infection. There is high mortality due to multisystem involvement that leads to heart arrhythmias, congestive heart failure, and death. Patients often present with psychosis/mania and delirium.

3. Hypothyroidism: Hashimoto thyroiditis is the most common form of chronic autoimmune thyroiditis. There are high serum concentrations of thyroid globulin antibodies and thyroid peroxidase antibodies. Patient's TSH is elevated and T4/T3 are low. Symptoms of hypothyroid disease include bradycardia, fatigue, weight gain, dry skin, and amenorrhea. Psychiatric symptoms are memory decline, depression, delirium, and catatonia [13].

B. Limbic encephalitis presents with neuropsychiatric symptoms (personality changes / florid psychosis, severe agitation, cognitive decline, emotional lability seizures and movement abnormalities).

1. Limbic encephalitis is an inflammatory autoimmune brain disorder. There is frequently a viral prodrome. Antibodies are produced against cell surface receptors (NMDR receptor or leucine rich glioma inactivated 1 LGI1) or intracellular antigens (glutamic acid decarboxylase).

2. Anti-NMDR encephalitis is the most common form of limbic encephalitis. It is paraneoplastic syndrome, and in 60% of patients an underlying malignancy such as small lung cell cancer or ovarian teratoma is found [14].

C. Wilson's disease is an autosomal recessive disorder impairing copper excretion by a mutation in the ATP7B gene on chromosome 13. Copper accumulates in the brain and liver. Psychiatric symptoms usually present in late adolescence with personality changes, irritability, anxiety, psychosis, and mania. Often there are parkinsonian symptoms, dysarthria, dystonia, resting and action tremor, ataxia, and chorea. Diagnosis is made by low ceruloplasmin (value less than 5 mg/dL) and 24-hour urine copper measurement (greater than 100 microgram/day); Kayser Fleisher rings may be seen on slit-lamp examination [15].

30.4 Conclusions

Psychiatrists in the general hospital are in a unique position to correctly identify and manage patients with delirium and other psychiatric disorders secondary to medical conditions. Patients, families, and staff must be educated on such conditions, aiming at improving patient outcomes and safety.

References

1. D. B. Arciniegas, S. C. Yudofsky, R. E. Hales, American Psychiatric Association, eds. *Textbook of Neuropsychiatry and Clinical Neurosciences*. 6th ed. American Psychiatric Association Publishing; 2018.

2. T. A. Stern, O. Freudenreich, F. A. Smith, G. Fricchione, J. F. Rosenbaum. *Massachusetts General Hospital Handbook of General Hospital Psychiatry*. 7th ed. Elsevier; 2018.

3. Jose R. Maldonado. Delirium. In H. Leigh, J. Streltzer, eds. *Handbook of Consultation Liaison Psychiatry*. 2nd ed. Springer International Publishing; 2015.

4. Jose Maldonado, Psychiatric aspects of critical care medicine: update. *Clinics Review*, 2017: 461–467.

5. J. J. Barry, S. Bajestan, J. L. Cummings, M. R. Trimble, American Psychiatric Association, eds. *Concise Guide to Neuropsychiatry and Behavioral Neurology*. 3rd ed. American Psychiatric Association Publishing; 2023.

6. Albert F. G. Leentjens, David Meagher, In J. L. Levenson, ed. *Textbook of Psychosomatic Medicine and Consultation*

Liaison Psychiatry. 3rd ed. American Psychiatric Association Pubishing; 2019.

7. Antoinette Ambrosino Wyszynski, Bernard Wyszynski, *Manual of Psychiatric Care for the Medically Ill*. 2nd ed. American Psychiatric Publishing; 2008.

8. S. Ahmad, ed. *Kaplan & Sadock's Pocket Handbook of Clinical Psychiatry*. 7th ed. Wolter Kluwer; 2024.

9. Jose Maldonado, Delirium pathophysiology: an updated hypothesis of the etiology of acute brain failure, *Int J Geriatric Psychiatry*. 2018;33:1428–1457.

10. TD Girard, Haldol and ziprasidone for the treatment of delirium in critical illness, *New Engl J Med*. 2018;379:2506–2516.

11. Mariela Herrera Rojas, Leopoldo Pozuelo, Fundamentals of consultation liaison psychiatry, *Neuropsychiatry, Nova*. 2019:83–105.

12. P. P. Pandharipande, T. D. Girard, J. C. Jackson, et al. Long-term cognitive impairment after critical illness. *New Engl J Med*. 2013:369:1306–1316.

13. Katrine E. Williams, Evaluation and Treatment of Endocrine Disorders with Neuropsychiatric Symptoms. In J. J. Barry, S. Bajestan, J. L. Cummings, M. R. Trimble, American Psychiatric Association, eds. *Concise Guide to Neuropsychiatry and Behavioral Neurology*. 3rd ed. American Psychiatric Association Publishing; 2023.

14. Scheherazade Le, Limbic Encephalitis. In J. J. Barry, S. Bajestan, J. L. Cummings, M. R. Trimble, American Psychiatric Association, eds. *Concise Guide to Neuropsychiatry and Behavioral Neurology*. 3rd ed. American Psychiatric Association Publishing; 2023.

15. Sandra A. Jacobson, *Laboratory Medicine in Psychiatry and Behavioral Science*. 2nd ed. American Psychiatric Association Publishing; 2023.

Chapter

31

Dementia

Jeffrey McBride and Lokesh Shahani

31.1 Introduction

As an increasing number of people are living longer and later into life than ever before, neurocognitive disorders including dementia are becoming a growing burden to patients, their families, and the health care system overall [1]. The term *major neuro-cognitive disorder*, or *dementia*, describes a collection of impairments in cognition from a previous level of functioning that can be the result of several different neuropathologic etiologies; it is usually a progressive decline in lucid sustained cognition. These deficits can present in a variety of cognitive domains including memory and learning, complex attention, executive functioning, language, perceptual-motor, and social cognition [2]. Impairments associated with dementia affect the person's independence to complete daily activities, their social functioning and relationships, and occupational tasks. Dementia differs from normal aging, which is not associated with considerable cognitive decline, despite sometimes presenting with small memory troubles that do not have a significant impact on the person's life [1].

31.2 Epidemiology and Course

About 5% of people above 65 years of age have dementia [3]. While some forms of dementia can present prior to 65 years of age, there is a known positive correlation between developing dementia and increasing age. For the general population, the prevalence of dementia increases to about 20% between 85 and 89 years of age, and it is about 30% for the group older than 90 years of age [3]. Despite some demographic studies showing a slight decline in the prevalence of dementia within each age group between 2010 and 2020, the absolute number of those with dementia continues to increase as more and more persons live to these elderly ages [4]. Currently there are about 7 million Americans with some form of dementia, and estimates indicate that by 2050 there will be more than 18 million Americans with dementia [1].

The different types of dementia have varying expected courses. Some, like Alzheimer's disease, usually cause a slow, gradual deterioration in functioning for about a decade, eventually leading to death [2]. Other types progress much quicker, whereas still others may have a generally stable and unchanging deficit, such as dementias related to head trauma. Cases with a younger age at diagnosis or a significant family history of dementias tend to have a quicker disease progression. Regardless of the course, these disorders have significant impact on patients and warrant intervention by providers and caregivers.

31.3 Etiologies and Pathophysiology

There are numerous possible etiologies for dementia; any process that has the potential to affect normal brain structure or neuropsychiatric functioning can contribute to the development of dementia. Since there is such a wide range of causes, it is important for the evaluating provider to perform a thorough workup to identify the most likely etiology in each patient, as this can provide valuable information about tailoring an individualized treatment and management plan. For those cases that can be attributed in part to vitamin deficiencies, metabolic changes, infections, or endocrine changes, appropriate workup and intervention can help minimize future progression of symptoms or even reverse some of the existing deficits. While a proper identification of the type of dementia is a primary goal of the clinician, the boundaries and clinical presentations of each form can overlap, making true identification extremely difficult. In addition, the presenting signs and symptoms can be similar to those observed in other disorders including delirium, pseudodementia, or even schizophrenia.

Affecting about 50–60% of those with dementia, the most prevalent etiology is Alzheimer's type [4]. Alzheimer's disease is more common in women compared to men, and it is estimated that half of all beds in American nursing homes are occupied by someone with Alzheimer's type dementia. While an official confirmed diagnosis of Alzheimer's type dementia requires neuropathologic examination, *probable* or *possible* Alzheimer's disease can be inferred with a good clinical exam and history and ruling out alternative etiologies of dementia.

While the first step in the pathophysiology for Alzheimer's disease is not known, there are likely multiple genetic and environmental factors that contribute to whether an individual will develop this form of dementia. About 40% of patients have a known family history of Alzheimer's disease, and some families have shown an autosomal dominant inheritance pattern [5]. Genes coding for amyloid precursor protein have been implicated in the pathophysiology of Alzheimer's disease, and people who have multiple copies of these genes are more likely to develop Alzheimer's disease within their lifetime.

Gross anatomical changes observed in Alzheimer's includes diffuse cortical degeneration and atrophy. The normal depth of cortical sulci can be markedly reduced and flattened. Tissue atrophy also leads to a considerable increase in ventricle size. Microscopic changes include amyloid senile plaques, and postmortem observation of the density of these plaques correlates with the severity of the disease. Additional findings include neurofibrillary tangles from phosphorylated tau protein, neuronal cell death, and up to a 50% decrease in synaptic connections [4].

The next most common category of dementia is vascular dementia, which accounts for about one-fifth of total cases. Compared to Alzheimer's disease, vascular dementia has a more stepwise progression, is more common in males than in females, is associated with hypertension, and typically affects the subcortical and basal ganglia, as it primarily impacts medium- and small-sized cerebral vessels. Vascular dementia is thought to be the result of multiple infarcts from arteriosclerotic plaques or other emboli leading to damage and atrophy of the affected areas. Recommendations for proper control of blood pressure, serum lipids, and any cardiac arrhythmia should be an appropriate part of any treatment plan in order to minimize the future risk of additional infarcts.

Lewy body disease shares many of the pathologic and clinical features of Alzheimer's disease, but there are a few key differences. Clinically, persons with Lewy body dementia are more likely to have early symptoms of hallucinations and Parkinsonian motor features but memory problems may be less prominent early in the course of the disease. Typical microscopic findings of cortical and midbrain tissue reveal Lewy inclusion bodies in the cytoplasm of neurons, which are primarily made of alpha-synuclein. The precise role that these inclusions play within the pathophysiology of Lewy body dementia is not known, and they can also be found in Parkinson's disease as well as multiple systems atrophy patients.

Another distinct group of dementia is frontotemporal dementia, of which Pick's Disease is the most typical example. As the name implies, this form of dementia shows a pattern of damage located in the frontal and temporal lobes of the brain. Microscopic examination of tissue of frontotemporal dementia also shows inclusion bodies, known as Pick bodies, whose major components are tau fibrils. One notable characteristic with this type of dementia is that it has an earlier age of onset with almost a fourth of cases beginning before 45 years of age [4]. Compared to other dementias, the early stages of Pick's disease are more likely to have impacts on the behavior and personality of the patient while preserving other cognitive functions. Emotional lability, withdrawing from family, excessive spending, increasingly vulgar language, and hypersexuality have all been associated with frontotemporal dementia.

Other neurodegenerative disorders, including Huntington's disease and Parkinson's disease, are also possible causes for a presenting dementia case. These diseases are mostly identified as progressive movement disorders, but they also are well associated with subcortical dementias and increased risk of co-occurring depression.

In addition, systemic infections are a significant risk factor for developing dementia. Persons living with HIV have a 15% chance of being diagnosed with dementia year-on-year [4]. Other infections that can lead to dementia include *Treponema pallidum*, *Cryptococcus*, and Creutzfeldt-Jakob disease.

Last, lingering cognitive deficits, and therefore a diagnosis of dementia, are a potential result of head trauma. Repeated physical hits to the head can lead to chronic traumatic encephalopathy and is a serious potential injury for some athletes, such as boxers and football players. This form of dementia is noted for increased risk of irritability, impulsivity, aggression, and speech difficulties.

31.4 Clinical Features

The age of onset, progression of disease, and even particular symptoms vary based on the specific etiology, genetic and environmental risk factors, clinical management, and other variables. With most forms of dementia, one of the earliest signs is usually forgetfulness, with trouble remembering recent events and details. If assessed by a clinician at this stage, the patient's family are usually the primary source of information detailing memory deficits, as the patient can be defensive, attempting to rationalize the problem, minimizing the severity of symptoms, or be generally unaware of the issue.

Changes in the personality of persons with dementia are common and can be quite distressing to the family [5]. These patients may become more socially withdrawn as they forget social engagements or become more isolated to try to hide their symptoms. Alternatively, those with frontal and temporal lobe involvements may be more likely to become more irritable and hostile, especially if paranoia is present [4]. Dementias impacting the cortex are more likely to affect a patient's language and calculation skills, whereas subcortical dementias are more likely to impact their mood and motor capabilities. In addition to these, there can be impacts on the patient's attention, executive functioning and processing speed, abstraction, and visuospatial skills. About one-fourth of those with dementia will experience hallucinations or delusions (usually paranoid and persecutory in theme). This psychosis is more prevalent in those with Alzheimer's or Lewy body type dementias.

Nocturnal worsening of symptoms is not unusual, as fewer external cues are present to reorient the patient. All these symptoms and presentations can contribute to an overall decreased independence and ability for those with dementia to take care of themselves. People with any form of dementia are at increased risk of having a superimposed delirium. Since the brain controls almost all aspects of a person's behavior, cognition, and emotion, and since dementia is a neuropsychiatric disease of the brain, dementia affects just about every facet of a person's life.

31.5 Risk Factors

As discussed in the preceding sections, there are numerous genetic factors that contribute to the different types of dementia. For instance, Down's syndrome is the result of trisomy 21, which is the chromosome that carries the amyloid precursor protein, which in turn helps explain why those with Down's syndrome are at an increased risk for developing Alzheimer's disease. Other genetic and psychosocial risk factors are wide ranging and include high blood pressure, diabetes, diet and vitamin deficiencies, head injuries, smoking status, alcohol use, lack of physical activity, obesity, depression, hearing or vision loss, lower level of education, marriage status, fewer close social contacts and loneliness, environmental toxins or pollution, economic disadvantages, low purpose in life, and even some personality traits such as high neuroticism and low conscientiousness [4].

Some risk factors for dementia are modifiable, and it is possible that minimizing one's risk factors may reduce the severity, or occurrence, of a future neurocognitive disorder. Physical activity and routine cognitive stimulation are seen as the most modifiable risk factors and can be the target of focus for clinicians. Especially for vascular dementias, prevention techniques and modification of risk factors may have a positive benefit.

31.6 Diagnosis and Workup

When a diagnosis of dementia is suspected, a full neurocognitive and medical workup is warranted. The diagnosis of dementia is made clinically, and the formally accepted criteria for all major neurocognitive disorders are laid out in DSM-5. The clinician should find evidence "of significant cognitive decline from a previous level of performance in one or more cognitive domain (complex attention," executive function, learning and memory, language, perceptual-motor, or social cognition)" [6]. The identified deficit must interfere with the independence in everyday activities and cannot occur solely in the context of a delirium. This usually requires a detailed conversation to gather information on the patient's daily routine including their ability to care for themselves, their hobbies and interests, personal finances, interactions with friends, and abilities to do tasks or errands. In order to get a complete and accurate assessment, the clinician may consider supplemental information from a knowledgeable informant or from prior documented neuropsychiatric testing.

Once a diagnosis of a major neurocognitive disorder is established, the clinician can utilize an array of different chemistry, imaging, and neuropsychological tests to assist in identifying the type of dementia present. Readily available chemistry tests include complete blood cell count, complete metabolic panel, liver panel, thyroid panel, vitamin B_{12} and folate levels, urinalysis, urine drug screen, HIV screening, rapid plasma regain test, and HgbA1c. In addition to chemistry tests, an electroencephalography, transthoracic echocardiogram, head computerized tomography, or a brain magnetic resonance imaging can be useful imaging modalities to help distinguish the type or cause of a particular case of dementia. Not every patient who receives a formal diagnosis of dementia is necessarily expected to complete all tests listed above, but the investigation of contributing factors is important, since between 10% and 15% of cases are potentially reversible [4].

31.7 Management and Treatment

While the behavioral and cognitive problems caused by the nonreversible dementias are generally seen as chronic and progressive, that does not mean that there are no options to try to improve the patient's condition. Both patients and families tend to respond well to psychosocial interventions including education, support groups, behavioral modification techniques, and psychotherapy [4].

Pharmacologic interventions can be used, including medications for mood, anxiety, psychosis, insomnia, and movements, but clinicians should be aware of the pharmacokinetic and pharmacodynamic changes that can exist within the elderly population as well as within certain forms of dementia. For instance, while benzodiazepines may be indicated for anxiety, there is an increased risk of paradoxical agitation within geriatric populations as well as an increased risk of falls. Antipsychotic medications are commonly prescribed medication for dementia patients who experience hallucinations or disorganized thought process, but these should be used with care, as these patients are likely more sensitive to neuroleptic medications. Moreover, the majority of antipsychotics carry black box warnings issued by the US Food and Drug Administration (FDA) regarding the risks associated with their use among patients with dementia.

Cholinesterase inhibitors are commonly used as a treatment strategy for those with mild and moderate neurocognitive disorders [8]. These medications, such as donepezil, rivastigmine, and galantamine, prevent the degradation of synaptic acetylcholine, increasing the downstream effects of acetylcholine in hopes to provide an improvement in memory and function. None of these medications have shown an ability to completely reverse or prevent the progression of symptoms, but they can be part of a comprehensive treatment plan that includes pharmacology and psychosocial interventions.

Memantine is an N-methyl-D-aspartate (NMDA) receptor antagonist and used for treatment of moderate to severe neurocognitive disorder [7]. Glutamate is the principal excitatory amino acid neurotransmitter in cortical and hippocampal neurons, and one of the receptors activated by glutamate is the NMDA receptor, which is involved in learning and memory.

31.8 Support for Caregivers

Caregivers of patients with dementia can suffer significant stress, particularly as cognitive function declines or behavioral symptoms worsen. Counseling and support groups can be beneficial. Caregivers are encouraged to get help in sharing the caregiving burden with other family members or paid caregivers. Respite care, daycare, and other day programs are available in most areas, often through the local agency on aging.

31.9 Conclusion

With the increasing population of older adults, there has been a rise in the patient population living with major neurocognitive disorder. Health care providers need to be proficient in identifying patients with neurocognitive disorder and in providing management and, when necessary, referring them to specialized treatment.

References

1. J. M. Zissimopoulos, B. C. Tysinger, P. A. St Clair, et al. The impact of changes in population health and mortality on future prevalence of Alzheimer's disease and other dementias in the United States. *The Journals of Gerontology. Series B, Psychological Sciences and Social Sciences* 2018; **73**:S38–S47.

2. J. C. Breitner. Mild cognitive impairment and progression to dementia: new findings. *Neurology* 2014; **82**:e34–e35.

3. V. A. Freedman, J. D. Kasper. Cohort profile: the National Health and Aging Trends Study (NHATS). *Int J Epidemiol* 2019; **48**:1044–1045g.

4. B. J. Sadock, V. A. Sadock, P. Ruiz, eds. *Kaplan & Sadock's Synopsis of Psychiatry.* 11th ed. Lippincott Williams & Wilkins; 2015.

5. D. Gallagher, R. Coen, D. Kilroy, et al. Anxiety and behavioral disturbance as markers of prodromal Alzheimer's disease in patients with mild cognitive impairment. *International Journal of Geriatric Psychiatry* 2011; **26**:166.

6. American Psychiatric Association. *Diagnostic and Statistical Manual of Mental Disorders.* 5th ed., text rev. APA Publishing; 2022.

7. P. Raina, P. Santaguida, A. Ismaila, et al. Effectiveness of cholinesterase inhibitors and memantine for treating dementia: evidence review for a clinical practice guideline. *Ann Intern Med* 2008; **148**: 379.

Psychiatric Care of the Medical Patient
Neuroleptic Malignant Syndrome and Serotonin Syndrome

Lindsey S. Pershern and Robert J. Boland

32.1 Neuroleptic Malignant Syndrome

32.1.1 Introduction

Neuroleptic malignant syndrome (NMS) is a life-threatening condition associated with using antipsychotic medications or other medications with similar pharmacodynamics. The classic symptoms include fever, muscle rigidity, autonomic instability, and delirium. Although uncommon, it is essential to recognize this condition quickly, as rapid management is critical.

The condition was first described shortly after the introduction of Chlorpromazine in the 1950s [1]. A 1960 French study of the syndrome gave the condition its name [2]. Early reports suggested sometimes alarming rates, mainly owing to unfamiliarity with the syndrome. However, the increasingly judicious use of antipsychotic medications and atypical antipsychotics has likely led to a decrease in the condition. Currently, the rate is about 0.01% to 0.02% of patients receiving antipsychotic medication [3].

The syndrome is more common in men than in women, with a ratio of about 1.47:1, and the sex difference is highest for younger ages [4]. Whether this is an independent risk factor or related to the frequency of antipsychotic use is not clear [3]. Postpartum women may also be at a greater risk for the syndrome.

Rapidly increasing an antipsychotic dose also increases the risk of NMS. However, there does not appear to be a relationship between the length of treatment on an antipsychotic and the development of NMS. First-generation ("typical") antipsychotics are thought to have a higher risk, and some data based on drug safety programs support this [5]. However, some meta-analyses have found no association between antipsychotic class and risk for NMS. Similarly, long-acting injectables are sometimes thought to carry a higher risk, although this is not supported by meta-analyses and registries [6, 7].

A rapid switch from one antipsychotic to another may increase the risk. Patients on anti-Parkinson's medications such as levodopa or amantadine are also at risk if they withdraw too quickly from these medications. Patients with dementia, particularly Lewy body dementia, have a more significant risk, given that these patients are already sensitive to antipsychotic side effects. Dehydration increases the risk of NMS in patients taking antipsychotics, presumably because it alters the distribution of the medication. Some reports suggest that catatonia can put a patient at a higher risk for NMS [8].

Table 32.1 Medications associated with NMS

Category	Examples
Antipsychotics	All antipsychotic agents, both typical and atypical, carry a risk.
Non-antipsychotic antidopaminergics	Antiemetics: metoclopramide, droperidol, promethazine Huntington's disease treatments: Tetrabenazine Antihypertensives: reserpine Antidepressants: amoxapine Contrast agents: diatrizoate
Dopaminergic agents (in withdrawal)	Levodopa, Amantadine, Tolcapone, and other dopamine agonists
Other medications with little or no dopaminergic effect	Lithium Phenelzine Dosulepin Desipramine Trimipramine

Several medical conditions may increase the mortality risk of NMS. These include respiratory problems and the severity of hyperthermia [6]. Older age is another risk factor. Alcohol use, central nervous system disease, and infections may also be risk factors [5].

32.1.2 Pathophysiology

We do not know the exact mechanism of NMS. However, it is associated with dopamine receptor blockade, and most causative agents have a dopamine-blocking effect. These include antipsychotic medications, non-antipsychotic antidopaminergic agents, and anti-Parkinson agents (when withdrawn). However, some agents with no known dopaminergic effect have been reported to be associated with NMS, such as lithium, certain tricyclic antidepressants, and other antidepressants (Table 32.1).

The exact pathophysiology is not fully understood. However, a sudden decrease in central dopaminergic activity is at the heart of NMS's symptoms. There are three main dopamine pathways in the brain, and disruption of these pathways can explain many of the symptoms of the disorder, including muscle rigidity (nigrostriatal), hyperthermia (tuberoinfundibular), and delirium (mesolimbic/cortical). In addition to the fact that antipsychotic drugs are the primary cause of the syndrome, other evidence includes imaging evidence of blocked D2 receptor binding during the acute phase of NMS. Furthermore, another study of patients with acute NMS showed low CSF levels of dopamine metabolites [9].

Not all NMS symptoms, however, are dopamine related. Sympathetic dysregulation also occurs. This dysregulation likely relates to the reciprocal relationship of dopamine and norepinephrine in the midbrain, with dopamine blockade resulting in a concomitant increase in noradrenergic activity.

Some theories also suggest that pathologies associated with malignant hyperthermia, such as calcium dysregulation in the musculoskeletal system, similarly occur in NMS [10].

There may be a genetic risk, and an increased prevalence has been reported in families after one member developed NMS [11].

None of these theories account for why most patients on antipsychotic or similar medications will not experience NMS, nor why a similar agent to the causative one can safely treat a patient with schizophrenia who has had an episode of NMS.

32.1.3 Clinical Presentation

The classic symptoms of NMS are the triad of fever, muscle rigidity, and altered mental status. In addition, patients show autonomic instability, including tachycardia, hypertension or unstable blood pressure, sialorrhea, diaphoresis, flushing, pallor, and incontinence. Other symptoms include dysphagia and mutism [3].

The particular combination of symptoms varies by patient, with muscle rigidity as the most common group of symptoms. The rigidity can be extreme and is sometimes called "lead pipe rigidity." Other motor symptoms may also occur, including tremor, chorea, akinesia, or dystonic movements. The most severe complication of the disorder are rhabdomyolysis and associated leukocytosis. This results from the disorder's rigidity and other musculoskeletal effects and can be severe enough to cause renal failure.

32.1.4 Clinical Course

The symptoms usually develop within hours to days of exposure to the offending drug but can occur weeks after. It is rare to see the syndrome begin more than a month after beginning an antipsychotic. Muscle rigidity is usually the first symptom, followed by fever and mental status changes. The mental status changes can range from minor sedation or agitation to delirium or coma.

32.1.5 Diagnosis

The diagnosis requires both a careful history and physical and laboratory testing. Most important to the history is eliciting a history of antipsychotic use. In the absence of such a history, one should look for another agent known to cause the disorder; clinicians have mistakenly assumed that a patient not on antipsychotics could not have the syndrome. The clinician should gear the physical exam toward observing or eliciting the signs and symptoms described above. Crucial to the exam is a thorough neurological exam, including a careful motor exam.

The most common laboratory findings are from rhabdomyolysis and leukocytosis caused by muscle breakdown. The most characteristic is elevated creatinine phosphokinase (CPK). However, this is not specific to the disease, and a normal CPK does not rule out NMS. Leukocytosis is another common finding and can be as high as 40,000 mm^3 with a left shift and elevated neutrophil/lymphocyte ratio. Other associated laboratory findings include iron deficiency, elevated transaminases, and evidence of metabolic acidosis.

Lumbar puncture or neuroimaging is often normal but can help exclude other causes. Electroencephalogram (EEG) is rarely performed but shows diffuse slowing, indicative of the global cerebral nature of the syndrome's effect.

The Diagnostic and Statistical Manual of Mental Disorders, Fifth Edition, Text Revision (DSM-5-TR) includes NMS under "Medication-Induced Movement Disorders and Other Adverse Effects of Medication." The diagnosis is descriptive, without specific diagnostic criteria. The International Classification of Diseases 11th Revision (ICD-11) includes NMS under the generic diagnosis of "Other specified Movement Disorders."

32.1.6 Differential Diagnosis

Many conditions can resemble, at least superficially, NMS. Worsening the dilemma is the fact that NMS is rare, making it easy to overlook. Most common are infections affecting the central nervous system (CNS), heat stroke, toxic encephalopathies, status epilepticus, and other causes of delirium. In most cases, the other disorder has some overlapping symptoms, but the absence of other key symptoms can help in the differential.

We can broadly divide the differential into two categories: acute dysautonomias, a group of similar syndromes of which NMS is one; and unrelated syndromes with some overlapping characteristics.

Acute Dysautonomias

Serotonin syndrome, described below, can also be confused with NMS. Patients with serotonin syndrome are less likely to have muscle rigidity, instead having tremor. The use of a selective serotonin reuptake inhibitor (SSRI) rather than an antipsychotic, a normal CPK, and leukocytes all help distinguish the two disorders.

Malignant hyperthermia can appear identical to NMS; however, the different history (of anesthesia agents) will distinguish the two syndromes.

Malignant catatonia is a rare syndrome that also can seem identical to NMS. Usually, catatonia has typical prodromal symptoms, including withdrawal, apathy, and automatisms. The differential is vital, as antipsychotic medications may be used to treat lethal catatonia.

Unrelated Syndromes

Heat stroke causes fever and delirium. However, the limbs are usually flaccid and do not show extrapyramidal signs. Also, the skin is usually dry, and the blood pressure is low. As patients on antipsychotics are prone to hyperthermia; this is a common mimicking syndrome.

Infections affecting the CNS include fever and mental status changes. In addition, there are usually prodromal signs of an impending infection. Laboratory analysis, including blood, urine, and CSF, can distinguish between the disorders.

Seizures have characteristic motor movements. Therefore, the focal changes on EEG can distinguish the disorder.

Various drugs, both medications and illicit substances, can have motor or cognitive effects, and antipsychotics can cause many muscle effects seen in NMS, including extrapyramidal symptoms and muscle rigidity. Usually, these symptoms are less severe than would be seen in NMS. Stimulant toxicity can include hyperthermia, mental status changes, and autonomic dysfunction. Withdrawal syndromes from alcohol or benzodiazepines can cause altered mental status and muscle rigidity. A careful history, examination for uncharacteristic symptoms, and laboratory evaluation are essential in each case.

Table 32.2 Supportive care for NMS

Management	Purpose	Examples
Hydration	Treat associated dehydration Decrease rhabdomyolysis Prevent renal failure	IV hydration
Cardiopulmonary stabilization	Decrease the likelihood of complications or organ failure	Antiarrhythmic medications Antihypertensives (clonidine, nitroprusside)
Fever management	Decrease hyperthermia and related complications	Antipyretics Cooling blankets Ice packs Ice water gastric lavage (when severe)
Anticoagulation	Prevent deep vein thrombosis	Heparin
Sedation	Treat agitation	Benzodiazepines

Various other disorders, including spinal cord injuries, acute hydrocephalus, porphyria, pheochromocytoma, and many other systemic illnesses, can overlap in symptoms. A thorough history, exam, and select laboratory tests can again help distinguish.

32.1.7 Treatment and Prognosis

There is no definitive treatment for NMS apart from stopping the causative agent. The worst cases occur when the disorder is not recognized quickly. By then the symptoms are often severe, and in these cases treatment should occur in an intensive care setting to allow constant monitoring and rapid intervention.

Stopping the offending agent is by far the most crucial step in managing the syndrome. This step involves identifying the agent, usually a dopamine receptor blocker. However, as discussed, in some cases an agent with no known dopamine effect could cause the disorder, and when in doubt, stopping all nonessential medications is a reasonable step. An exception to this is the class of anti-parkinsonian medications such as levodopa, as it may be the withdrawal syndrome causing the disorder. In that case, the clinician should restart or increase the medication.

Additional treatment involves aggressive supportive care to address the complications of the disorder.

Supportive Care

Supportive care includes hydration, cardiopulmonary stabilization, fever management, and treating or preventing other harmful symptoms. Table 32.2 lists supportive measures and their rationale.

Therapeutic Treatments

There is little support for specific agents to treat NMS. However, some agents are commonly used. Unfortunately, this data is limited, and no randomized controlled studies support any medication.

Dantrolene is commonly used, given its effectiveness with malignant hyperthermia. It is most likely helpful for severe NMS cases [12]. It can lessen muscle rigidity and hyperthermia and can work rapidly. It is usually given in doses of 1–2.5 mg/kg/dose IV, repeated as needed until symptoms subside, to a maximum of 10 mg/kg/day [13]. This regimen can be continued at the same dose every 6 hours or in a 0.25 mg/kg/hour continuous infusion for 48–72 hours. Opinions vary on how quickly, once started, the medication can be discontinued. It is usually prudent to taper the medication slowly once the patient shows improvement.

Dopamine agonists, such as bromocriptine or amantadine, may help counteract the dopamine blockade. Bromocriptine is given in doses of 2.5–5 mg every 8 hours [14]. Amantadine is given at 100 mg twice daily for as long as 3 weeks [15]. As these medications do not have an IV formulation, and many patients with NMS cannot safely take oral medications, it can be given through a nasogastric tube.

Several other medications have reports of being helpful, although these are anecdotal. These include apomorphine, carbamazepine, bupropion, and dexmedetomidine.

Electroconvulsive therapy (ECT) may have some use as a last resort in patients not responding to other treatments [16]. However, there is limited data to support this, and experts base this recommendation on an analogy with ECTs efficacy for malignant catatonia and case reports.

Prognosis

Originally, NMS was a highly fatal syndrome, with more than one-third of patients dying from it. The cause of death is usually a fatal arrhythmia, disseminated intravascular coagulation, or renal or cardiopulmonary complications. Currently, the mortality rate is closer to 10%. The odds of survival depend on how quickly the disorder is recognized and treated [17].

Most patients will recover completely from NMS. The time until recovery depends on how quickly the clinical team begins treatment. In the case of early recognition and treatment, recovery can take from a couple of days to 1 or 2 weeks. Delayed intervention can lengthen the recovery time by weeks. Delays may also result in residual symptoms, such as catatonic or parkinsonian symptoms. If prolonged, renal or cardiovascular effects could also have long-term consequences.

32.1.8 Example Case

Mr. Jones is a 70-year-old man with a history of schizophrenia beginning in his 20s, who was admitted to an internal medicine service for fever, muscle rigidity, and inattention. The staff at the nursing home where he resides reported an exacerbation of his schizophrenia 1 month ago when he experienced intense delusions despite adherence to his usual quetiapine treatment. At that time, his psychiatrist discontinued the quetiapine and started risperidone at 3 mg/day, increasing to 5 mg/day the next day. Mr. Jones's delusions responded after several days. However, 2 days before admission, the staff noted he seemed lethargic and ate little. The next day the staff found him in bed, rigid, weak, and not responding to questions, and his psychiatrist discontinued his risperidone. The next day, the staff found his temperature to be 38.5°C, so they sent him by ambulance to the hospital.

In the emergency department, his temperature was 38°C, and his pulse was 120 bpm. His examination was significant for profound rigidity in his lower extremities, with severe cogwheel rigidity in his upper extremities. He was confused, anxious, and unable to articulate meaningful information. Laboratory values were significant for a WBC of 18,700/uL (87% polymorphonucleocytes) and a creatine phosphokinase level of 318 units/L. His spinal fluid, including culture, was unremarkable, as were blood cultures. He was admitted to the medical intensive care unit and received supportive treatment, including hydration and cooling blankets, and a regimen of dantrolene (initial dose 120 mg IV and 100 mg per nasogastric tube every 8 hours). His symptoms improved, his fever subsided, his rigidity lessened by the next day, and he returned to the internal medicine service. By the next week, he was talking coherently and no longer confused.

32.2 Serotonin Syndrome

32.2.1 Introduction

Serotonin syndrome is the term used to describe the condition associated with excessive serotonergic activity in the CNS. It was first described in the literature in the 1960s and has also been referenced as "serotonin toxicity." It can occur with therapeutic medication use of multiple serotonergic medications, inadvertent interactions between medications/substances, and intentional overdose. The manifestation of excessive serotonin activity occurs on a spectrum from mild symptoms of toxicity to severe, life-threatening reaction. Moderate and severe cases usually require emergent care. With increased prescribing of antidepressants in the last 20 years, the incidence of identified cases of serotonin syndrome is also increasing. It is estimated that cases presenting to emergency, inpatient, and outpatient settings rose by 18% between 2002 and 2016 [18]. Although the condition can be life-threatening, most cases do not require hospitalization and resolve with discontinuation of the serotonergic medication(s). It is likely that mild cases are missed or attributed to another cause, making the true prevalence difficult to estimate. Patients who are on medications that increase serotonin are at risk of developing serotonin syndrome, regardless of the medication's mechanism of action. The primary risk factor for serotonin syndrome is the use of serotonergic medications, regardless of patient age, ethnicity, or gender. Patients who are medically ill, especially those on multiple centrally acting medications, may be at an increased risk of developing moderate to severe serotonin syndrome [19]. The yearly estimated incidence of serotonin syndrome fatality in patients taking serotonergic medications is 100 deaths per 7,300 diagnosed cases [19].

32.2.2 Pathophysiology

Medications that increase serotonin act by increasing serotonin synthesis or release, reducing serotonin uptake or metabolism, or by direct activation of the serotonin receptor. At present, at least 15 serotonin receptors have been cloned, and others have been identified in genome project databases. The majority of symptoms associated with serotonin syndrome are likely due to the activation of two specific receptors: 5-HT1A, a metabotropic receptor found in high density in limbic system structures (hippocampus, amygdala) and present in astrocytes and glia; and 5-HT2A, a metabotropic receptor found in highest amounts in the cortex [18]. Medications that have been associated with the development of serotonin syndrome include SSRIs; serotonin and norepinephrine reuptake inhibitors; tricyclic antidepressants; monoamine oxidase inhibitors (MAOIs) (including linezolid); synthetic opioids such as meperidine, tramadol, fentanyl, and methadone; dextromethorphan; chlorpheniramine/brompheniramine; herbal supplements St John's Wort, L-tryptophan, SAMe, and panax ginseng; and diet supplements that include fenfluramine and sibutramine [20, 21, 22]. Methylene-dioxymethamphetamine, cocaine, amphetamine, and LSD increase serotonin and can lead to serotonin syndrome, most commonly in combination with another serotonergic agent or in overdose. Although there is a concern for additional risk with medications that modulate the serotonin system through other mechanisms, mirtazapine, trazodone, lithium, ondansetron, and triptans have not been frequently mentioned in published cases of serotonin syndrome [20].

The most common cause of serotonin syndrome is the coadministration of multiple substances that increase serotonin, including prescribed medications, herbal supplements, and illicit substances. MAOIs are the most common medication involved in published cases, specifically those of severe serotonin syndrome. Overuse or overdose of serotonergic medications increases patient risk, as well as concurrent use with medications that inhibit CYP 2D6 and 3A4 [21].

32.2.3 Clinical Presentation

The symptoms of serotonin syndrome fall into three categories: neuromuscular hyperactivity, autonomic instability, and psychomotor/neurocognitive changes [18–28]. Manifestations of neuromuscular hyperactivity include tremor, hyperreflexia, rigidity, and clonus. Clonus is the involuntary rhythmic contraction in response to a stimulus, typically more pronounced in the lower extremities in serotonin syndrome, and a distinguishing feature. Autonomic instability symptoms include mydriasis, diaphoresis, hypertension, tachycardia, elevated temperature, and tachypnea. Psychomotor/neurocognitive changes in serotonin syndrome can include anxiety, agitation, excitement, restlessness, and confusion. In severe cases, symptoms can progress to include seizures, rhabdomyolysis, organ failure, hyperthermia, and/or delirium [22, 23, 24].

32.2.4 Clinical Course

The onset of serotonin syndrome occurs most typically within 6–24 hours of ingestion of the precipitating medication, whether newly prescribed or taken at an increased dose. Variations in the time course of onset of symptoms have been linked to the unique pharmacokinetic and pharmacodynamic properties of the offending agent(s) [18, 22]. The temporal association between exposure to an agent that can increase serotonin in the CNS and the onset of symptoms can aid in accurate diagnosis.

Symptoms of serotonin syndrome should also be considered based on severity and time progression. Mild (early) symptoms, including nervousness, insomnia, diarrhea, tremor, and pupil dilation, may be misattributed to normal side effects, discontinuation, or other clinical causes [18]. In these cases, fever is not common [19, 20]. Early detection is important, as untreated serotonin toxicity can escalate quickly. As the condition progresses, patients can develop hyperreflexia, diaphoresis, agitation, restlessness, or clonus (including ocular clonus). With progression, patients may develop fever, myoclonic jerking, confusion, or delirium. Laboratory abnormalities in serotonin syndrome are nonspecific and related to secondary medical complications [18]. Patients with severe symptoms will require hospitalization. Untreated serotonin syndrome can be associated with seizures, shock, and death. Potentially fatal complications of serotonin syndrome include rhabdomyolysis with or without associated acute renal failure and disseminated intravascular coagulation [20, 22, 23]. In a recent systematic review, the most common complication present in 56 serotonin syndrome fatality cases were cardiac, including arrhythmias and carido pulmonary arrest [25].

32.2.5 Diagnosis

Identification and diagnosis of serotonin syndrome require a complete and accurate medication, dietary supplement, and substance use history. The clinical manifestations of serotonin toxicity can be highly variable, with the consistent feature of exposure to serotonergic substances combined with the identification of signs and symptoms through a physical exam with particular focus on signs of muscle rigidity, reflexes, and autonomic instability. There is no gold-standard diagnostic test for serotonin syndrome. The clinical diagnosis can be guided by several proposed diagnostic criteria, specifically the Sternbach, Radomski, and Hunter criteria. Although some have regarded the Hunter criteria as more sensitive and specific, a systematic review in 2020 showed the superiority of the Sternbach and Radomski criteria for identifying serotonin syndrome in 411 published cases [24]. The three criteria systems can be helpful guides in making the diagnosis. The classic triad of symptom domains is consistent across each set of criteria, with variations in the number of symptoms and descriptions of symptoms as major or minor. All three require the presence of serotonergic medications, and Sternbach and Randomski criteria require the absence of an antipsychotic agent [26–28]. Sternbach defined 10 symptoms of serotonin syndrome, requiring the presence of 3 symptoms for the diagnosis [28]. Randomski categorizes mental, neurological, and vegetative symptoms as major and minor. Using these criteria, the diagnosis requires four major criteria or three major and two minor symptoms [27]. The Hunter criteria propose five symptom combinations as criteria, with the diagnosis made if a patient is on a serotonergic agent and exhibits one condition. These include spontaneous clonus, inducible clonus + agitation or diaphoresis, ocular clonus + agitation or diaphoresis, ocular clonus or inducible clonus + hypertonia + temperature > 38 degrees C, and tremor and hyperreflexia [26].

32.2.6 Differential Diagnosis

The diagnosis of serotonin syndrome is often missed or misdiagnosed [18–23]. This is due to the overlap of symptoms with other potential diagnoses, making the comprehensive approach to the patient with suspicious symptoms very important. Laboratory and other diagnostic studies are used to rule out alternative explanations of symptoms of serotonin syndrome, but the clinical history is critical to differentiating from conditions that may present similarly. The differential diagnosis should include infections (meningitis, encephalitis, tetanus, sepsis), substance intoxication or withdrawal phenomenon (alcohol, benzodiazepines, stimulants) including delirium tremens, anticholinergic toxicity, thyroid storm, heat stroke, malignant hyperthermia and NMS [18].

The most challenging syndromes to differentiate from serotonin syndrome are listed in Table 32.3. As discussed in this chapter, NMS can be differentiated by the medication

Table 32.3 Differential diagnosis of serotonin syndrome

Condition	History	Time course	Vital signs	Clinical symptoms
Serotonin syndrome	Exposure to excessive serotonin via combined serotonergic medications, overdose, use of serotonergic substances (illicit or herbal)	<24 hours	Hypertension, tachycardia, tachypnea, hyperthermia	Diaphoresis, hyperreflexia/clonus, agitation, increased bowel sounds, mydriasis, increased tone
Malignant hyperthermia	Exposure to anesthetics or succinylcholine during surgery; family history is a risk factor	During anesthesia or within 1 hour post-op	HTN, tachycardia, tachypnea, hyperthermia	Diaphoresis, *bradyreflexia*, agitation, *decreased bowel sounds, muscle rigidity, normal pupil size*
Neuroleptic malignant syndrome	Exposure to dopamine antagonists	Hours to days	HTN, tachycardia, tachypnea, hyperthermia	Diaphoresis *"Lead pipe" rigidity, decreased bowel sounds, bradyreflexia normal pupil size*
Anticholinergic toxicity	Exposure to anticholinergic medications	Hours to weeks	Tachycardia, tachypnea, hyperthermia	*Dry mouth,* blurred vision, *decreased bowel sounds,* mydriasis, flushing, urinary retention, *Normal muscle tone*

Clinical symptoms distinguishing from serotonin syndrome are in italics.

history and prominent neurological differences, although overlap in pharmacology may complicate the diagnosis. Of note, the two most utilized sets of criteria require that patients are not taking "neuroleptic" medications concurrent with serotonergic medications [27, 28].

32.2.7 Treatment, Prognosis, and Prevention

When identified early, most cases of serotonin syndrome are self-limited and do not require medical intervention beyond stopping the serotonergic medication(s) or substance [18–23]. In these cases, symptoms typically resolve within 24–72 hours of discontinuation of the offending agent, with slightly longer periods needed for longer-acting medications including irreversible MAOIs and fluoxetine. With more severe cases that involve hyperthermia, autonomic instability, neurocognitive changes, rhabdomyolysis, or other complications, patients will require hospitalization. The priorities of management include supportive care, management of agitation, body temperature, vital signs, and consideration of the need for additional treatment. Intensive care may be required for more severe cases that do not respond to standard measures or due to medical complications including hyperthermia, seizures, metabolic or electrolyte disturbances, renal failure, or delirium. Although there is no specific antidote for excessive serotonin activity in the CNS, benzodiazepines are commonly used effectively for agitation and tremor, and cyproheptadine, a 5HT-2A antagonist, can be administered with some expectation of benefit [22, 23]. For severe symptoms, patients may require neuromuscular paralysis, sedation, and intubation. Long-term prognosis is favorable when diagnosed and treated early. For moderate to severe cases, prognosis depends on the effective identification and management of the complications of serotonin syndrome. Death from serotonin syndrome is rare [24].

Many cases of serotonin syndrome could be avoided with closer attention to medication regimens involving serotonergic medications and screening for signs and symptoms of toxicity [20, 23]. Prescribers need to be aware of the risks of medications that can increase serotonin and screen for the use of herbal and illicit substances that can potentiate the risks of medications prescribed for both psychiatric and nonpsychiatric conditions [19, 20]. When making changes to medication regimens, prescribers should follow recommendations regarding washout periods, especially when involving MAOIs. In addition to physician prescribing practices, electronic medical records can aid in the identification of potential interactions and the use of multiple medications with similar mechanisms of action. Providing education for patients on the signs and symptoms of excessive serotonin can be helpful in early identification [23].

References

1. Ayd FJ. Fatal hyperpyrexia during chlorpromazine therapy. *J Clin Exp Psychopathol* 1956; 17: 189–192.

2. Delay J, Pichot P, Lemperiere T, et al. [A non-phenothiazine and non-reserpine major neuroleptic, haloperidol, in the treatment of psychoses]. *Ann Med Psychol (Paris)* 1960; 118(1): 145–152.

3. Berman BD. Neuroleptic malignant syndrome: a review for neurohospitalists. *Neurohospitalist* 2011; 1: 41–47.

4. Gurrera RJ. A systematic review of sex and age factors in neuroleptic malignant syndrome diagnosis frequency. *Acta Psychiatr Scand* 2017; 135: 398–408.

5. Schneider M, Regente J, Greiner T, et al. Neuroleptic malignant syndrome:

evaluation of drug safety data from the AMSP program during 1993–2015. *Eur Arch Psychiatry Clin Neurosci* 2020; **270**: 23–33.

6. Guinart D, Misawa F, Rubio JM, et al. A systematic review and pooled, patient-level analysis of predictors of mortality in neuroleptic malignant syndrome. *Acta Psychiatr Scand* 2021; **144**: 329–341.

7. Misawa F, Okumura Y, Takeuchi Y, et al. Neuroleptic malignant syndrome associated with long-acting injectable versus oral second-generation antipsychotics: Analyses based on a spontaneous reporting system database in Japan. *Schizophr Res* 2021; **231**: 42–46.

8. Funayama M, Takata T, Koreki A, et al. Catatonic stupor in schizophrenic disorders and subsequent medical complications and mortality. *Psychosom Med* 2018; **80**: 370–376.

9. Ueda M, Hamamoto M, Nagayama H, et al. Biochemical alterations during medication withdrawal in Parkinson's disease with and without neuroleptic malignant-like syndrome. *J Neurol Neurosurg Psychiatry* 2001; **71**: 111–113.

10. Gurrera RJ. Is neuroleptic malignant syndrome a neurogenic form of malignant hyperthermia? *Clin Neuropharmacol* 2002; **25**: 183–193.

11. Ortiz JF, Wirth M, Eskander N, et al. The genetic foundations of serotonin syndrome, neuroleptic malignant syndrome, and malignant hyperthermia: is there a genetic association between these disorders? *Cureus* 2020; **12**: e10635.

12. Kuhlwilm L, Schönfeldt-Lecuona C, Gahr M, et al. The neuroleptic malignant syndrome: a systematic case series analysis focusing on therapy regimes and outcome. *Acta Psychiatr Scand* 2020; **142**: 233–241.

13. PDR.net. Dantrium Capsules (dantrolene sodium) dose, indications, adverse effects, interactions… from PDR.net, www.pdr .net/drug-summary/Dantrium-Capsules-dantrolene-sodium-1213 (accessed February 15, 2023).

14. PDR.net. Parlodel (bromocriptine mesylate) dose, indications, adverse effects, interactions… from PDR.net, www.pdr.net/drug-summary/Parlodel-bromocriptine-mesylate-1808.330 (accessed February 15, 2023).

15. PDR.net. Amantadine Hydrochloride Capsules (amantadine hydrochloride) dose, indications, adverse effects, interactions… from PDR.net, www.pdr .net/drug-summary/Amantadine-Hydrochloride-Capsules-amantadine-hydrochloride-1475 (accessed February 15, 2023).

16. Rajan R, Sage M. Successful emergency treatment of refractory neuroleptic malignant syndrome with electroconvulsive therapy and a novel use of dexmedetomidine: a case report from California in the era of COVID-19. *J ECT* 2021; **37**: 71–73.

17. Tao M, Li J, Wang X, et al. Malignant syndromes: current advances. *Expert Opin Drug Saf* 2021; **20**: 1075–1085.

18. Scotton WJ, Hill LJ, Williams AC, Barnes NM. Serotonin syndrome: pathophysiology, clinical features, management, and potential future directions. *Int J Tryptophian Res* 2019; **12**: 1–14.

19 Sparado A, Scott KR, Koyfman A, Long B. High risk and low prevalence diseases: aerotonin syndrome. *Am J Em Med* 2022; **61**: 90–97.

20. Foong A, Grindrod KA, Patel T, Kellar J. Demystifying serotonin syndrome (or serotonin toxicity). *Can Fam Physician* 2018; **64**(**10**): 720–727.

21. Boyer EW, Shannon M. The serotonin syndrome. *N E J Med* 2005; **352**(**11**): 1112–1120.

22. Levenson, JL. *Textbook of Psychosomatic Medicine and Consultation: Liaison Psychiatry*. 3rd ed. American Psychiatric Association Publishing; 2019.

23. Ables AZ, Nagubilli R. Prevention, diagnosis and management of serotonin syndrome. *Am Fam Physician* 2010; **81** (**9**): 1139–1142.

24. Werneke U, Truedson-Martiniussen P, Wikström H, Ott M. Serotonin syndrome: a clinical review of current

controversies. *J Integrat Neurosci* 2020; **19**(4): 719–727.

25. Prakash S, Rathore C, Rana K, Prakash A. Fatal serotonin syndrome: a systematic review of 56 cases in the literature. *Clin Toxicol* 2020; **59**(2): 89–100.

26. Dunkley EJ, Isbister GK, Sibbritt D, Dawson AH, Whyte IM. The Hunter serotonin toxicity criteria: simple and accurate diagnostic decision rules for serotonin toxicity. *QJM* 2003; **96**: 635–642.

27. Radomski JW, Dursun SM, Reveley MA, Kutcher SP. An exploratory approach to the serotonin syndrome: an update of clinical phenomenology and revised diagnostic criteria. *Medical Hypotheses.* 2000; **55**: 218–224

28. Sternbach H. The serotonin syndrome. *Am J Psychiatry* 1991; **148**(6): 705–713.

Appendix

This section includes a series of tables containing practical information on the most commonly utilized pharmacological agents in psychiatry. It includes data regarding the usual dose range, side effects, and precautions, in order to facilitate the process involved in choosing a certain medication. In that sense, a few points should be emphasized:

1. Given the scope of the present book, the information included in these tables is not comprehensive, and the list of side effects and precautions is not exclusive. The reader should refer to the respective manufacturer's full information for prescribers for a full list of details regarding possible adverse reactions, additionally recommended monitoring/precautions, and peculiarities regarding the safety and recommended adjustments (when applicable) involving the use of the respective medications in especial populations and situations (children, elderly, women in reproductive age, pregnancy/lactation, renal impairment, liver impairment), as well as drug interactions.

2. The "usual dose ranges" provided are based on available literature data and the authors' clinical experience. In several cases, the maximum approved dose for a certain agent exceeds the usual dose range provided, and certain patients might need lower or higher doses than the ones included in these tables. Similarly, information on FDA approval included in some of these tables is not comprehensive, and medical knowledge/evidence on psychiatric treatments is in continuous advance. Again, the reader should refer to the updated respective manufacturer's full information for prescribers for additional details regarding dose range, recommendations for titration, and black box warnings.

3. This book is not intended to provide diagnostic or treatment information for patients and families and is not intended as a substitute for consultation with a licensed practitioner. Please consult with your own physician or health care specialist regarding the suggestions and recommendations made in this book.

4. The publisher and the author make no guarantees concerning the level of therapeutic success associated with following the treatment strategies contained in this and other sections of this book, and assume no responsibility for any negative outcomes associated with following these strategies or for any eventual inaccuracies or errors included in the present book.

Table A.1 Commonly used antidepressants

Antidepressant	Usual Dose Range	Mechanism of Action	Notable Side Effects
Bupropion	Bupropion: 225–450 mg daily divided in 3 dosages Bupropion SR: 200–450 mg daily divided in 2 doses Bupropion XL: 150–450 mg daily	NDRI	Insomnia, agitation, anxiety Abdominal pain, tinnitus, rash, hypertension More significant lowered threshold for seizures Reported cases of Stevens-Johnson syndrome (extremely rare)
Citalopram Paroxetine Sertraline Escitalopram Fluoxetine Fluvoxamine	20–40 mg daily 20–50 mg daily 50–200 mg daily 10–20 mg daily 20–80 mg daily Once daily with extended release or divided into 2 times if immediate release 100–300 mg daily	SSRI	Citalopram: sedation and fatigue Paroxetine: constipation, dry mouth, sedation, weight gain Sertraline: possible undesirable activation especially in early dosing Fluoxetine: agitation and anxiety, especially in early dosing Fluvoxamine: sedation and fatigue
Levomilnacipran Desvenlafaxine Duloxetine Venlafaxine	40–120 mg daily 50 mg daily 40–60 mg daily Once daily with extended release or divided into 2–3 times if immediate release 75–225 mg daily	SNRI	Tachycardia, palpitations, increase in blood pressure, urinary hesitancy or retention, nervousness, insomnia Venlafaxine: dose-dependent increase in blood pressure
Mirtazapine	15–45 mg at night	SN-RAn	Increased appetite, weight gain, sedation, abnormal dreams, confusion, flu-like symptoms (may indicate low white blood cell count), change in urinary function, hypotension

Vilazodone	20–40 mg daily	multimodal	Less sexual dysfunction side effects when compared with SSRIs or SNRIs
Vortioxetine	5–20 mg daily	multimodal	Nausea, vomiting, constipation, sexual dysfunction
Clomipramine	100–200 mg daily	TCA	Blurred vision, urinary retention, constipation, increased appetite, weight gain, dry mouth, unusual taste in mouth, fatigue, sedation. Hyperthermia, paralytic ileus, orthostatic hypotension, arrhythmias, QTc prolongation, sudden death, hepatic failure, EPS symptoms, increased intraocular pressure
Desipramine	100–200 mg daily		
Nortriptyline	75–150 mg daily		

Potential side effects common to most antidepressants include gastrointestinal symptoms such as decreased or increased appetite, nausea, vomiting, constipation, diarrhea, dry mouth. Also, insomnia, sedation, tremors, agitation, headache, dizziness, sweating, weight gain or weight loss, and sexual dysfunction can be observed. Risk of bruising/bleeding, hyponatremia, and SIADH (rare).

Rare but dangerous side effects also common to antidepressants are seizures, induction of hypomania/mania, and activation in suicidality (short-term studies didn't show increased risk of suicidality compared to placebo in ages older than 24 years).

Some (but not all) peculiarities regarding side effect profile of specific antidepressants are listed in the "Notable Side Effects" column of the table.

This list of side effects and recommendations is not exclusive. Readers should consult manufacture's prescription guidelines for additional information regarding dosage, side effects, precautions, and use in special populations (children, elderly, medically ill patients, pregnant and lactating patients) before prescribing medications.

NDRI, Norepinephrine-Dopamine reuptake inhibitor; *SNRI*, serotonin, norepinephrine receptor antagonist; *SNRI*, serotonin-norepinephrine reuptake inhibitor; *SSRI*, selective serotonin reuptake inhibitor; *TCA*, tricyclic antidepressant.

Table A.2 Commonly used mood stabilizers

Medication	Usual Dose Range (PO)	Comments*	Side Effects/Precautions*
Lithium Carbonate	600–1800 mg/day, usually divided BID or TID Lithium ER is usually divided BID	Start with 300 mg BID or TID. Obtain a level 5–7 days after each dose change; increase dose gradually, based on levels and treatment response; therapeutic level usually between 0.8–1.2 MEq/L (for acute mania) and 0.6–0.8 MEq/L (for maintenance)	Can cause gastrointestinal discomfort and, in the long term, hypothyroidism, diabetes insipidus, and impairment in kidney function. Risk of toxicity, which can include severe vomiting, diarrhea, altered mental status, ataxia, acute kidney failure, and death; risk of teratogenicity (use with caution in women in reproductive age). In case of suspected toxicity, hold medication, obtain level immediately, and provide emergency medical attention
Divalproex	500–2000 mg/day, usually divided BID; Divalproex ER can be given as single daily dose; dose adjustment necessary when switching from immediate release to ER due to differences in bioavailability	Start with 250 mg daily or BID. Increase dose gradually. Fast titration or a higher starting dose (1000 mg/day) can be used with close monitoring, especially in inpatient settings, for the management of severe mania. No necessary correlation between serum level and effect, but usually aimed at levels above 45 micrograms/ml; levels should be checked to ensure it is not at toxic values (usually above 125 micrograms/ml). Monitor liver enzymes and CBC	Can cause gastrointestinal discomfort, drowsiness, ataxia, liver toxicity, thrombocytopenia/ blood discrasia, alopecia; important risk of teratogenicity (avoid in women in reproductive age); risk of acute hepatitis, pancreatitis, and hyperammonemia. Risk of drug interactions

Lamotrigine	25–200 mg/day, usually given once a day	Start with 25 mg/day for 2 weeks, then increase to 50 mg/day for 2 weeks, then increase to 100 mg/day for 1 week. Can increase to 150–200 mg/day after 1–2 weeks	Risk of rash, including Stevens-Johnson syndrome, especially when medication is titrated fast. Risk of hemophagocytic lymphohistiocytosis (rare). Dose adjustments necessary if combined with enzyme inducers or valproic acid
Carbamazepine	400–1200 mg/day, usually divided TID or BID (Carbamazepine ER)	Start with 200 BID; increase gradually; therapeutic level usually at 4–12 mg/L (for epilepsy; no consensus about optimal levels for mood stabilization). Monitor liver enzymes, CBC, and electrolytes	Risk of rash (including Stevens-Johnson syndrome), gastrointestinal discomfort, drowsiness, ataxia, liver toxicity, hyponatremia, blood dyscrasia, and heart problems (rare); risk of teratogenicity (use with caution in women in reproductive age). Risk of drug interactions. May require dose increase over time, as medication induces its own metabolism. Should not be used in individuals with the HLA-B*1502 allele (screen patients with Asian ancestry). May worsen angle-closure glaucoma
Oxcarbazepine	600–1800 mg/day, usually divided BID	Start with 300 mg BID; increase gradually; Monitor liver enzymes, CBC, and electrolytes	Risk of hyponatremia and rash. Other side effects and precautions are similar to carbamazepine, but overall it is better tolerated; significantly lower risk of drug interactions compared to carbamazepine.

* Abrupt discontinuation of mood stabilizer can exacerbate mood symptoms or precipitate seizures, in the case of anticonvulsants. This list of side effects and recommendations is not exclusive. Readers should consult manufacture's prescription guidelines for additional information regarding dosage, side effects, precautions, and use in special populations (children, elderly, medically ill patients, pregnant and lactating patients) before prescribing medications.

BID, Twice a day; *PO*, orally; *QAM*, in the morning; *QHS*, at bedtime; *TID*, three times a day.

Table A.3 Commonly used atypical antipsychotics

Medication	Usual Dose Range (PO)	Special Comments*
Risperidone	0.5–4 mg/day, usually divided BID	Start with a total of 0.5–1 mg/day. Increase dose gradually. Risk of hypotension
Olanzapine	5–20 mg/day, usually as single dose QHS	Higher risk of excessive sedation and metabolic syndrome
Clozapine	300–600 mg/day, divided BID	Medication not routinely managed by nonspecialists. Needs to be started at low dose (12.5–25 mg/day) and titrated slowly over the course of 2 weeks to a target dose of 300 mg/day. Risk of seizures and of leukopenia; needs close CBC monitoring; risk of sedation and metabolic syndrome
Quetiapine	150–800 mg/day, usually divided BID; extended-release form usually given as single daily dose at night	Start with 25–50 mg QHS. Increase dose gradually. Optimal dose varies according to indication
Ziprasidone	40–160 mg/day, usually divided BID	Higher risk of QTc prolongation; lower risk of metabolic syndrome
Aripiprazole	2–30 mg/day, given as single daily dose	Partial dopamine agonists. More metabolic friendly; low QTC prolongation risk; antidepressant augmentation, use lower doses; risk of akathisia and impulse control issues, including (but not limited to) gambling and compulsive buying
Brexpiprazole	0.5–3 mg/day, given as single daily dose	
Cariprazine	1.5–6 mg/day, given as single daily dose	
Lurasidone	40–160 mg/day, given as single daily dose	More metabolic friendly; low QTc prolongation risk; risk of akathisia
Asenapine	10–20 mg/day, usually divided BID	Given sublingual. Risk of hypotension

* Potential side effects common to almost all atypical antipsychotics include sedation, hypotension/orthostasis, blood discrasia, QTc prolongation, seizures, and extra-pyramidal side effects (EPS) such as parkinsonism, akathisia, dystonia, and tardive dyskinesia associated with prolonged use. Risk of neuroleptic malignant syndrome (rare). Overall, risk of EPS is lower than with typical antipsychotics. Risk of metabolic syndrome. Patients need to be regularly monitored with regards to abnormal movements (AIMS scale), weight gain, blood sugar/hemoglobin A1C, and lipid panel. Some (but not all) peculiarities regarding side effect profile of specific agents are listed in the "Special Comments" column of the table. Other than Brexpiprazole (approved by the FDA for agitation associated with dementia due to Alzheimer's disease), atypical antipsychotics are not approved for use in patients with dementia-related behavioral symptoms.
* List of side effects and recommendations is not exclusive. Readers should consult manufacture's prescription guidelines for additional information regarding dosage, side effects, precautions, and use in special populations (children, elderly, medically ill patients, pregnant and lactating patients) before prescribing medications.
AIMS, Abnormal Involuntary Movement Scale; BID, twice a day; PO, orally; QAM, in the morning; QHS, at bedtime; TID, three times a day.

Table A.4 Commonly used typical antipsychotics

Medication	Usual Dose Range (PO)	Special Comments*
Haloperidol	5–20 mg/day, given as single dose at bedtime or divided BID	Start with 2.5–5 mg QHS. Higher risk of EPS and QTc prolongation
Chlorpromazine	100–400 mg/day, usually divided TID	Start with small dose (10–25 mg tid). Increase dose gradually. Higher risk of excessive sedation and hypotension
Trifluoperazine	4–10 mg/day, usually divided BID	Start with 1–2 mg BID
Perphenazine	12–32 mg/day, usually divided BID or TID	Start with 4–6 mg TID

* Potential side effects common to almost all typical antipsychotics include sedation, falls, hypotension/orthostasis, blood dyscrasia, QTc prolongation, seizures, and extra-pyramidal side effects (EPS) such as parkinsonism, akathisia, dystonia, and tardive dyskinesia associated with prolonged use. Risk of neuroleptic malignant syndrome (rare). Overall, risk of EPS is higher than with atypical antipsychotics. Risk of weight gain and metabolic syndrome. Patients need to be regularly monitored with regards to abnormal movements (AIMS scale), CBC, weight gain, blood sugar/hemoglobin A1C, and lipid panel. Some (but not all) peculiarities regarding side effect profile of specific agents are listed in the "Special Comments" column of the table. Typical antipsychotics are not approved for use in patients with dementia-related behavioral symptoms.

* List of side effects and recommendations is not exclusive. Readers should consult manufacture's prescription guidelines for additional information regarding dosage, side effects, precautions, and use in special populations (children, elderly, medically ill patients, pregnant and lactating patients) before prescribing medications.

AIMS, Abnormal Involuntary Movement Scale; *BID*, twice a day; *PO*, orally; *QAM*, in the morning; *QHS*, at bedtime; *TID*, three times a day.

Table A.5 Benzodiazepines and other commonly used anti-anxiety and sleep-inducer medications

Medication	Usual Dose Range (PO)	Class	Special Comments*
Diazepam	2–10 mg daily, usually divided BID	Benzodiazepine	Start with 2–5 mg daily
Chlordiazepoxide	30–100 mg daily, usually divided TID or QID	Benzodiazepine	Start with 5 mg once a day or BID
Lorazepam	1–6 mg daily, usually divided BID or TID	Benzodiazepine	Start with 0.5–1 mg BID; better choice than other benzodiazepines for patients with liver impairment
Clonazepam	0.5–4 mg daily, usually divided BID or TID	Benzodiazepine	Start with 0.25–0.5 mg BID
Alprazolam	0.5–6 mg daily, usually divided TID. Alprazolam ER can be used once a day	Benzodiazepine	Risk of rebound anxiety, especially if used PRN or once or twice a day (immediate release). Might cause lower sedation but higher potential for abuse than other benzodiazepines
Temazepam	7.5–30 mg QHS	Benzodiazepine	Approved for short-term insomnia treatment. Better choice than other benzodiazepines for patients with liver impairment
Oxazepam	30–90 mg daily, used divided TID or QID	Benzodiazepine	Better choice than other benzodiazepines for patients with liver impairment. Not frequently used
Zolpidem	5–10 mg QHS (immediate release) 6.25–12.5 mg QHS (continuous release)	"Z" drug	Recommended maximum dose for women is 5 mg QHS (immediate release) and 6.25 mg QHS (extended release). FDA approved for short-term insomnia treatment
Eszopiclone	1–3 mg QHS	"Z" drug	Start with 1 mg QHS; use lowest effective dose
Suvorexant	5–20 mg QHS	Orexin antagonist	Use lowest effective dose. Risk of drowsiness and other sleep-related symptoms. Monitor for worsening in
Lemborexant	5–10 mg QHS	Orexin antagonist	depression, suicidality, and other psychiatric symptoms. Use with caution in patients with history of substance abuse/ dependence. Use with caution in patients receiving other CNS depressors

Trazodone	Antidepressant	25–200 mg QHS	Risk of sedation, falls, hypotension/orthostasis, and priapism (rare). Used off-label for the treatment of insomnia (not FDA approved for that indication)
Buspirone	Azapirone	20–60 mg daily, usually divided BID or TID	Nonaddictive; latency of effect (2–4 weeks). Approved for generalized anxiety disorder. Risk of serotonin syndrome (rare), especially when combined with antidepressants
Gabapentin	Anticonvulsant	300–1800 mg daily, usually divided TID	Wide dose range. Used off-label for the treatment of anxiety (not FDA approved for that indication). Risk of seizures if abruptly discontinued (needs to be gradually tapered off). Risk of sedation and respiratory depression. Monitor for increased suicidality. Use with caution in patients with renal impairment and in those receiving other CNS depressors
Hydroxyzine	Antihistaminic	25–50 mg TID or QID	Often given PRN for anxiety. Start with 10–25 mg TID and adjust dose based on response/tolerability. Can be used for insomnia (off-label). Risk of sedation, anticholinergic effects, seizures, and QTc prolongation

* Potential side effects common to all benzodiazepines and "Z" drugs include sedation, falls, respiratory depression, and risk of abuse/dependence. Avoid prolonged use and use minimally effective dose. Use with caution in patients receiving other CNS suppressors, especially opioids, and in those with history of substance use disorder. Risk of withdrawal symptoms if discontinued abruptly after continuous use for more than 2–3 weeks. Needs to be tapered off gradually. Certain benzodiazepines (diazepam, chlordiazepoxide, lorazepam, and oxazepam) are often used for management of acute alcohol withdrawal syndrome. Different dose ranges and protocols are available for that particular indication.
* This list of side effects and recommendations is not exclusive. Readers should consult manufacture's prescription guidelines for additional information regarding dosage, side effects, precautions, and use in special populations (children, elderly, medically ill patients, pregnant and lactating patients) before prescribing medications.
AMS, Abnormal Involuntary Movement Scale; BID, twice a day; PO, orally; QAM, in the morning; QHS, at bedtime; QID, four times a day; TID, three times a day.

Index